Cancer
Esophagus

As the Genius of Science extends the horizon of
WHAT WE CAN DO

We are increasingly confronted by the questions of
WHAT WE SHOULD DO

Cancer Esophagus

Editor in Chief

Praful Desai MS FRCS FACS
Senior Surgical Oncologist
Former Director and Chief of Surgery
Tata Memorial Hospital
Breach Candy Hospital and Bombay Hospital, Mumbai

Co-editor

Ratna Parikh MS FACS FAIS
Consultant Surgical Oncologist
Breach Candy Hospital and
Bharatiya Arogya Nidhi Hospital, Mumbai

Editorial Assistant

Ishan Thakkar

Foreword

Tehemton Erach Udwadia

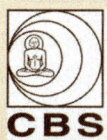

CBS Publishers & Distributors Pvt Ltd

New Delhi • Bengaluru • Chennai • Kochi • Kolkata • Mumbai
Bhopal • Bhubaneswar • Hyderabad • Jharkhand • Nagpur • Patna • Pune
Uttarakhand • Dhaka (Bangladesh) • Kathmandu (Nepal)

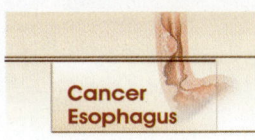

ISBN: 978-93-89261-83-7

Copyright © Editors and Publisher

First Edition: 2020

Published by Satish Kumar Jain and produced by Varun Jain for

CBS Publishers & Distributors Pvt Ltd
4819/XI Prahlad Street, 24 Ansari Road, Daryaganj, New Delhi 110 002, India.
Ph: 23289259, 23266861, 23266867   Website: www.cbspd.com
Fax: 011-23243014   e-mail: delhi@cbspd.com; cbspubs@airtelmail.in.

Corporate Office: 204 FIE, Industrial Area, Patparganj, Delhi 110 092
Ph: 011-4934 4934   Fax: 011-4934 4935 e-mail: publishing@cbspd.com; publicity@cbspd.com

Branches

- **Bengaluru:** Seema House 2975, 17th Cross, K.R. Road, Banasankari 2nd Stage, Bengaluru 560 070, Karnataka
  Ph: +91-80-26771678/79   Fax: +91-80-26771680 e-mail: bangalore@cbspd.com
- **Chennai:** 7, Subbaraya Street, Shenoy Nagar, Chennai 600 030, Tamil Nadu
  Ph: +91-44-26680620/26681266   Fax: +91-44-42032115   e-mail: chennai@cbspd.com
- **Kochi:** 68/1534, 35, 36, Power House Road, Opp KSEB, Power House, Ernakulam 682 018, Kochi, Kerala
  Ph: +91-484-4059061-65   Fax: +91-484-4059065 e-mail: kochi@cbspd.com
- **Kolkata:** 6/B, Ground Floor, Rameswar Shaw Road, Kolkata 700 014, West Bengal
  Ph: +91-33-22891126, 22891127, 22891128   e-mail: kolkata@cbspd.com
- **Mumbai:** 83-C, Dr E Moses Road, Worli, Mumbai 400018, Maharashtra
  Ph: +91-22-24902340/41   Fax: +91-22-24902342 e-mail: mumbai@cbspd.com

Representatives

- **Bhopal** 0-8319310552 • **Bhubaneswar** 0-9911037372 • **Hyderabad** 0-9885175004 • **Jharkhand** 0-9811541605
- **Nagpur** 0-9421945513 • **Patna** 0-9334159340 • **Pune** 0-9623451994 • **Uttarakhand** 0-9716462459
- **Dhaka (Bangladesh)** 01912-003485 • **Kathmandu (Nepal)** 01912-003485

Printed at: Rashtriya Printers, Dilshad Garden, Delhi, India

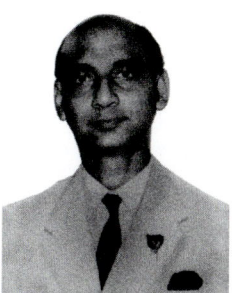

Dr Ernest Borges

Dr Ernest Borges was one of the more famous and outstanding surgeons of his times from mid 1940's till his passing. Starting his surgical career in Ahmednagar, he made his way to the Tata Memorial Hospital, Mumbai. He distinguished himself as an outstanding surgeon in oncology and his fame as a cancer surgeon spread rapidly not only in western India, but patients gravitated to him from many parts of India. His expertise in surgery for esophageal cancer (an extremely common disease in India) was outstanding and many surgical colleagues made their way to the Tata Memorial Hospital from all parts of India to watch and learn from him, the fineness and techniques of esophageal surgery and anastomosis in particular.

Dr Praful Desai had the good fortune to be associated with him for more than a decade and grasp the nuances of this difficult surgery. Knowledge is for onward transmission and this humble effort of the author is to transmit his experience in esophageal surgery which the author hopes may be of some help and benefit to surgeons and patients involved with cancer of the esophagus. Many different approaches and techniques for this procedure are now available. The author hopes that the techniques outlined are feasible and doable even in smaller hospitals in various parts of our country with ease and minimal requirement of sophisticated equipment.

This compilation is therefore gratefully dedicated to Dr Ernest Borges, an extraordinary surgeon of his times, with outstanding expertise in surgery of esophageal cancer.

Foreword

Dr Praful Desai has inherited his passion for the surgery and treatment of cancer breast and cancer esophagus from his mentor and legendry Chief Dr Ernest Borges. This was from the time we were both co-residents at the Tata Memorial Hospital in 1958, full sixty years back. This passion and his immense experience, work and study in these two areas has its outpouring in the previous book on cancer breast and this current one on cancer esophagus.

Cancer esophagus, a very virulent malignancy, has a varied geographic incidence, even in the same country, is more common in the developing world, as it is in India. Sadly, it is hardly ever diagnosed till it is well advanced, for the esophagus is insensible, uncomplaining, entirely silent. Being the only organ to traverse all three domains, neck, thorax and abdomen, with no serosal lining, poor vasculature, prolific lymphatic drainage, it does not lend itself readily to curative treatment. Whether the histopathology is the commoner squamous cell carcinoma or adenocarcinoma, which is rapidly increasing in incidence in the West, the prognosis remains dismal at a 5 year mortality of over 80% due to loco-regional failure and early dissemination. Hence, the need for a current and comprehensive book on Cancer Esophagus, with rapidly evolving newer modalities for early diagnosis, treatment and improved cure rates.

As Heneage Ogilvie wrote in the BMJ in 1947 for cancer esophagus "Radical Surgery can hardly get more radical, for the limitations now set are due to Charles Mayo's stipulation that among the results of successful surgery should be a live patient. If therefore, we are to get more cures it can only be by finding more patients in stage 1, the stage of silence". What was true in 1947 stands true today— education and awareness for prophylaxis and early diagnosis is the key to cancer esophagus.

This volume is authored by the cream workers, who have devoted their entire lives to their specific fields and every chapter is a storehouse of their personal expertise, as also their evaluation of current practice and progress. The range of chapters is all encompassing and holistic, from epidemiology, anatomy, pathology, every mode of diagnosis which gives a final platform for planning, decision-making and ideal treatment management. Operative procedures which range from traditional hand-sewn anastomosis to laparoscopic and robotic surgery are described with appropriate illustrations, so are current and evolving adjuvant therapy, their role, indications and value pragmatically discussed.

The true thrust of this book is that while surgery is the bed-rock of cancer management, it is supported, augmented and at times replaced by what is today termed "adjuvant therapy" which may in the foreseeable future be "definitive therapy". This will include sophistication in chemotherapy, radiation, immunotherapy and way beyond. For instance in Barrets esophagus cancer gene variants are more common, suggesting regular endoscope surveillance of this group worthwhile, as also making their targeted therapy a possibility. Cancer research in gene-therapy, molecular biology, nano-technology, is well funded, and progressing among other thrust areas, as is research in futuristic fields of eventual cure of cancer which today may appear almost in the realm of science fiction. On the other hand just as bacteria can mutate to resist newer antibiotics, will cancer cell evolve to outwit newer therapy? Like the battle against infection, will the battle against cancer be unending? Is it on the cards that newer therapy against cancer will displace the role of surgery in several areas of cancer? It may be worth recalling the prediction of John Hunter who lived more than three centuries ahead of his time, experimented, taught, practiced "scientific surgery" in 18th Century "With the advance in knowledge, surgery will become knifeless and bloodless", for, "operation is a reflection on the healing are; it is a tacit acknowledgement of the insufficiency of surgery. It is like an armed savage who attempts to get that by force what a civilized man would get by stratagem". With bated breath we await the future stratagem on the ongoing relentless battle against all cancer.

Without emotion or embarrassment, we discreetly brush under the carpet the fact that cancer esophagus, as all other cancers in India and other developing countries impact a horrendous burden on over one-third the vast population which is below the poverty line. The Lancet Commission on Global Surgery estimates this impoverished population at over 5 billion, 70% of the world population. With no access to surgery, no health insurance, their physical, emotional misery and suffering is compounded by the financial ruin of their entire family, as a result of illness. The profession cannot redress this seemingly insoluble national problem. Fortunately, over the last few years giant steps have been taken with astonishingly ambitious, well-planned and workable health schemes for all marginalized poor, notably the Ayushman Bharat Scheme. Tata Memorial Center and other organizations have long back set-up satellite peripheral cancer centers, but far more needs to be done, done with the same dedications, passion and determination as is shown in our battle against cancer into the future. Billions are spent on research for help and cure of future cancer patients, but sadly these benefits may not reach the majority of people merits at least as much attention, concern and empathy as the salvaging of future generations. Medicine and surgery, over and above becoming more and more a science, supposedly, have a humanitarian core. As Martin Luther King Junior wrote "Of all the forms of inequality, injustice in health care is the most shocking and inhumane."

I heard Dr Praful Desai say, very many years ago, in his conference Chairman's speech at an International Oncology Conference in Mumbai, which drew the foremost oncologists from all over world, "I am merely the string that holds all these pearls together". Dr Desai has spent a lifetime being the string that holds pearls together, whether during his long tenure as Director Tata memorial Hospital and Center, or his literary assays like his books. To collect and hold the very best talent together and derive the best from each one of them, is the ultimate quality of leadership.

Tehemton Erach Udwadia
MS FRCS (Eng) FRCS (Edin) FACS FAMS
Emeritus Professor of Surgery
Grant Medical College and JJ Hospital
Consultant Surgeon
Head of the Department Minimally Access Surgery
Hinduja and Breach Candy Hospitals, Mumbai

Contributors

Aagre Suhas Vilasrao
MD (Medicine) DM (Medical Oncology)
Consultant, Medical Oncology
Asian Cancer Institute
Mumbai

Advani Suresh
MD FICP FNAMS
Director, Medical Oncology
Jaslok Hospital and Research Centre
Mumbai

Agarwal Jai Prakash
MD
Professor and Head
Department of Radiation Oncology
Tata Memorial Hospital
Mumbai

Arneja Sarabjeet Kaur
MD
Head
Department of Surgical Pathology and Cytology
Breach Candy Hospital
Mumbai

Balasubramaniam Ganesh
PhD (Epidemiology)
Assistant Professor
Tata Memorial Hospital
Mumbai

Chitale Mihir
MBBS FCPS DNB (Surgery)
Galaxy Care Laparoscopic Institute
Pune

Desai Praful
MS FRCS FACS
Senior Surgical Oncologist
Former Director and Chief of Surgery
Tata Memorial Hospital
Breach Candy Hospital and Bombay Hospital
Mumbai

Deshpande Ramakant
MS FICS FAIS DHA
Consultant Surgical Oncologist
Asian Institute of Oncology
Breach Candy Hospital and Jaslok Hospital
Mumbai

Espuniyani Prriya
MS DNB (Thoracic)
Consultant Surgical Oncologist
Asian Institute of Oncology
Mumbai

Jathar Advait
MBBS MS
Galaxy Care Laparoscopic Institute
Pune

Kohli Anirudh
MD DNB DMRD
Department of Radiology
Breach Candy Hospital
Mumbai

Laskar Sarbani Ghosh
MD DNB DMRT
Professor, Radiation Oncology
Tata Memorial Hospital
Mumbai

Majeed Tanveer Abdul
MS (G Surg) DNB (Surg Oncology) MRCSEd (UK) MRCPS (Glas)
MNAMS FAIS FICS
Consultant Surgical Oncologist
Asian Cancer Institute
Mumbai

Manchekar Manoj
MBBS MS
Galaxy Care Laparoscopic Institute
Pune

Panse Mangesh
MBBS MS
Galaxy Care Laparoscopic Institute
Pune

Parikh Anuj
MBBS
Kasturba Medical College
Manipal

Parikh Purvish M
MD DNB FICP PhD ECMO
Director of Precision Oncology
Asian Cancer Institute
Mumbai

Parikh Ratna
MS FACS FAIS
Consultant Surgical Oncologist
Breach Candy Hospital and
Bharatiya Arogya Nidhi Hospital
Mumbai

Parikh Samir
MD DM DNB (Gastroenterology)
Consultant Gastroenterologist
Lilavati Hospital and
Medical Research Center
Mumbai

Puntambekar Aishwarya
MBBS
Galaxy Care Laparoscopic Institute
Pune

Puntambekar Shailesh
MS
Medical Director
Laparoscopic Oncosurgery
Galaxy Care Laparoscopic Institute
Pune

Sathe Ravindra
MBBS MS
Galaxy Care Laparoscopic Institute
Pune

Shrivastava Shyam Kishore
MD DNBR
Director, Radiation Oncology
Apollo Hospitals
Navi Mumbai

Preface

Esophageal cancer is a common disease in India, often diagnosed late in majority of patients. Esophagus is the only organ which traverses three anatomical regions; the neck, the thorax and the upper abdomen, ending at the cardia of the stomach. A major consequence of this anatomy results in profuse lymphatic drainage of the esophagus in the neck, the thorax and the abdomen which can result in lymph node metastasis far away from the primary site of the disease, which impacts on the extent of surgical approach needed in a given patient.

Surgery has remained steadfast as a major therapeutic approach up until the 1970s before the advent of chemotherapy and radiotherapy. The morbidity and mortality after surgery by low volume surgeons and low volume hospitals is a cause of concern, proven by recorded data in the literature; however, appropriately selected patients for surgery by experienced surgeons in large volume hospitals result in a satisfactory and pleasing outcome for both the surgeon and the patient. Rigorous and prolonged training with experienced surgeons are mandatory. Esophageal surgery ranks with that of the brain, liver and lung in its complexity and precision needed for a successful outcome without complications which can entail prolonged stay, significant morbidities and even mortalities.

Cancer of the esophagus is, therefore, best managed by a team of specialists involving a surgeon, a chemotherapist and a radiotherapist. Such facilities are not easily available in India due to socio-economic reasons. This collation, also refers to appropriate case selections for a surgical approach (including techniques); indications for chemoradiotherapy, preoperative and postoperative issues, complications and their management.

The authors hope that this compilation will be useful to all colleagues involved in treatment of cancer of the esophagus in their own environment.

Praful Desai
Ratna Parikh

Contents

Historical Overview

Praful Desai, Ratna Parikh

"Nothing illumines the human mind more than the perusal of history"

There is no greater saga in the history of mankind than the epic of medicine. A precise understanding of the nuances of a disease process is dependent on the knowledge of its etiology, its evolution, its progress and finally the therapy response for its control and cure. The perusal of history therefore, is an important and vital factor in assessing and understanding the intricacies of a given disease. Lessons from history are therefore, a major source of inspiration, helps to inculcate a sense of humility, makes one realize the limits of medicine and the fact that any truth is relative, never absolute.

It is interesting to know that esophageal cancer dates back to ancient Egyptian times, Circa 3000 BC.[1] It was described in China over 2000 years ago as YE GE, which means dysphagia and belching.[2] It was known to be a fatal disease and it was believed, "Those discovered to suffer from esophageal cancer in the autumn, will not live through the next summer."[2]

GALEN in the 2nd century described "Fleshy Growths" as a cause of obstruction of the esophagus with cachexia and a fatal outcome.[2] The history of development of esophageal resection has thus been long and difficult. "The tales of men repeatedly losing to a stronger adversary yet persisting in the unequal struggle until the nature of the problem became apparent and the war was won."[3]

The progress to safe and satisfactory surgery and anastomosis was slow and arduous. The reasons for this are strong:

1. The esophagus has a deep anatomic location.
2. It traverses three anatomic areas, viz. the neck, the chest and the upper abdomen.
3. Profuse lymphatic supply owing to its length is conducive to frequent lymph nodal metastasis to the neck, the chest and even the abdomen. The author has the experience of a histologically proven metastasis in the right inguinal region from an esophageal cancer.
4. The absence of a serosal coat.
5. The absence of serosa is compensated by a strong esophageal mucosa and an adequate muscle coat.
6. The anastomosis is often located in areas where postoperative infection is dangerous and can spread rapidly as in the chest or the upper abdomen.

The earliest report on esophageal intervention is credited to the Mayo brothers who published their experiences on lye strictures of the esophagus, esophageal bougienage and the management of impacted foreign body in the esophagus.[4] Dr. Henry Ellis Jr. spent 20 years at the Mayo Clinic and worked on the anatomy and physiology of the organ. The early history of esophageal resection is prolonged and tinged with frequent failures and only occasional successes. Czerny, Torek, Ivor Lewis and many other outstanding surgeons of the time struggled to unlock the mystery of esophageal cancer and its surgical treatment.

ED Churchill wrote in 1960[5] "Surgeons have travelled a long road to bring their craft to its present position. The road can be measured by milestones of triumph and progress; also by tombstones of tragedy and prejudice. The journey cannot be described as a particularly sentimental one but rather as a struggle in which stern realism has usually obscured any elements of romance. Only the words of those who have lighted the way remains to show the romance of surgery. They are the words of earnest men, the strength of those convictions exceeded the techniques available for its expression. These men stand poles apart from today's 'bright boys' who are so facile in wielding the techniques they have inherited."

Resection was first carried out for cervical esophageal growths, then for the lower end growth (including the cardia) and finally thoracic esophageal growths. The prolonged saga of esophageal resection is divided into three distinct eras:[6]

1877–1912: No attempt, to restore continuity between pharynx and stomach (except for carcinoma of the cervical esophagus)

1913–38: Continuity restored usually at a subsequent operation, by a presternal tube of skin, stomach, jejunum or an external rubber tube

1938 onwards: Excision and immediate restoration of continuity in neck or chest.

Table 1.1	Timeline for esophageal surgery	
Year	**Author**	**Event**
1870	**Theodor Billroth[7]**	Cervical resection and anastomosis in dog
1877	**Czerny[8]**	First esophageal resection for a cervical tumor-local excision and a feeding cervical esophagostomy
1886	**Mikulicz[9] (Pupil of Billroth)**	Reconstructed the cervical esophagus by use of skin flaps (11 months survival)
1888	**Nassiloff [10] (St. Petersburg)**	Extrapleural route (to reduce risk of pleural infection) for upper thoracic esophageal resection. Approached from posterior part of the thorax by resecting four ribs in cadavers
1891	**Von Hacker[11]**	Replaced segment of the cervical esophagus in dogs by a horizontal bridge of skin. Unsuccessful in a patient
1898	**Ludwig Rehn[12] (Germany)**	First surgeon to approach esophagus through the chest by an extrapleural route
1901	**Dobromysslov[13]**	First successful transpleural resection with immediate restoration of continuity carried out in dogs
1903	**Mikulicz and Fauré[14]**	Attempted a left transpleural approach before Czery but without success
1907	**Roux[15] (Lausanne)**	Used a loop of jejunum as the lower part of a presternal conduit, the upper part made from a skin tube

Contd...

Table 1.1	Timeline for esophageal surgery *(Contd...)*	
Year	**Author**	**Event**
1908	Voelker[16] (Heidelberg)	First successful resection of a carcinoma at the lower end of the thoracic esophagus by the abdominal route. Left subcostal incision. The esophagus pulled down into the abdomen. The carcinoma resected and an esophagogastric anastomosis created
1911	Sir Arbuthnot Lane[17] (Guys Hospital)	Successfully resected cancer of the upper esophagus and back of the larynx, continuity restored by a skin flap
1911	Kelling Dresden[18]	Used the transverse colon to replace the esophagus. This staged operation was almost successful
1913	Torek[19]	The first successful resection of a mid-esophageal carcinoma by a left transpleural approach
1913	Denk[20]	First transhiatal esophagectomy in cadavers
1913	Zaaijer[21] (Leiden)	Performed two successful staged transpleural resections of cancer at the lower end of the esophagus
1913	Willey Meyer[22]	Used the greater curvature of the stomach to make a long tube to reach high in the chest. This was used to bypass an inoperable carcinoma and also to replace the lower esophagus after resection
1922	Kummell[23]	First attempt at gastric transposition
1933	Grey Turner[24]	Transhiatal esophagectomy
1933	Oshawa[25] (Kyoto)	Performed the first successful transthoracic esophagectomy and primary esophagogastric anastomosis for esophageal cancer
1934	Heneage Ogilvie,[26] O'Shaughnessy and Raven[27]	Published a masterly paper on the techniques for surgical exposure of the esophagus
1938	Garlock[28]	Three consecutive successful resections with the Torek technique
1946	Ivor Lewis[29]	Ivor Lewis esophagectomy
1978	Orringer[30]	Reintroduced transhiatal esophagectomy after Turner's dismal outcomes in 1933
1978	Belsey[31]	Advocated the use of ascending, transverse and descending segments of colon for esophageal replacement
1979	McKeown[32]	Three phase total esophagectomy operation with anastomosis in the neck

Franz Torek (1861–1938)[33] is one of the early pioneer surgeons in thoracic surgery (Fig. 1.1). In 1913 he performed the first thoracic esophagectomy for a mid-esophageal cancer, on a 67 years old woman, who survived for 12 years (Fig. 1.2). The proximal end of the esophagus was brought out through a cervical incision; the cancer resected and the remainder of the esophagus was tunneled under the skin to make an esophagostomy on the anterior chest wall at the 2nd interspace. A gastrostomy was also performed and the patient was fed through the gastrostomy tube for the first 8 postoperative days and later received nutrition orally. The meal passed from the proximal esophageal stoma through

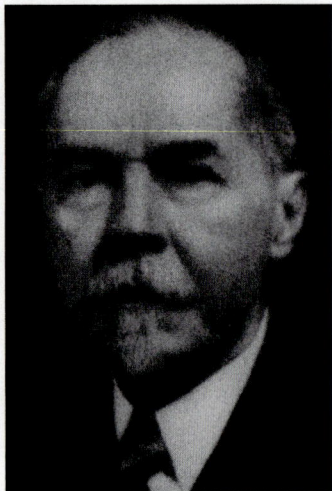

Fig. 1.1: Franz Torek (1861–1938)

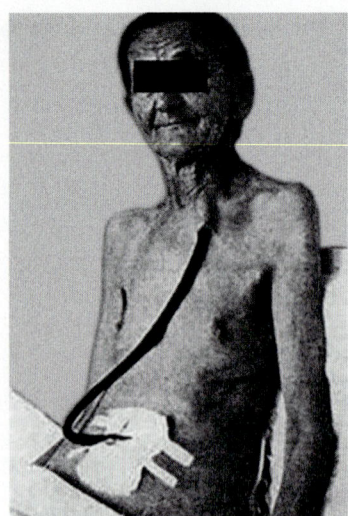

Fig. 1.3: Franz Torek's patient who had undergone the first successful resection of a carcinoma of the middle third of the esophagus in 1913. The meal passed from the proximal esophageal stoma through an external tube to the gastrostomy

and his contributions, Dr. Torek will be remembered and be an inspiration to those who follow after. He was one of America's great surgeon." Torek operation was reported from 1936 to 1943 by Muir, Alison, Franklin and Brock.[34]

Ivor Lewis (1895–1982) (Fig. 1.4): In August 1944, the Welsh surgeon described a two stage esophagectomy including a laparotomy to

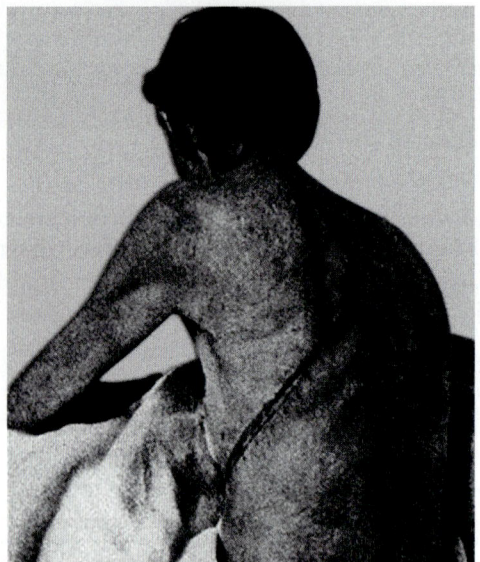

Fig. 1.2: Cachectic lady (due to disease) with an abdomino-thoracic incision after completion of esophageal resection. Incision was marked with silver nitrate the day before the operation

an external tube to the gastrostomy (Fig. 1.3). The other way was to create a presternal tube of skin, stomach, jejunum or colon to restore continuity. Torek's operation was a major surgical breakthrough proving that eso-phageal cancer could be cured surgically; Carl Eggers wrote in his obituary: "Because of his personality, his sterling character, his work

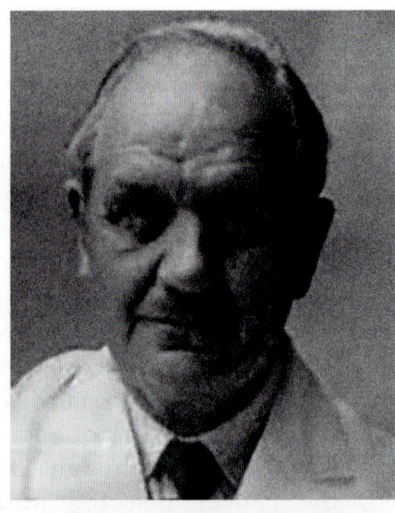

Fig. 1.4: Ivor Lewis (1895–1982)

mobilize the stomach followed by a right sided thoracotomy and an immediate right intrathoracic gastroesophageal anastomosis by pulling up the mobilized stomach. This involved two standardized incisions. The Ivor Lewis procedure gained popularity and is currently the most commonly utilized approach for mid-esophageal resections worldwide.[2]

Further evolution of surgical techniques has led to the description of a hybrid, minimally invasive and a robotic approach.

CHEMORADIOTHERAPY FOR ESOPHAGEAL CANCER

Since the beginning of the 20th century, radiotherapy and surgery have played important roles for the treatment of esophageal cancer. Exner[35] first described the treatment of esophageal cancer with radium in 1904. Adding cytotoxic chemotherapy to radiotherapy for additive or synergistic effect was described as early as 1968.[36]

The Indian Scenario

Though published data on esophageal resection surgery is hard to find in India, the earliest published report about resection of the esophagus is from TATA MEMORIAL HOSPITAL, in mid 1940's by the late Dr. Ernest Borges and Dr. Jussawalla. By the early 50's esophageal resections were frequently performed in Bombay and larger institutes in Kolkata and major medical centers in the south (Adyar, Coimbatore, Vellore and other centers). Currently, many centers in India perform esophageal resection for cancer, as it is an extremely common disease. However, most patients present late when effective surgery is not feasible and only palliative relief is offered by chemoradiotherapy and supportive treatment.

REFERENCES

1. Guy D Eslick. Esophageal Cancer: A Historical Review.

2. Raymond Hunt. Historical Review: Surgical treatment of carcinoma of the esophagus. Thorax 1991;46:528–35.

3. Elmslie RG. Perspectives in the development of esophageal surgery. In: Jamieson GG, (Ed.) Surgery of the esophagus. London: Churchill-Livingstone, 1988:3–8.

4. W Spencer Payne, Arthur Olsen—The Esophagus.

5. Churchill ED. In: Foreword to Hochberg LA. Thoracic Surgery before the 20th century. New York: Vantage Press, 1960.

6. Historical Review: Surgical treatment of carcinoma of the esophagus. Thorax 1991;46:528–35.

7. Billroth CAT. Uber die resektion des esophagus. Arch Klin Chir 1871;13:65–9.*

8. Czerny V. Neue Operationen; resektion des esophagus. Zentr Chir 1877;4:433–4.*

9. Mikulicz J Von. Ein Fall von Resektion des Carcinomatosen Esophagus mit plastichen Ersatz des exeidirten Stuckes. Prag Med Wochenschr 1886;11:93–4.*

10. Nassiloff II. Esophagotomia et resetcio oesophagi endo-thoracica. Vrach St Peterberg 1888;9:481–2.*

11. Hacker Von. Uber Resektion und Plastik am Kebsabschnitt der Spieserohre, inbesondere beim Carcinom. Arch Klin Chir 1908;87:257–323.*

12. Rehn L. Operationen an dem brustabschnitt der speiserohre. Verh Dtsch Ges Chir 1898;21; 448–70.*

13. Dobromysslov WD. Ein Fall von transpleuraler Osophagotomie im Brustabschnitte. Zbl Chir 1901;1:18.*

14. Fauré JL. Cancer de la portion thoracique de l'oesophage. Extirpation du neoplasme par la voie mediastinin posterior droite. Combinée a une incision cervicale. Bull Mem Soc Chir 1903;29:122–34.*

15. Roux C. L'Esophago-jejuno-gastrome, nouvelle operation pour retrecissement infrachisable de l'oesophage. Semaine Méd 1907;27:37.*

16. Voelcker. Uber Extirpation der Cardia wegen Carcinoms. Verh Dtsch Ges Chir 1908;37; 126–9.*

17. Lane WA. Excision of a cancerous segment of the esophagus: restoration of the esophagus by means of a skin flap. Br Med J 1911;1:16–7.

18. Kelling. Esophagoplastik mit hilfe des querkolon. Zbl Chir 1911;38;1209–12.*

19. Torek F. The first successful case of resection of the thoracic portion of the esophagus for carcinoma. Surg Gynecol Obstet 1913;16:614–7.
20. Denk W. Zur Radikaloperation des Oesophaguskarzinoms. Zentralbl Chir 1913;40;1065–8.*
21. Zaaijer JH. Erfolgreiche transpleurale Resektion eines Cardia-carcinoms. Beitr Klin Chir 1913;83; 419.*
22. Meyer W. Esophagoplasty. Ann Surg 1913;58: 289–95.
23. Kummell HJ. Ueber intrathorakale ooesophagus plastic. Beitr Klin Chir 1922;126:264–77.†
24. Turner GG. Some experiences in the surgery of the esophagus. N Engl J Med 1931;205:657–74.
25. Oshawa T. The surgery of the esophagus. Arch Jap Chir 1933;10:604–95.
26. Ogilive WH. Intrathoracic reconstruction of lower esophagus. Br J Surg 1938;26:10–22.
27. O'Shaughnessy L, Raven RW. Surgical exposure of the esophagus. Br J Surg 1934;22:365–77.
28. Garlock JH. The surgical treatment of the thoracic esophagus. Surg Gynecol Obstet 1938; 66;534–48.
29. Lewis I. Surgical treatment of carcinoma of the esophagus. Br J Surg 1946;34:18–31.
30. Orringer MB. Transhiatal esophagectomy without thoracotomy for esophageal carcinoma. In: Delarue NC, Wilkins EW, Wong J, (Eds.) International trends in general thoracic surgery. Vol 4. St Louis: Mosby, 1988:200–9.
31. Belsey RHR. Reconstruction of the esophagus with left colon. J Thorac Cardiothorac Surg 1965; 49:33–55.
32. McKeown KC. The surgical treatment of carcinoma of the esophagus. J R Coll Surg Edinb 1985;30:1–14.
33. Attila D, Seymour Schwartz. Franz John A. Torek. Ann Thorac Surg 2008;85:1497–9.
34. Eggers C, Franz JA Torek 1861–1938. Ann Surg 1939;110:797–9.
35. Exner A. Veber die behandlung von oesophagus karzinomen mit ardiumstrahlen. Wien Klin Wochenschr. 1904;17:514.¶
36. Neuner G, Patel A. Chemoradiotherapy for esophageal cancer. Gastrointest Cancer Res. 2009 Mar–Apr;3(2):57–65.

*References 7–16, 18, 20, 21 cited from Raymond Hurt. Historical review: Surgical treatment of carcinoma of the esophagus. Thorax 1991;46:528–35.

†Reference 23 cited from Vishesh J, Shilpa S. Transposed intrathoracic stomach: Functional evaluation. African Journal of Pediatric Surgery 2012:9;3:210–6.

¶Reference 36 cited from G Neuner, A Patel. Chemoradiotherapy for esophageal cancer. Gastrointest Cancer Res 2009 Mar–Apr;3(2):57–65.

2

Surgical Anatomy

Ratna Parikh, Praful Desai

The esophagus has a deep anatomic location and is the only organ which traverses three anatomic regions; the neck, the thorax and the upper abdomen. It commences at the lower edge of the cricoid cartilage (C_6 vertebra) and ends at the esophagogastric junction by merging with the cardia, about 40 cm from the incisor teeth. For anatomic and clinical convenience, the esophagus is divided into an upper, middle and lower segment (Figs 2.1 and 2.2). Squamous cell carcinoma is the predominant histology in the cervical, upper and middle third esophagus (above the pulmonary vein), whereas Adenocarcinoma predominates in the distal esophagus.

The anatomical relationship of the cervical esophagus is shown in Fig. 2.3. As seen in the cross section, the left border of the esophagus

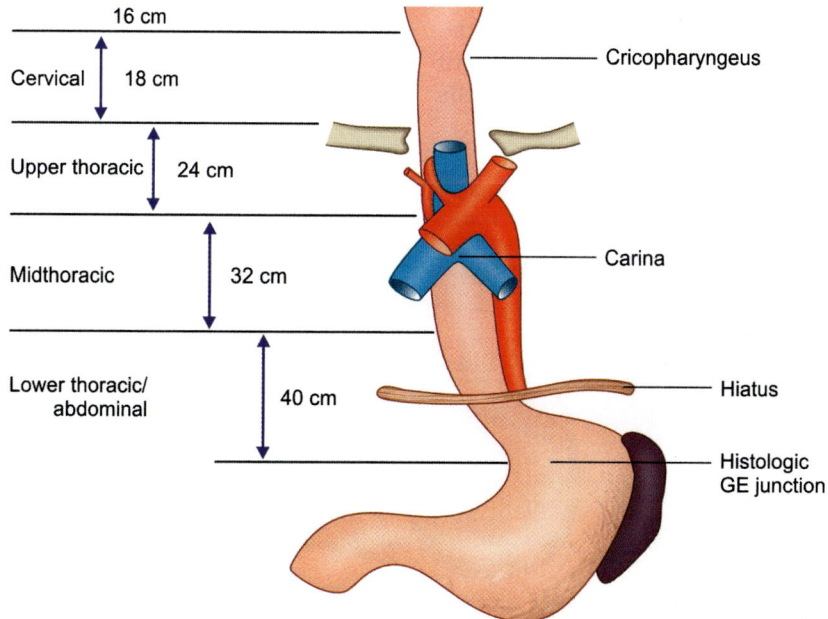

Fig. 2.1: Anatomical divisions of the esophagus

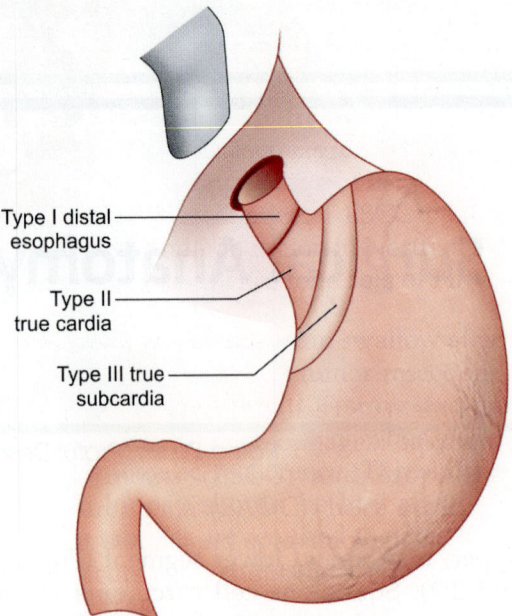

Type I distal esophagus

Type II true cardia

Type III true subcardia

Fig. 2.2: Conventional Siewarts classification is useful for therapy planning for gastroesophageal junction tumors. Type I tumors are considered adenocarcinomas of the distal esophagus and type II and III lesions are classified as gastric cancers (cardia and subcardia). Recent guidelines include gastroesophageal junction tumors under the esophageal cancer staging classification

extends beyond the trachea; hence, it is approached via a left sided cervical incision. It is important to know that the recurrent laryngeal nerve ascend on either side in the tracheoesophageal groove. The surgeon must therefore be careful during mobilization of the cervical esophagus.

The thoracic esophagus traverses through the superior and posterior mediastinum. Below the tracheal bifurcation, the esophagus curves to the right. Hence, mid esophageal lesions are approached through a right thoracotomy (Ivor Lewis procedure). Figure 2.4 shows the relationship of the esophagus with the descending aorta lying more to its right than anteriorly. The right wall of the esophagus is adjacent to the right parietal pleura; therefore, in the event of a perforation or postoperative anastomotic leak, a right sided pleural effusion is more likely. During mobilization of the esophagus the parietal pleura may be inadvertently nicked. This needs to be identified and sutured lest it may produce a pneumothorax of the right chest of varying severity. If this is of significant severity an intercostal drainage tube insertion is safer and worthwhile to prevent lung dysfunction. The thoracic duct crosses behind the esophagus from the seventh to the fifth thoracic vertebrae and then continues along its left border. It needs to be carefully identified to prevent injury and should be carefully sutured to avoid leakage in the chest, if injured.

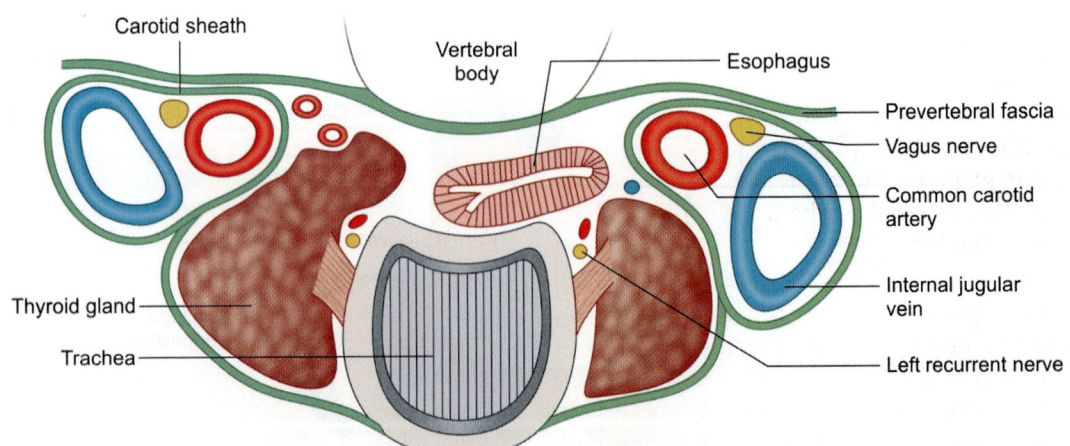

Carotid sheath

Vertebral body

Esophagus

Prevertebral fascia

Vagus nerve

Common carotid artery

Internal jugular vein

Thyroid gland

Trachea

Left recurrent nerve

Fig. 2.3: Anatomic relationship of the cervical esophagus

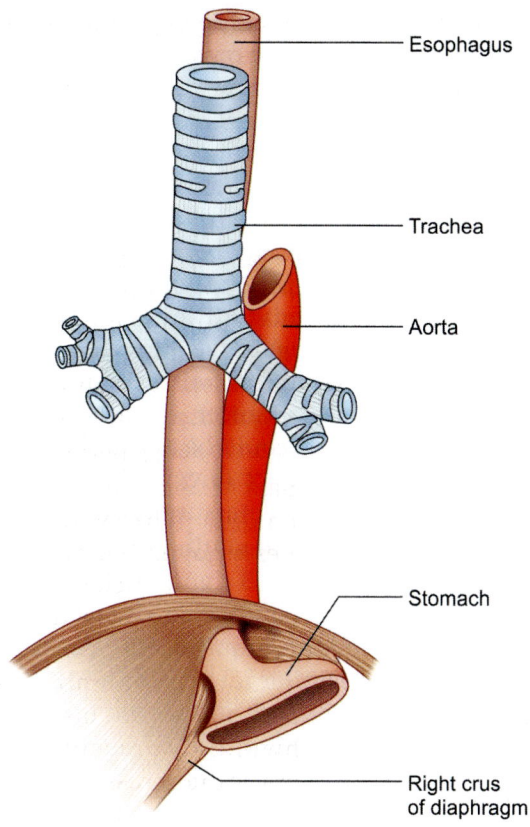

Fig. 2.4: Anatomy of the esophagus

through a left thoracoabdominal incision the median arcuate ligaments are divided for mobilizing the prepared stomach tube into the thorax for an esophagogastric anastomosis.

The esophagus has an inner and outer longitudinal muscle layer. Though the muscle layer coverage is important for a safe anastomosis, the more important layer is the strong esophageal mucosa, which holds the anastomotic sutures with greater safety. Because of the longitudinal muscle layer, anastomotic techniques require great care and very appropriate use of the strong mucosal layer. Esophageal muscle stitches, should be taken transversely because of its longitudinal anatomy.

The inferior thyroid artery supplies the upper third of the esophagus, while the multiple small esophageal branches of the aorta supply the major segment of the esophagus. It is important to keep in mind that most of these arteries are small and need to be carefully handled (Fig. 2.5). Branches of the gastric and inferior phrenic arteries supply

The lower esophagus deviates towards the left behind the pericardial sac and then passes through the esophageal hiatus to the left of the midline. Hence the lower esophagus is best approached through a left thoracoabdominal incision. Anastomotic leaks and perforations of the lower third of the esophagus result in a left sided pleural effusion. The abdominal esophagus is only 2.5 cm long and it grooves the posterior surface of the liver. It is covered by the peritoneum in front and on the left.

The mechanism of the cardia prevents the normal gastric contents from regurgitating into the esophagus. Following esophageal resection and esophagogastrostomy patients can develop reflux or aspiration pneumonia as the esophagogastric junction is resected. During mobilization of the esophagus

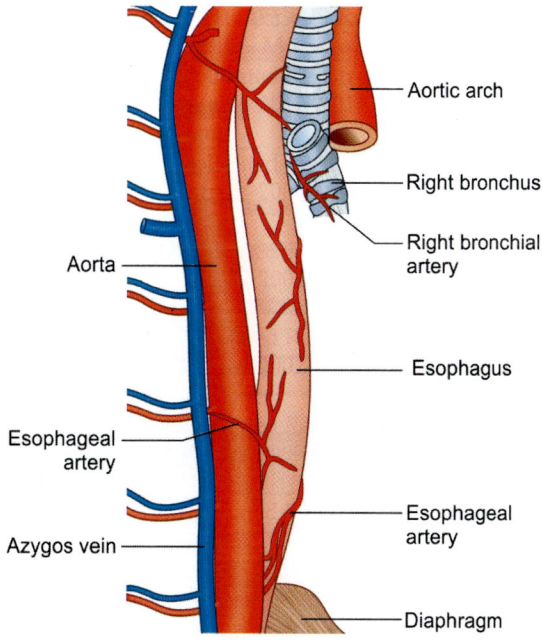

Fig. 2.5: Vascular anatomy of the esophagus. Tiny branches from the aorta, which supply the esophagus

the lower segment of the esophagus. Extensive posterior mobilization of the esophagus should be avoided as it may compromise this blood supply which can result in anastomotic disruption and significant postoperative complications. Blind mobilization of the esophagus during transhiatal resections should therefore be gently executed to avoid damage to these tiny vessels which provides significant vascularity. These vessels are the mainstay of a safe and successful esophageal resection. In a long segment adherent disease, blind digital dissection must be avoided to prevent any major complications. The venous drainage of the cervical esophagus is into the brachiocephalic vein via the inferior thyroid veins. The left side of the thoracic esophagus

drains into the brachiocephalic vein via the left hemiazygos system, while on the right, drainage is through the azygos system into the superior vena cava.

Lymphatic drainage of the esophagus is longitudinal. The lymphatic vessels in the submucosa may traverse for a long distance superiorly and inferiorly before penetrating the muscle layers to join the lymphatics in the adventitia. Even adventitial lymphatics, which usually drain into the adjacent lymph nodes, have a longitudinal arrangement; hence, in esophageal cancer, the first lymph node to be involved could be at a distant site from the primary tumor (Fig. 2.6). This does not necessarily exclude a surgical approach for its management and the primary

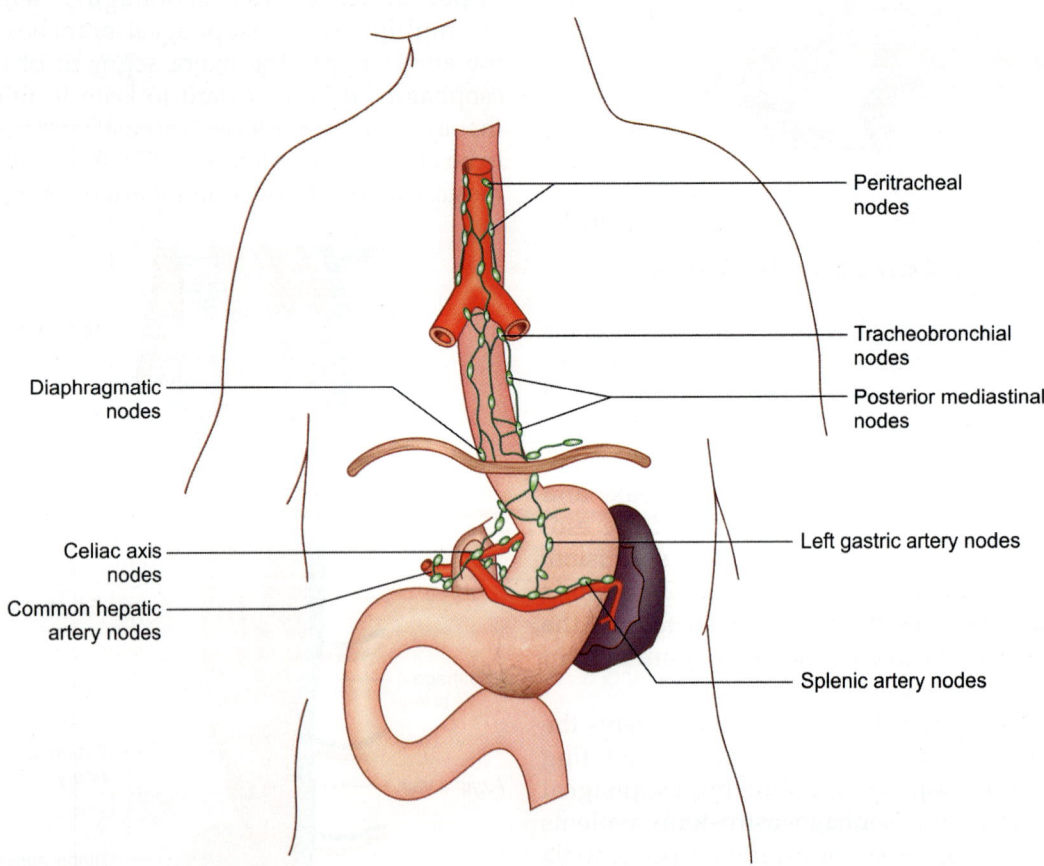

Fig. 2.6: Profuse lymphatic drainage of the esophagus, which is conducive for even distant metastasis

esophageal cancer should be treated on its merits; vis-à-vis a resection or chemo-radiotherapy as indicated in a given case.

In patients with cancer of the esophagus, mediastinal infiltration can obliterate the peri-esophageal fat planes in relation to the tumor. Anastomosis of the esophagus to the stomach, small bowel or colon is prone to leakage from the suture line. The reason may be poor blood supply at the ends, the absence of a strong serosal layer, the friability and the longi-tudinal anatomy of the muscle layer. Nature however, has compensated this by giving the esophagus a strong mucosal layer. It is therefore imperative to include this strong mucosal layer in the anastomotic technique. Most surgeons use "all coats" interrupted sutures during the anastomosis.

BIBLIOGRAPHY

1. The Esophagus: A Synopsis of Surgical Anatomy, 12th edition - Lee McGregor.
2. Cancer of the Esophagus - DeVita, Hellman and Rosenberg's Principle and Practice of Oncology 10th edition.

3

Esophageal Cancer and its Associated Factors – An Epidemiological Overview

B Ganesh

Introduction

The Global cancer burden is estimated to have risen to 18.1 million new cases and 9.6 million deaths in 2018. One in 5 males and one in 6 females worldwide develop cancer during their lifetime, and one in 8 males and one in 11 females die from the disease. Worldwide, the 5-year prevalence is estimated to be 43.8 million. The increasing cancer burden is due to several factors, including growing population, ageing and the changing prevalence of certain causes of cancer linked to socioeconomic development. This is particularly true in rapidly growing economies, where a shift is observed from cancers related to poverty and infections, to cancers associated with lifestyles more typical of industrialized countries. Effective prevention efforts may explain the observed decrease in incidence rates for some cancers, such as lung cancer (in males in Northern Europe and North America) and cervical cancer (in most regions apart from Sub-Saharan Africa). However, the new data show that most countries are still faced with an increase in the absolute number of cases requiring therapy and care.

Esophageal cancer (EC) is a relatively rare disease; however, in some areas they have a much higher incidence than others; China, Iceland, India, Japan and United Kingdom, appear to have a higher incidence, including the region around the Caspian Sea. In India the incidence rates vary across the country. High incidence of cancer of esophagus has been reported from Caspian littoral of Iran, central and East Asia and certain areas of China.[1]

WORLD SCENARIO

Estimates of Cancer Burden

As per the estimates of Globocan (2018), the major cancer types are the lung, female breast, and colorectum. These are the top three cancer types in terms of incidence, and are ranked within the top five in terms of mortality (first, fifth, and second, respectively). Together, these three cancers are responsible for one third of cancer incidence and mortality burden worldwide. Cancers of the lung and female breast are the leading types worldwide in terms of the number of new cases; for each of these types, approximately 2.1 million cases are estimated in 2018, contributing about 11.6% of the total cancer incidence burden.[2] Colorectal cancer (1.8 million cases, 10.2% of the total) is the third most commonly diagnosed cancer; prostate cancer is the fourth (1.3 million cases, 7.1%), and stomach cancer is the fifth (1.0 million cases, 5.7%) in incidence rates. Lung cancer is also responsible for the largest number of deaths (1.8 million deaths, 18.4% of the total), because of the poor prognosis for this cancer worldwide, followed by colorectal cancer (0.88 deaths, 9.2%), stomach cancer (0.78 deaths, 8.2%), and liver cancer (0.78 deaths, 8.2%). Female breast cancer ranks as the fifth leading cause of death (0.62 deaths, 6.6%) because the prognosis is relatively favorable, at least in more developed countries.[2]

Esophageal cancer is predominant in developing countries compared to developed countries. It may be added that the high-risk area of Caspian littoral is a part of an infamous 'Asian esophageal cancer belt' that stretches from the eastern part of the Caspian littoral in Iran via Turkmenistan to the northern provinces of China.[3] The ethnic background of the high-risk area of Iran includes Persian (including people of Sistani and Baloochi ethnicity who have migrated from south east of Iran seeking work) and the Turkmen scattered from north of Khorasan to east of the Caspian Sea. This registry shut down in the late 1970's. The registry reported a very high incidence (truncated rate of 150 cases per 100,000) with a sex ratio of one and in some parts higher incidence among females.[4] Although there was no report of incidence according to the ethnic group living in the area, an extension of the registry in other parts of the Caspian littoral revealed that the areas closer to the central part of the Caspian littoral (primarily Persian ethnicity) had a lower incidence.[5] The breakdown of incidence based on ethnicity is not available; however, based on data from case-control and other analytical studies, the highest incidence is seen among those of Turkmen ethnicity.[5]

Geographic variations in incidence

Cancer incidence worldwide among men is more than in women; with World age-standardized incidence rates of 219 and 183 per 100,000, respectively, in 2018;[2] male incidence rates vary almost fourfold across the different regions of the world; in 2018, rates ranged from 98 per 100,000 in South Central Asia to 364 and 571 per 100,000 in Western Europe and Australia and New Zealand, respectively.

Similarly in Asia, the rates in men were 170.6 and 139.6 in women, which are higher than those seen in South-Central Asia in both the sexes. In general, the rates higher in Europe and North America compared to other areas imply geographic variation in cancer occurrence across the world.

Although cancer is often considered to be more prevalent in the developed world, in fact, 56% of all cancers (excluding non-melanoma, skin cancer) occur in the less developed countries and 44% in more developed countries.[6]

Esophageal Cancer

World Scenario

Incidence rates

Esophageal cancer is the eighth most common cancer worldwide, with an estimated 5,72,034 new cases in 2018 (3.2% of the total), and the sixth most common cause of death from cancer with an estimated 5,08,585 deaths (5.3% of the total); these figures include both adeno-carcinoma and squamous cell carcinoma subtypes.[2]

Geographic variation–World

Around 80% of the cases worldwide occur in less-developed regions. Esophageal cancer incidence rates worldwide in males are more than double of those in females (Fig. 3.1). In both sexes there is more than 20-fold difference in incidence between different regions of the world, with rates ranging from 1.6 per 100,000 in Western Africa to 17.9 per 100,000 in Eastern Asia in males, and 0.8 per 100,000 in Micronesia/Western Africa to 7.1 per 100,000 in Eastern Africa in females.[2]

Incidence rates–World Comparison

Incidence of esophageal cancer varies across the world as seen among male and female as seen in Fig. 3.2[7] for some selected countries; it

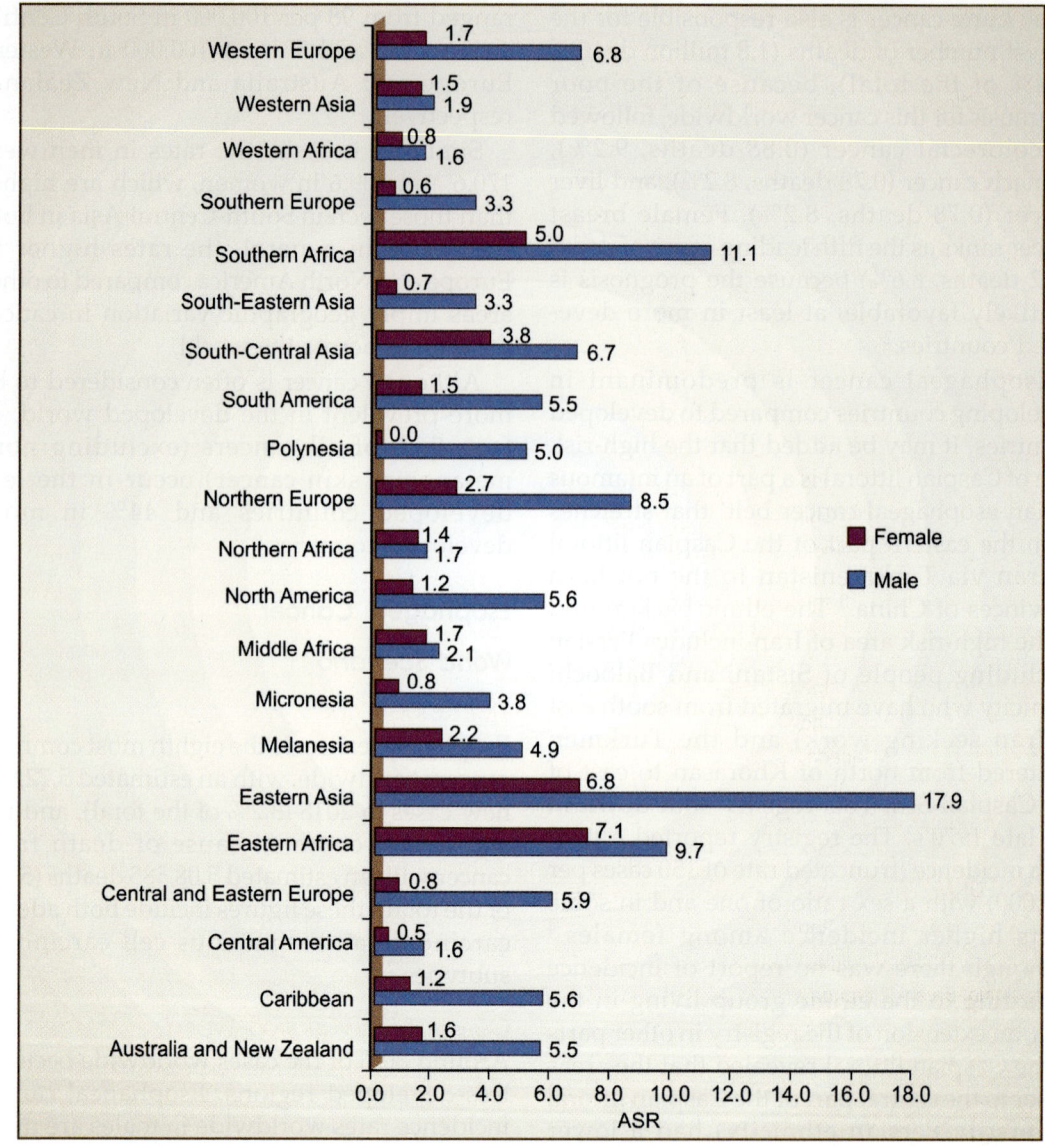

Fig. 3.1: Estimated incidence rates for esophagus cancer across world regions, 2018

is seen that rates are highest in China, Cixian country among males (162.8) and among females (101.9). In India, rates are highest in Bengaluru, in urban registries; however, it is uniformly higher in all north-eastern regions of India, led by Mizoram, India.[8]

Migration effects

The difference in incidence of esophageal cancer among the host and migrant population can be seen as migrant effect in CI5, IARC.[7] The Japanese, Niigata show incidence of 15.8 and 2.0 incidence rates in males and females respectively, but the migrant Japanese in US, Hawaii show the rates in level with the host population, i.e. 3.9 in males and 0.5 in females which is similar as in the US, San Francisco males and females; further similar observation can be seen of Chinese migrants, wherein Cixian,

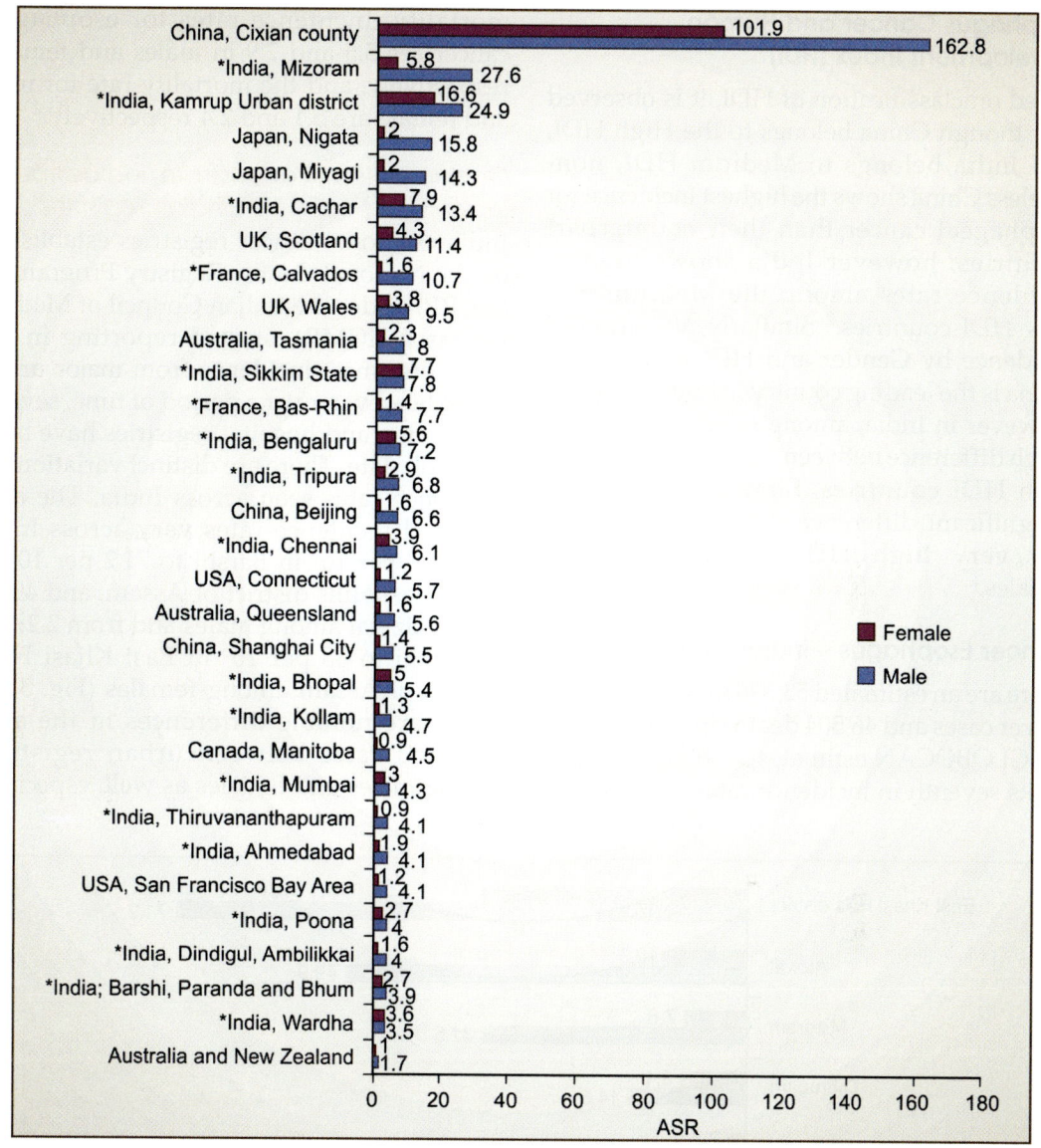

Fig. 3.2: Incidence rate (ASR per 10⁵) for esophageal cancer in Individual Registries - World comparison (*Source:* Forman et al. 2013, Cancer Incidence in Five Continents (CI5), Volume 10, IARC, www.ci5.iarc.fr)

China shows 162.8 and 101.9 in males and females respectively, while the Chinese in US, Hawaii, the rates are 2.7 and 0.4 in males and females respectively. The large variation in time for migrants to adopt the host population's cancer risk suggests that risk factors have organ-specific effects, or operate at different times in life. The persistent difference in cancer incidence several generations after migration supports the idea that living in the host country is not, alone, sufficient to modify cancer risk for all cancer sites to the level of the host population. Although the migration effect can be partially explained by known etiologic factors, a large proportion of the changing risk remains.

Esophagus Cancer and Human Development Index (HDI)

Based on classification of HDI, it is observed that though China belongs to the High HDI, and India belongs to Medium HDI, nonetheless China shows the highest incidence for esophageal cancer than their counterpart countries; however India shows highest incidence rates among the Medium and Low HDI countries.[2] Similarly, variation of incidence by Gender and HDI reveals that China is the leading country in both the sexes. However in India, among males there is not much difference between India and low/very high HDI countries. Similarly, there are insignificant differences between India and low/very high HDI countries among females.[2]

Cancer Esophagus – Indian Scenario

There are an estimated 52,396 new esophageal cancer cases and 46,504 deaths in India, as per the GLOBOCAN estimates 2018.[2] Esophagus ranks seventh in incidence rates and sixth in mortality. Incidence rates for esophageal cancer are 5.5 and 2.9 in males and females respectively, and the mortality rate for male and female are 5.1 and 2.4 respectively.[2]

Geographical Variation in incidence of esophageal cancer in Indian registries

Indian national cancer registries established by the National Cancer Registry Programme (NCRP) under the Indian Council of Medical Research (ICMR), started reporting in the 1980s on cancer incidence from major urban areas; however, over a period of time, several population and hospital registries have been setup till date. There are distinct variations in incidence rates seen across India. The age-adjusted incidence rates vary across India from 4.0 per 10^5 in Barshi to 71.2 per 10^5 in East Khasi Hills district of Assam, and 49.9/10^5 in Aizwal among males and from 2.2/10^5 in Barshi to 33 per 10^5 in East Khasi Hills district of Assam among females (Fig. 3.3).[8] There are notable differences in the age-adjusted rates between urban registries among males and females as well, especially

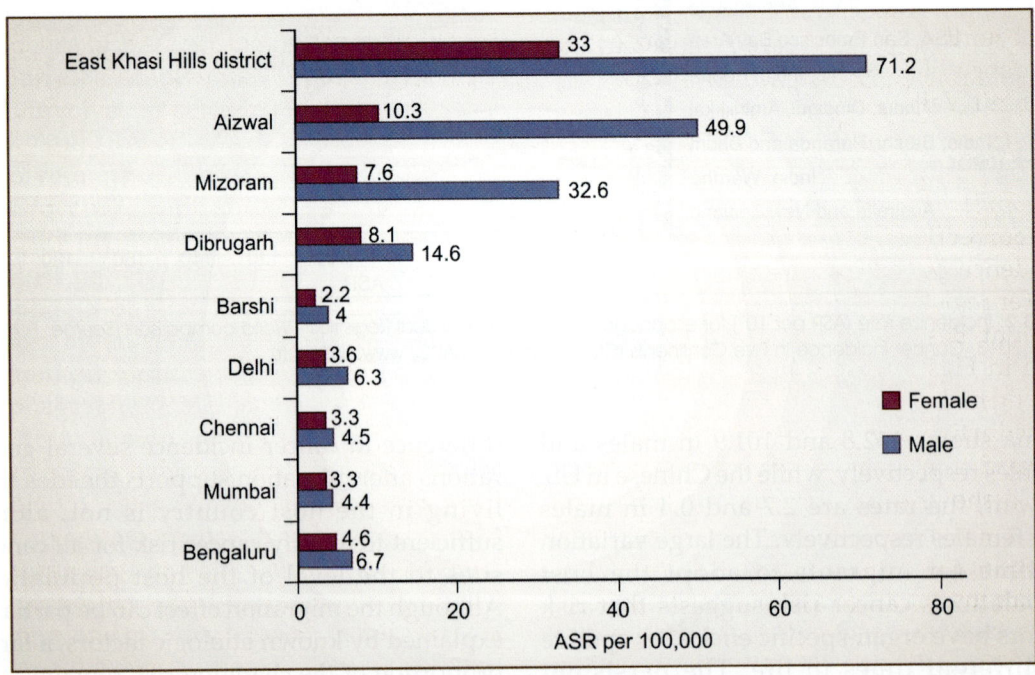

Fig. 3.3: Incidence rates of esophageal cancer in Indian population registries; *Source:* NCDIR, (2016a)

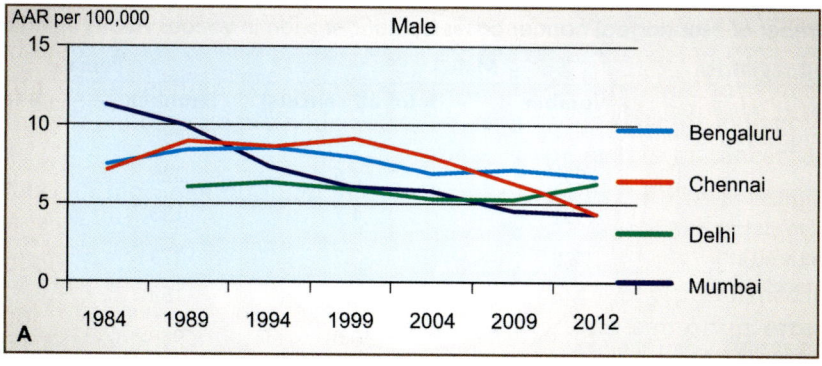

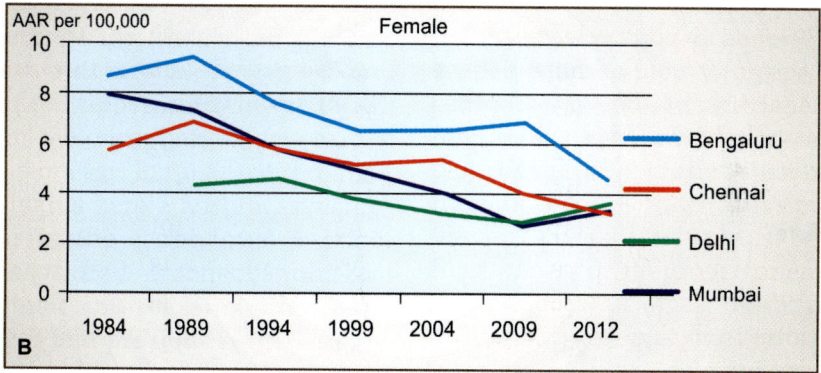

Figs 3.4A and B: Incidence rates of esophageal cancer in Indian PBCRs over the decades (*Source:* NCDIR, PBCR Reports 1984–2014)

in the north-east registries. However, the high incidence of esophagus cancer observed in Kashmir Valley.[9]

Time-Trends: Esophageal Cancer in India

Population based cancer registries (PBCR): To correctly assess the trend of cancer incidence over the years, population based cancer registries should be always taken into account. Based on the data on time trends, as seen in Figs 3.4A and B, it is observed that among males, the rates in Mumbai has shown a distinctive decline while Delhi shows an upward trend among females. Figures 3.4A and B shows only moderate upward trends except a significant decline in Bengaluru and a moderate upward trend in Delhi.[8,10,11] Variations in different areas are subject to the methods of data collection and the precision with which they are recorded by the investi-

gators. The PBCR is the only avenue by which we can access the variation of a country or a state.

Hospital based cancer registries (HBCR): The esophageal cancer frequencies differ between hospital registries and that seen in population based registries. To demonstrate this, the following table is elucidated from India of different HBCR in India. Table 3.1 show that Guwahati hospital recorded the highest number of esophagus cancer cases (1973) among males, followed by Chandigarh (649), Srinagar (597) and Mumbai (528); similarly among females Guwahati (989), followed by Chandigarh (478), Srinagar (461) and Mumbai (285). There is a male-preponderance in all the registries. North-east shows the highest number of cancer cases seen in a single institution.[12]

Table 3.1	Number of esophageal cancer cases by gender seen in various HBCRs in India			
Hospital based registries	Male		Female	
	Number	% (of all cancers)	Number	% (of all cancers)
Mumbai	528	3.6	285	2.6
Bengaluru	298	7.6	225	4.7
Chennai	191	4.7	133	3.0
Thiruvananthapuram	428	3.7	173	1.5
Dibrugarh	244	13.6	159	8.9
Guwahati	1973	15.0	989	10.5
Chandigarh	649	6.7	478	6.3
New Delhi	137	3.1	86	2.4
Kochi	161	2.7	52	1.1
Srinagar	597	11.2	461	12.1
Kannur	172	4.4	92	2.6
Silchar	316	11.1	147	7.4
VIMS - Bangalore	131	6.3	101	5.1
RCC - Raipur	49	3.7	18	1.0
ICC - Neyyoor	29	4.8	18	2.4
RCC - Nagpur	204	8.1	124	4.9
CCICH - Kottayam	65	3.9	12	0.7

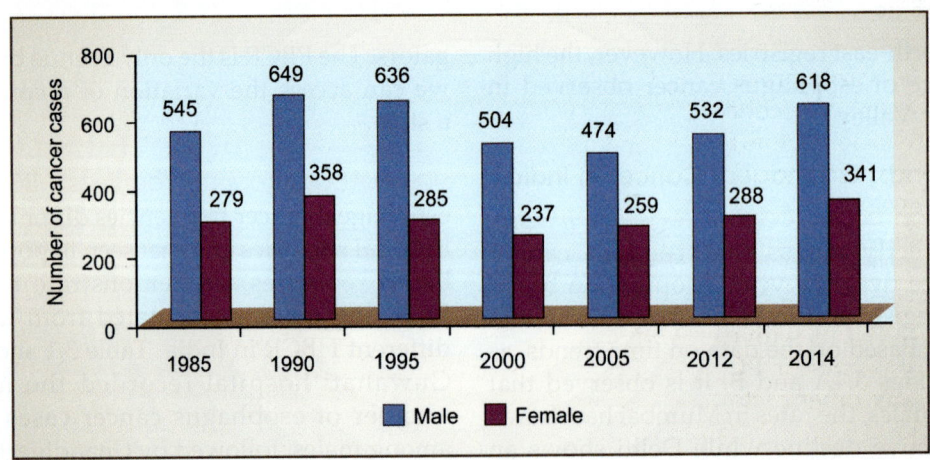

Fig. 3.5: Distribution of esophageal cancers in Tata Memorial Hospital (TMH) 1985–2014 (*Source:* Annual Reports of Hospital cancer registries, 1985–2014. Tata Memorial Hospital, Mumbai, India)

Trends in HBCRs

It is seen in Fig. 3.5 that cases seen in TMH over the years has not shown any remarkable increase or significant difference among male and female cases over the period.[13–19]

It has been observed that esophageal cancer cases have increased over the period for both the sexes in Bengaluru, Chennai, Thiruvananthapuram and Dibrugarh hospital registries.[20–25] Probably because more patients

Site\Year	1985	1990	1995	2000	2005	2012	2014	Total
Table 3.2								
Cervical Esophagus	20	19	14	6	4	1	2	66
U/3 Esophagus	102	112	113	97	90	84	112	710
M/3 Esophagus	419	567	446	283	203	210	288	2416
L/3 Esophagus	268	293	307	233	149	203	271	1724
Overlapping Esophagus	2	–	–	–	–	–	–	2
Esophagus No's	13	16	41	122	287	322	286	1087
Total	**824**	**1007**	**921**	**741**	**733**	**820**	**959**	**6005**

Table 3.2 Number of esophageal cancer cases by subsites seen in TMH-1985–2014

are now treated locally in their own environment.

TMH being a premier Cancer Institute in the country it is possible to classify the cases by subsites from the Hospital Cancer Registry data. From Table 3.2 it is seen that middle one-third and lower one-third esophagus are commonly affected subsites in the esophagus as seen in Tata Memorial Hospital.[13-19]

RISK FACTORS

A risk factor is anything that will increase the chance of developing a disease (cancer). Different cancers have varied risk factors, some are however preventable. Factors like smoking, drinking alcohol, dietary deficiencies, etc. are major factors for the development of esophageal cancer (EC).[26] Age, family history are other important risk factors. Some are more likely to increase the risk of adenocarcinoma while some increase the risk of squamous cell carcinoma. Having a risk factor is not synonymous with development of EC; there are patients of EC without any risk factors. Many other factors can increase the risk of developing EC; these are elucidated below.

Age

Age increases the risk for esophageal cancer; the disease is more common after the age of 50. Less than 15% of cases occur in patients younger than 55.[27]

Gender and Race

The risk of development of EC is three times higher in male than females.[28] EC rate disparities are pronounced for Blacks and Whites. In a study on black-white esophageal cancer incidence, mortality, relative survival rates, histology and trends for the time period 1991–2000 showed, the age-adjusted rate of EC in Black Americans is twice that of Whites (8.63 vs 4.39 per 100,000, $p<0.05$). The age-adjusted mortality for blacks, although showing a declining trend, was nearly twice that of Whites (7.79 vs 3.96, $p<0.05$). Though survival is poor overall it was twice more than the Blacks. Squamous cell carcinoma is common in Blacks and white females, whereas adenocarcinoma was more common among white males ($p < 0.001$).[29]

Family History

Family history (FH) and risk of upper gastrointestinal (UGI) cancers has been reported rarely; the data on UGI cancer survival are sparse. In a large case-control study, it was reported that increased esophageal squamous cell carcinoma (ESCC) risk was associated with a FH of any cancer, FH of any UGI cancer and FH of esophageal cancer.[30] This data provided strong evidence that shared susceptibility is involved in esophageal carcinogenesis and also suggest a role in prognosis.

Gastroesophageal Reflux Disease (GERD)

The stomach secretes acid and enzymes to help digest food. In some individuals, acid regurgitates from the stomach into the lower part of the esophagus. This is gastro-esophageal reflux disease (GERD). This can cause symptoms such as heartburn or retro-sternal pain; however, in some individuals reflux does not cause any symptoms at all. People with GERD have a slightly higher risk of getting adenocarcinoma of the esophagus. This risk seems to be higher in people who have more frequent symptoms. GERD is very common condition, and most of the people who have it do not go onto develop eso-phageal cancer. GERD can also cause Barrett's esophagus (discussed below), which is linked to an even higher risk.[31]

Barrett's Esophagus

Prolonged reflux can damage the inner lining of the esophagus. This causes the squamous cells that normally line the esophagus to be replaced with gland cells. These gland cells usually look like the cells that line the stomach and the small intestine, and are more resistant to stomach acid. This condition is known as Barrett's (or Barrett) esophagus. The longer someone has reflux, the more likely it is that they will develop Barrett's esophagus. Most people with Barrett's esophagus have had symptoms of heartburn, but many have no symptoms at all. People with Barrett's eso-phagus are at a much higher risk than people without this condition to develop adenocarci-noma of the esophagus.[31]

Tobacco and Alcohol

Tobacco use is quite common in India and is used in different forms. Pan, a preparation consisting of green betel-leaf containing sliced betel nut, slaked lime and some spicy ingre-dients, is a common form of chewing habit in India. Pan is chewed with or without tobacco. Bidi, an Indian cigarette, containing 0.2–0.3 gm of tobacco is rolled in a dried leaf, i.e temburni leaf. Doll (1971)[33] in his extensive review of both prospective and retrospective studies on esophageal cancer stated "Tobacco smoking to be casually associated with esophageal cancer consistently in all the studies."

The use of tobacco products, including cigarettes, cigars, pipes, and chewing tobacco, is a major risk factor for esophageal cancer. The more a person uses tobacco and the longer it is used, the higher the cancer risks. Someone who smokes a pack of cigarettes a day or more has at least twice the chance of getting adeno-carcinoma of the esophagus than a non-smoker, and the risk does not go away if tobacco use stops. The link to squamous cell esophageal cancer is even stronger, but this risk decreases for people who quit tobacco. In a recent study from Jammu region of India, the risk was highest for those who indulged in tobacco-snuffing.[34]

Table 3.3 shows the various risks of tobacco chewers and smokers reported by studies conducted in India.[32,35–45] The relative risk of esophageal cancer patients varied from 1.3[45] to 3.5 for tobacco chewers and from 1.7 to 6.4 among smokers. It is seen that a combined habit of tobacco chewing and smoking increases the risk multi-fold.; the risk reported ranged from 2.837 to 13.2,[45] proving that chewing acts synergistically with smoking in enhancing the risk.

Hookah Smoking, Nass-chewing

Although cigarette smoking is an established risk factor for esophageal squamous cell carcinoma (ESCC), there is little information about the association between other kind of smoking and smokeless tobacco products, including hookah and nass, and ESCC risk. In Kashmir Valley, India, hookah smoking, nass chewing, and ESCC are common. A case control study was undertaken to investigate the association of hookah smoking, nass use, and several other habits with ESCC.[46] For hookah smoking (OR = 1.85; 95% CI, 1.41–2.44) and nass chewing (OR = 2.88; 95% CI, 2.06–4.04) were associated with ESCC risk.

Author	Chewing	Smoking	Chew + Smoke
Sanghvi et al 1955[32]	3.5	2.9	5.3
Paymaster et al 1968[35]	1.9	2.5	3.1
Jussawalla & Deshpande 1971a[36]	2.5	2.9	6.2
Paymaster et al 1973[37]	2.1	1.9	2.8
Jayant el at 1977[38]	2.5	2.2	6.2
Jussawalla 1971b[39]	2.9	2.6	5.6
Jussawalla 1981[40]	2.8	5.3	—
Notani & Jayant 1987[41]	1.5	3.2	3.3
Notani 1988[42]	1.6	4	6.3
Rao et al 1989[43]	1.3	1.7	1.6
Ramesh 1993[44]	2.6	6.4	13.2
Ganesh et al 2009[45]	1.3	2.0	—

Table 3.3 Relative risk of esophageal cancer of tobacco chewers and smokers

Alcohol Habits

Alcohol consumption increases the risk for esophageal cancer and is known to affect the squamous cell type more than the adenocarcinoma of the esophagus.[45,47] The combined habit of smoking and alcohol multiplies the risk. A 1.8-fold excess risk for alcohol drinkers was observed in this study;[45] there was a clear dose-response relationship in those with the habit.

Although alcohol drinking is considered as an important risk factor for esophageal cancer, the magnitude of the association might be varied among geographic areas. In a review of four cohort and nine case-control studies in a Japanese population, it was concluded that there is convincing evidence that alcohol drinking increases the risk of esophageal cancer in the Japanese population.[48] Combining smoking and drinking alcohol raises the risk of esophageal cancer much more than using either alone. Vioque et al (2008)[49] in a case-control study in Spain reported that alcohol consumption may not be significantly associated with ESCC in high-risk rural areas.

In another study from China, alcohol drinking among males significantly increased the risk for ESCC (OR = 2.20) and observed increasing ESCC risks with decreasing age at behavior initiation as well as with increasing duration and intensity of alcohol intake, which were particularly evident among current smokers;[50] in contrast, neither smoking nor alcohol drinking was associated with ESCC risk among females. Alcohol drinking showed a monotonic dose-response relationship with ESCC risk among men, and this relationship was particularly evident among smokers. Very detailed case control study by Sankarnarayanan et al (1991) was conducted in Kerala, where they found that tobacco chewing, bidi, cigarette smoking, alcohol and snuff consummation were risk factors for esophageal cancer.[51] The dose-response relationship was also shown in this study for all risk factors.

Obesity

People who are overweight or obese have higher chances of developing adenocarcinoma of the esophagus. This is in part explained by the fact that people who are obese are more likely to have gastroesophageal reflux. The incidence of esophageal adenocarcinoma has increased dramatically in the developed world in the last half century. Approximately over the same period there has been an increase in the prevalence of obesity. Multiple epidemiological studies and meta-analyses have confirmed that obesity, especially abdominal (visceral obesity), is a risk factor for gastroesophageal reflux, Barrett's esophagus and esophageal adenocarcinoma.[52]

Dietary Habits

Certain substances in the diet may increase esophageal cancer risk. For example, there have been suggestions, as yet not well proven, that a diet high in processed meat may increase the chance of developing esophageal cancer. This may help explain the high rate of this cancer in certain parts of the world with such dietetic habits. Diet high in fruits and vegetables are known to reduce the risk whereas meat eaters are prone to higher risk for esophageal cancer. There are studies from India and western countries as well; fruits and vegetables provide a number of vitamins and minerals that may help prevent cancer.[28] Red meat, lamb, and boiled meat were directly associated with the risk of ESCC, whereas total white meat, poultry, fish, and liver were mainly protective against this malignancy.[53]

Drinking very hot liquids frequently may increase the risk for the squamous cell type of esophageal cancer[45, 54, 56] among others; this may be the result of a long-term damage the liquids can inflict on the cell lining the esophagus. In one of the earliest studies from India, the risk for smokers and chewers were higher among non-vegetarian group compared to the vegetarian group.[43] This study conducted at Tata Memorial Hospital, Mumbai, India, included 442 cases of esophageal cancer and 1628 hospital controls. Among the beverages, tea drinking, common in India, showed a fourfold excess risk for esophageal cancer. However fresh-fish showed a 20% reduction in risk for esophageal cancer.[45]

It may be observed from Table 3.4, that fruits, fresh-fish, vegetables, vegetarian diet are protective factors for esophageal cancer; however red chilli powder, tea drinking (hot), salted tea, use of very spicy food, pickled vegetables, wheat, corn, maize consumption and pork are risk factors for esophageal cancer. A diet high in fruits and vegetables is linked to a lower risk of esophageal cancer; the exact reasons for this are not clear, but fruits and vegetables have a number of vitamins and minerals that may help prevent cancer.[41,43–45,55–61]

Frequently drinking very hot liquids (temperatures of 149° F or 65° C - much hotter than a typical cup of coffee) may increase the risk for the squamous cell type of esophageal cancer. This might be the result of long-term damage to the cells lining the esophagus from hot liquids. The Odds ratio of drinking very hot green tea for ESCC risk was 2.15 compared with never drinking tea (Yang et al 2018); Very hot tea drinking significantly increases the risk

Table 3.4 Selected Indian and International studies on diet and esophageal cancer		
Author name	**Protective dietary item**	**Risk factor**
Notani & Jayant (1987)[41]	Vegetables, fruits, fish, buttermilk	Red chilli powder, tea drinking
Rao et al (1989)[43]	Vegetarian diet	—
Kumar et al (1992)[55]	—	Salted tea
Ramesh (1993)[44]	—	Use of very spicy food
Joint Iran IRAC (1977)[56]	Fresh fruit, green vegetables, fish protein	—
Tuyns et al (1987)[57]	Animal protein, polyunsaturated fats, citrus fruits, oil intake	—
Li et al (1989)[58]	—	Wheat, corn
Cheng et al (1992)[59]	—	Pickled vegetables
Van Rensberg et al (1985)[60]	—	Maize consumption
Yu Y et al (1993)[61]	—	Pork, corn, surface water use
Ganesh et al 2009[45]	Fresh fish	Tea (hot)

of ESCC among Chinese men, which is particularly evident among alcohol drinkers. Similar findings were observed in an Indian study by Ganesh et al 2009.[45, 62] Besides these there are other risk factors such as achalasia, tylosis, Plummer-Vinson syndrome injury to the esophagus (lye, a chemical found in strong industrial and household cleaners), history of other cancers, HPV virus, found only in Asian and South African patients and not in any other parts of the world.

Achalasia

In this condition, the muscle at the lower end of the esophagus (the lower esophageal sphincter) does not relax appropriately. Swallowed food and liquids do not pass normally into the stomach and tend to collect in the lower esophagus, which becomes distended over time. The lining of the esophagus in that area undergoes chronic irritation due to stasis of food for a long-time. People with achalasia have a risk of esophageal cancer. On an average, the cancers are detected 15–20 years after achalasia cardia develops.

Tylosis

This is a rare, inherited disease that causes an excess growth of the superficial layer of skin on the palms of hands and soles of the feet. People with this condition also develop small growths (papillomas) in the esophagus and have a very high-risk of developing ESCC. People with tylosis need to be watched closely to diagnose esophageal cancer early. This requires regular monitoring with an upper endoscopy.

Plummer-Vinson Syndrome

People with this rare syndrome also called Paterson-Kelly syndrome have webs in the upper part of the esophagus, typically along with anemia, tongue irritation (glossitis), brittle fingernails and sometimes a large thyroid gland or an enlarged spleen. A web is a thin membrane extending out from the inner lining of the esophagus that causes an area of narrowing. Most esophageal webs do not cause any symptoms, but larger ones can cause dysphagia, which can lead to chronic irritation in that area from the trapped food. About 1 in 10 people with this syndrome eventually develop ESCC of the lower esophagus or cancer in the hypopharynx.

Workplace Exposures

Exposure to chemical fumes in certain workplaces may lead to an increased risk of esophageal cancer. For example, exposure to the solvents used for dry cleaning may lead to a greater risk of esophageal cancer. Some studies have found that dry cleaning workers may have a higher rate of esophageal cancer but not all studies have found this link. Farmer/gardener and workers with exposure to dust had a significant excess risk in a Taiwanese study.[63]

Injury to the Esophagus

Lye is a chemical found in strong industrial and household cleaners. Lye is a corrosive agent that can burn and destroy cells. Accidentally drinking from a lye-based cleaner bottle can cause a severe chemical burn in the esophagus. As the injury heals, the scar tissue can result in narrowing of the esophagus (stricture). People with these strictures have an increased risk of ESCC, which often occurs many years (even decades) later.

Human Papilloma Virus (HPV) Infection

HPV is a group of more than 100 related viruses. They are called papilloma viruses because some of them cause a type of growth called a papilloma (or wart). Infection with certain types of HPV is linked to a number of cancers including throat, anal and cervical cancer. Signs of HPV infection have been found in one-third of esophageal cancers from patients in parts of Asia and South Africa. But signs of HPV infection have not been found in esophagus cancers from patients in the other areas including the US.

Cancers are the second most common cause of non-accidental deaths in Iran, following cardiovascular deaths. Mazandaran, near the Caspian littoral, north of Iran have identified several-high incidence areas for ESCC in the world. A high prevalence of HPV DNA in different anatomical sites of ESCC patients from the Mazandaran region in North of Iran provided more evidence for a role of HPV in this cancer.[64]

Histology Type

Cancer of the esophagus has two main histopathologic subtypes, esophageal squamous cell carcinoma (ESCC) and esophageal adenocarcinoma (EADC), have strikingly different clinical and epidemiologic features. ESCC occurs throughout the esophagus and is the most common histological subtype globally; over 90% of cases in traditionally high-risk regions of Eastern Asia and Eastern and Southern Africa are ESCC.[65] The incidence of ESCC is decreasing worldwide. In some high-risk areas in Asia the decrease was preceded by economic development and improvements in diet, whereas in high-income countries the decrease followed reductions in cigarette smoking. In contrast, the incidence of EADC continues to increase in many high and middle income countries, especially among white men. EADC develops in the lower third of the esophagus, primarily because of gastroesophageal reflux disease (GERD) and obesity. About 90% of esophageal cancers worldwide are Squamous Cell Carcinomas (SCC), mostly occurring in defined high-incidence areas of low and middle resource countries. Historically, the highest incidences are reported in regions of Central Asia. One such region is Kashmir Valley in Northern India.

Nitrosamines

Until date, more than twenty kinds of nitrosamines have been reported to play an important role in inducing EC in animals. N-nitro compounds and precursors are present in salted vegetables and preserved fish in high incidence areas such as Cixian and China.[66]

SUMMARY

In India, esophageal cancer is the most common malignancy involving the gastrointestinal tract in Karnataka, Tamil Nadu, Kerala and Assam.[67] In Kashmir, esophageal cancer has the highest incidence. There is scarcity of epidemiological studies of this malignancy.[68] Esophageal cancer has a peculiar geographical distribution and shows marked differences in incidence within a particular geographical region. The global cancer estimates indicate that esophageal cancer is basically a cancer common in developing and less developed countries. The rates seen are highest in China and in India, especially in the north-eastern states; however esophageal cancer is associated with various risk factors like lifestyle, diet, etc. which need to be spelt and provide leads for possible reduction and control of occurrence of esophageal cancer.

The national trend of esophageal carcinoma shows an increasing incidence over the past two decades. Alcohol consumption and smoking are major risk factors. Squamous cell carcinoma is the dominant histological type. Late presentation, is characteristic in most patients; conventional management does not have significant impact on survival. Early diagnosis and treatment is advocated but remains an uphill task. In view of this grim situation, prevention will be the key to reduce

I would like to hereby acknowledge Mr Mahadev Bhise, Ms Sushama Saoba and Mrs Sandhya Cheulkar of the department for the assistance provided in compiling the data required for the manuscript, and also the staff of the department. I would like to thank Dr RA Badwe, Director, Tata Memorial Centre, Dr AK D'Cruz, Director, Tata Memorial Hospital, and Dr S Chiplunkar, Director, Advanced Centre for Treatment, Research and Education in Cancer, for their support.

the incidence and mortality of esophageal cancer, by tobacco-use cessation, dietary preferences, reduction in alcohol drinking and other such risk-related issues which increases the risk of esophageal cancer.

It is known that the incidence of esophageal cancer is more so in the developing countries that includes India. However, with the possible factors for prevention that has been alluded to earlier, it is necessary, imperative and important that this cancer needs more attention and research for better outcomes in terms of its benefits to the population at large.

REFERENCES

1. Kamangar F, Malekzadeh R, Dawsey SM, Saeidi F. Esophageal cancer in Northeastern Iran: a review. 2007.

2. GLOBOCAN 2018. International Agency for Research on Cancer. http://gco.iarc.fr/...

3. Sagar PM. Aetiology of cancer of the Esophagus: geographical studies in the footsteps of Marco Polo and beyond. Gut 1989;30(5):561.

4. Mahboubi E, Kmet J, Cook PJ, Day NE, Ghadirian P, Salmasizadeh S. Esophageal cancer studies in the Caspian Littoral of Iran: the Caspian cancer registry. British journal of cancer 1973;28(3):197.

5. Hormozdiari H, Day NE, Aramesh B, Mahboubi, E. Dietary factors and esophageal cancer in the Caspian Littoral of Iran. Cancer research 1975; 35(11 Part 2);3493–8.

6. Ferlay J, Soerjomataram I, Dikshit R, Eser S, Mathers C, Rebelo M, Bray F. Cancer incidence and mortality worldwide: sources, methods and major patterns in GLOBOCAN 2012. International journal of cancer 2015;136(5): E359–86.

7. Forman D, Bray F, Brewster DH, Gombe Mbalawa C, Kohler B, Piñeros M, Steliarova-Foucher E, Swaminathan R and Ferlay J, (Eds) 2013. http://ci5.iarc.fr/CI5-X/Default.aspx

8. NCDIR. Three-Year Report of Population Based Cancer Registries 2012–2014. Incidence, Distribution, Trends in Incidence Rates and Projections of Burden of Cancer (Report of 27 PBCRs in India), NCDIR-NCRP, ICMR, 2016a.

9. Khuroo MS, Zargar SA, Mahajan R, Banday M. A. High incidence of Esophageal and gastric cancer in Kashmir in a population with special personal and dietary habits. Gut 1992;33(1): 11–5.

10. NCDIR. Time Trends in Cancer Incidence Rates 1982–2010, NCDIR-NCRP, ICMR, 2013a.

11. NCDIR. Three-Year Report of Population Based Cancer Registries 2009–2011, NCDIR-NCRP, ICMR, 2013b.

12. NCDIR. Consolidated Report of Hospital Cancer Registries 2012–2014. An Assessment of the Burden and Care of Cancer Patients, NCDIR-NCRP, ICMR, 2016b.

13. HBCR. Hospital Cancer Registry (Eds.) Desai PB, Rao RS, Rao DN, Shroff PD. Annual Report-1985, Tata Memorial Hospital, Mumbai, 1988.

14. HBCR. Hospital Cancer Registry (Eds.) Desai PB, Rao RS, Rao DN, Shroff PD. Annual Report-1990, Tata Memorial Hospital, Mumbai, 1992.

15. HBCR. Hospital Cancer Registry (Eds.) Dinshaw KA, Rao DN, Shroff PD. Annual Report-1995, Tata Memorial Hospital, Mumbai, 1998.

16. HBCR. Hospital Cancer Registry (Eds.) Dinshaw KA, Rao DN, Ganesh B. Annual Report-2000, Tata Memorial Hospital, Mumbai, 2004.

17. HBCR. Hospital Cancer Registry (Eds.) Dinshaw KA, Ganesh B. Annual Report-2005, Tata Memorial Hospital, Mumbai, 2008.

18. HBCR. Hospital Cancer Registry (Eds.) Badwe RA, Ganesh B. Annual Report-2012, Tata Memorial Hospital, Mumbai, 2016.

19. HBCR. Hospital Cancer Registry (Eds.) Badwe RA, Ganesh B. Annual Report-2014, Tata Memorial Hospital, Mumbai, 2017.

20. NCDIR. Consolidated Report of Hospital Based Cancer Registries 2012–2014. NCDIR-NCRP ICMR, 2016.

21. NCDIR. Consolidated Report of Hospital Based Cancer Registries 2007–2011. NCDIR-NCRP ICMR, 2013.

22. NCDIR. Consolidated Report of Hospital Based Cancer Registries 2004–2006. NCDIR-NCRP ICMR, 2009.

23. NCDIR. Consolidated Report of Hospital Based Cancer Registries 2001–2003. NCDIR-NCRP ICMR, 2007.

24. NCDIR. Consolidated Report of Hospital Based Cancer Registries 1999–2000. NCDIR-NCRP ICMR, 2005.

25. NCDIR. Consolidated Report of Hospital Based Cancer Registries 1984–1993. NCDIR-NCRP ICMR, 2001.

26. Wynder EL, Bross IJ. A study of etiological factors in cancer of the esophagus. Cancer 1961;14(2), 389–413.

27. Ferlay J, Shin HR, Bray F, Forman D, Mathers C, Parkin DM. GLOBOCAN 2008 v2.0, Cancer

incidence and mortality worldwide: IARC Cancer Base No. 10. 2010. Lyon, France: International Agency for Research on Cancer available at: http://globocan. iarc. fr.[Accessed 22 November 2011].

28. Pohl H, Wrobel K, Bojarski C, Voderholzer W, Sonnenberg A, Rösch T, Baumgart DC. Risk factors in the development of esophageal adeno-carcinoma. The American journal of gastroenterology 2013;108(2):200.

29. Baquet CR, Commiskey P, Mack K, Meltzer S, Mishra SI. Esophageal cancer epidemiology in blacks and whites: racial and gender disparities in incidence, mortality, survival rates and histology. Journal of the National Medical Association 2005;97(11):1471.

30. Gao Y, Hu N, Han X, Giffen C, Ding T, Goldstein A, Taylor P. Family history of cancer and risk for esophageal and gastric cancer in Shanxi, China. BMC cancer 2009;9(1):269.

31. Asanuma K, Iijima K, Shimosegawa T. Gender difference in gastro-esophageal reflux diseases. World journal of gastroenterology 2016;22(5): 1800.

32. Sanghvi LD, Rao KCM, Khanolkar VR. Smoking and chewing of tobacco in relation to cancer of the upper alimentary tract. British medical journal 1955;1(4922):1111.

33. Doll R. Esophageal cancer: A Preventable Disease?, In Monograph No. 1, International Seminar on epidemiology of Esophageal cancer Bangalore, India, 1971;3–8.

34. Sehgal S, Kaul S, Gupta BB, Dhar MK. Risk factors and survival analysis of the esophageal cancer in the population of Jammu, India. Indian journal of cancer 2012;49(2):245.

35. Paymaster JC, Sanghvi LD, Gangadharan P. Cancer in the gastrointestinal tract in Western India: Epidemiologic study. Cancer 1968;21(2): 279–88.

36. Jussawalla DJ, Deshpande VA. Evaluation of cancer risk in tobacco chewers and smokers: an epidemiologic assessment. Cancer 1971a;28(1): 244–52.

37. Paymaster JC, Gangadharan P, Nagaraj Rao D. Some high risk groups of the esophagus in cancer detection and prevention: Proceedings of the second international symposium of cancer detection and prevention. Bologna (Ed.) Cesare Maltoni Excerpta Medica, Amsterdam 1973.

38. Jayant K, Balakrishnan V, Sanghvi LD, Jussawalla DJ. Quantification of the role of smoking and chewing tobacco in oral, pharyngeal, and Esophageal cancers. British journal of cancer 1977;35(2):232.

39. Jussawalla DJ. Epidemiological assessment of aetiology of esophageal cancer in Greater Bombay. In Monograph No.1, International Seminar on Epidemiology of esophagus cancer Bangalore, India, 1971b.

40. Jussawalla DJ. Esophageal cancer in India. Journal of cancer research and clinical oncology, 1981;99(1–2);29–33.

41. Notani PN, Jayant K. Role of diet in upper aerodigestive tract cancers 1987.

42. Notani PN. Role of alcohol in cancers of the upper alimentary tract: use of models in risk assessment. Journal of Epidemiology & Community Health 1988;42(2):187–92.

43. Rao DN, Sanghvi LD, Desai PB. Epidemiology of esophageal cancer. In Seminars in surgical oncology. New York: John Wiley & Sons, Inc. 1989;5(5):351–4.

44. Ramesh C. Esophageal cancer: An epidemiological study in India. Ph.D. Thesis. Acta Universitatis Tamperensis Ser. A, Vol. 385, Univ. of Tampere, Finland, 1993.

45. Ganesh B, Talole SD, Dikshit R. Tobacco, alcohol and tea drinking as risk factors for esophageal cancer: A case-control study from Mumbai, India. Cancer epidemiology 1996;33(6):431–4.

46. Dar NA, Bhat GA, Shah IA, Iqbal B, Kakhdoomi MA, Nisar I, Shah SA. Hookah smoking, nass chewing, and Esophageal squamous cell carcinoma in Kashmir, India. British journal of cancer 2012;107(9):1618.

47. Sharma MK, Gour N, Pandey A, Wallia D. Epidemiological study of risk factors for oral, laryngeal and esophageal cancers at a tertiary care hospital in India. Asian Pac J Cancer Prev, 2011;12(5):1215–8.

48. Oze I, Matsuo K, Wakai K, Nagata C, Mizoue T, Tanaka K, Tsugane S. Alcohol drinking and esophageal cancer risk: an evaluation based on a systematic review of epidemiologic evidence among the Japanese population. Japanese journal of clinical oncology 2011;41(5):677–92.

49. Vioque J, Barber X, Bolumar F, Porta M, Santibáñez M, de la Hera MG, Moreno-Osset E. Esophageal cancer risk by type of alcohol drinking and smoking: a case-control study in Spain. BMC cancer 2008;8(1):221.

50. Yang X, Chen X, Zhuang M, Yuan Z, Nie S, Lu M, Ye W. Smoking and alcohol drinking in relation to the risk of esophageal squamous cell carcinoma: A population-based case-control study in China. Scientific reports 2017;7(1): 17249.

51. Sankaranarayanan R, Duffy SW, Padmakumary G, Nair SM, Day NE, Padmanabhan TK. Risk factors for cancer of the Esophagus in Kerala, India. International journal of cancer 1991;49(4): 485–9.

52. Long E, Beales IL. The role of obesity in Esophageal cancer development. Therapeutic advances in gastroenterology 2014;7(6):247–68.

53. De Stefani E, Deneo-Pellegrini H, Ronco AL, Boffetta P, Correa P, Aune D, Mendilaharsu M, Acosta G, Silva C, Landó G, Luaces ME. Meat consumption, cooking methods, mutagens, and risk of squamous cell carcinoma of the eso-phagus: a case-control study in Uruguay.Nutr Cancer 2012;64(2):294–9.

54. Lin J, Zeng R, Cao W, Luo R, Chen J, Lin Y. Hot beverage and food intake and esophageal cancer in southern China. Asian Pac J Cancer Prev 2011;12(9):2189–92.

55. Kumar R, Nende P, Wacker CD, Spiegelhalder B, Preussmann R, Siddiqui M. Caffeine odesive Nitroso compounds-1 Nitrosatable precursors from caffeine and their potential relevance in the etiology of oesphageal and gastric cancer in Kasmir India. Carcinogenesis 1992;Vol.13(11): 2179–82.

56. Joint Iran-International Agency for Research on Cancer Study Group. Esophageal cancer studies in the Caspian littoral of Iran: results of popu-lation studies-a prodrome. Journal of the National Cancer Institute 1977;59(4):1127–38.

57. Tuyns AJ, Riboli E, Doornbos G, Péquignot G. Diet and esophageal cancer in Calvados (France)1987.

58. Li JY, Ershow AG, Chen ZJ, Wacholder S, Li GY, Guo W, Blot WJ. A case?control study of cancer of the esophagus and gastric cardia in Linxian. International journal of cancer 1989;43(5): 755–61.

59. Cheng KK, Lam TH, Day NE, Duffy SW, Fok M, Wong J. Pickled vegetables in the aetiology of Esophageal cancer in Hong Kong Chinese. The Lancet 1992;339(8805):1314–8.

60. Van Rensburg SJ, Bradshaw ES, Bradshaw D, Rose EF. Esophageal cancer in Zulu men, South Africa: a case-control study. British journal of cancer 1985;51(3):399.

61. Yu Y, Taylor PR, Li JY, Dawsey SM, Wang GQ, Guo WD, Li B. Retrospective cohort study of risk-factors for esophageal cancer in Linxian, People's Republic of China. Cancer Causes & Control 1993;4(3):195–202.

62. Yang X, Ni Y, Yuan Z, Chen H, Plymoth A, Jin L, Ye W. Very hot tea drinking increases eso-phageal squamous cell carcinoma risk in a high-risk area of China: a population-based case-control study. Clinical epidemiology 2018;10:1307.

63. Huang SH, Wu IC, Wu DC, Wu CC, Yang JF, Chen YK, Wu MT. Occupational risks of esophageal cancer in Taiwanese men. The Kaohsiung journal of medical sciences 2012; 28(12):654–9.

64. Yahyapour Y, Shamsi-Shahrabadi M, Mahmoudi M, Motevallian A, Siadati S, Shefaii S, Keyvani H. High-risk and low-risk human papilloma-virus in esophageal squamous cell carcinoma at Mazandaran, Northern Iran. Pathology & Oncology Research 2013;19(3):385–91.

65. Mao WM, Zheng WH, Ling ZQ. Epidemiologic risk factors for esophageal cancer development. Asian Pac J Cancer Prev 2011;12(10):2461–6.

66. Morita M, Kumashiro R, Kubo N, Nakashima Y, Yoshida R, Yoshinaga K, Toh Y. Alcohol drinking, cigarette smoking, and the develop-ment of squamous cell carcinoma of the esophagus: epidemiology, clinical findings, and prevention. International journal of clinical oncology 2010;15(2):126–34.

67. Chitra S, Ashok L, Anand L, Srinivasan V, Jayanthi V. Risk factors for esophageal cancer in Coimbatore, southern India: a hospital-based case-control study. Indian journal of gastro-enterology: official journal of the Indian Society of Gastroenterology 2004;23(1):19–21.

68. Khan NA, Teli MA, Haq MMU, Bhat GM, Lone MM, Afroz F. A survey of risk factors in carcinoma esophagus in the valley of Kashmir, Northern India. Journal of cancer research and therapeutics 2011;7(1):15.

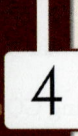

4

Clinical Assessment and Investigations

Praful Desai, Ratna Parikh

INTRODUCTION

Cancer of the esophagus, though easy to diagnose based on its symptomatology and simple investigations, still remains one of the more difficult disease to control and cure in the field of oncology. Depending on the type and extent of the disease, the therapy will either involve chemoradiotherapy or a surgical approach based on the data retrieved after appropriate pre-therapy investigations. Occasionally a combination therapy may have to be considered when indicated. The surgical management for esophageal cancer involves prolonged training with experts in the field and compares in its precision and difficulty similar to surgery of the brain, liver or lung malignancies. It is necessary to emphasize that a 5–7 years of preceptorship is needed with an experienced esophageal surgeon before attempting esophageal surgery.

In an era of combination therapeutic approaches for most cancers, a combined team of surgeons, chemotherapists and radiotherapists is mandatory before the final therapeutic decision. There is proven data that morbidities and mortalities after esophageal surgery is inversely proportional to the surgical experience; or simply stated, more the experience (individual and hospital) less the morbidity and mortality for the patient.

Appropriate preoperative data with complete medical evaluation of the patient is mandatory; the risks involved are directly dependent on the data retrieved by the pre-therapy workup.

Clinical Presentation

Most patients present with a short history of dysphagia for solids and weight loss. Advanced lesions with tracheoesophageal fistula will present with persistent cough and even vomiting, if the obstruction is near complete. The esophagus is a distensible organ and hence, patients often present in late stages, where occasionally, the esophagus assumes severe dilatation often reminiscent of a long-standing achalasia cardia. Symptoms and signs of metastatic disease will relate to the clinical location of the metastasis, like a palpable liver for liver metastasis and cough or hemoptysis for lung metastasis. Presence of any significant back pain should be carefully assessed to exclude any spine (vertebral) metastasis, though uncommon.

Pre-Therapy Workup

Irrespective of the therapy which may involve surgery or chemoradiotherapy as aforementioned, a routine hematologic, renal and hepatic assessment is necessary. A thorough evaluation of the cardiopulmonary status is also mandatory. The overall nutritional status of the patient is an important factor and needs to be appropriately corrected as post-operative anastomotic disruption can result despite a good anastomosis, due to poor nutritional status (low protein and albumin) of the patient.

Clinical Examination

Clinical examination with particular attention to lymph nodal areas of the neck, supra-clavicular regions, axillae and even the inguinal region is mandatory. The author has seen a proven lymph node metastasis in the right inguinal nodal area. Examination of the oral cavity, the pharynx, the vocal cords and its mobility are of importance. A hoarse voice and a paralyzed cord are indicative of an advanced disease involving the recurrent laryngeal nerve in the mediastinum, which excludes any surgical approach on the esophagus. A careful abdominal examination is important to exclude liver enlargement, a common site of metastatic spread.

Investigations

A routine X-ray chest and a Barium swallow are the initial simple investigations, which almost clinches the diagnosis (Figs 4.1 and 4.2). This should be avoided if there is a clinical evidence of an obvious near complete obstruction or a suspect tracheoesophageal fistula. Endoscopy with a tissue biopsy of an obvious lesion is the next logical step to histologically confirm the diagnosis (Fig. 4.3).

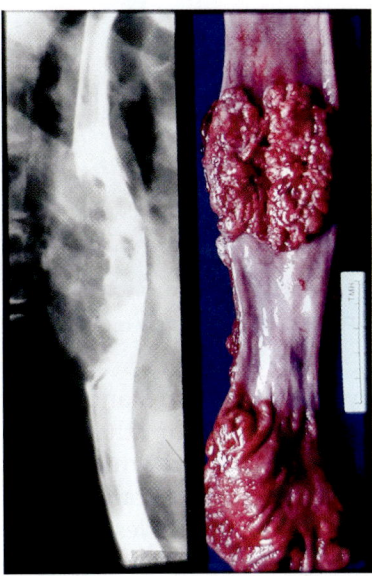

Fig. 4.2: Barium swallow of a large proliferative lesion in the esophagus and resected specimen of the same patient

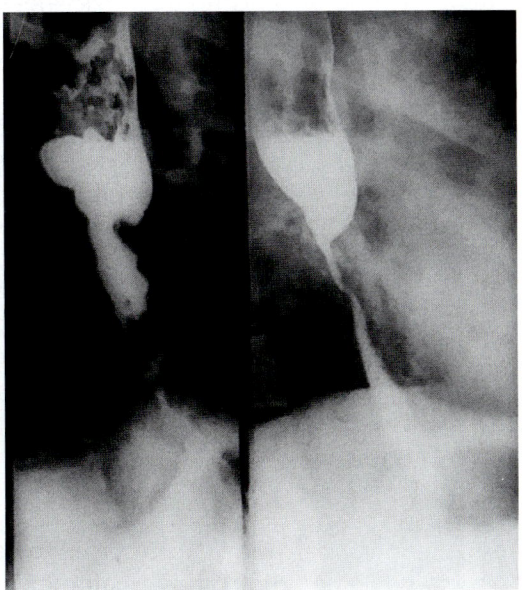

Fig. 4.1: Barium swallow study showing a proliferative mid-esophageal growth and in contrast a stricturous lesion in mid and lower third esophagus

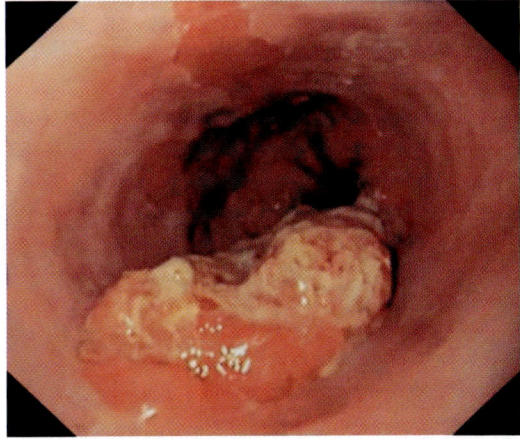

Fig. 4.3: Endoscopic image showing Barrett's mucosa with a polypoidal ulcerated lesion (adenocarcinoma)

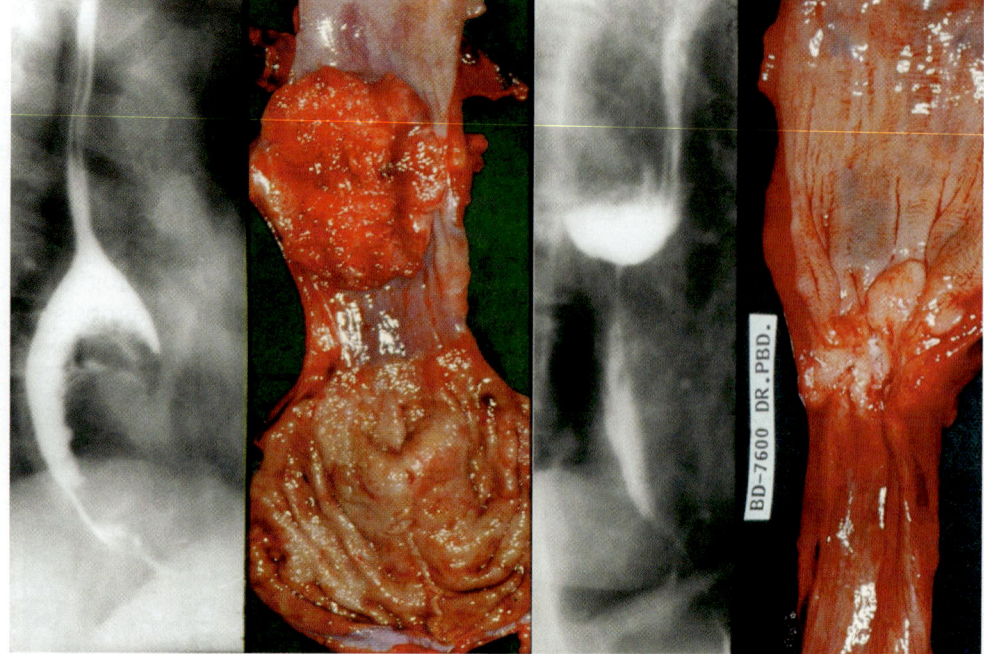

Fig. 4.4: Barium swallow and resected specimens of proliferative and stricturous esophageal lesions

It is very vital that the distance of the lesion from the incisors or the pharynx is appropriately recorded which also aids in planning the therapy. A careful endoscopic evaluation of the type of lesion is extremely important in treatment planning. Esophageal cancers are either proliferative or stricturous lesions (Fig. 4.4). Occasionally it may have a combined type of morphology. The therapeutic response to chemoradiation in a

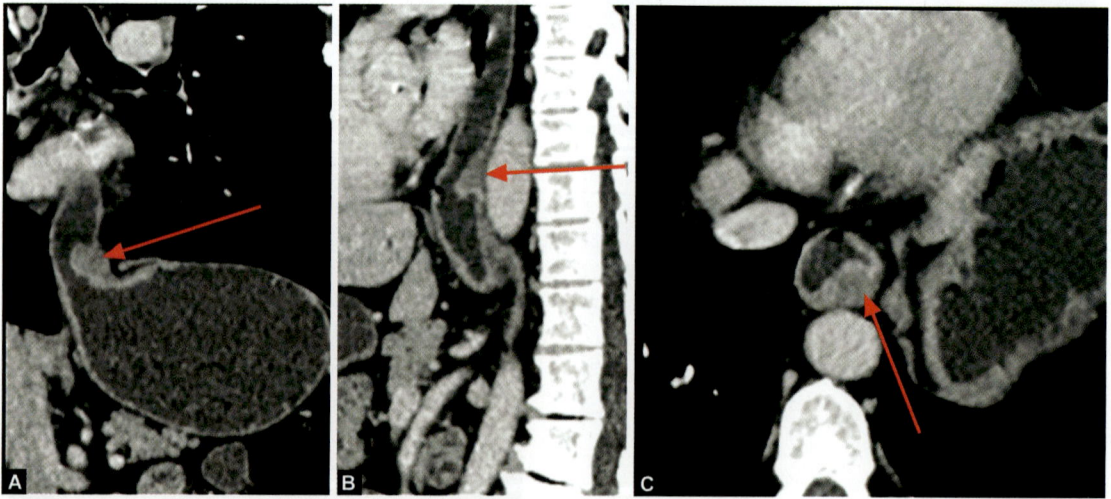

Figs 4.5A to C: CT Scans in coronal, sagittal and axial sections demonstrate an intraluminal nodular mass in the distal esophagus representing a primary esophageal neoplasm (*Courtesy* Dr Anirudh Kohli)

proliferative lesion is generally extremely favorable and contra wise the response to a strictured lesion is generally poor.

Endoscopic ultrasound is increasingly used in many centers to delineate the nodal burden, which can help in clinical staging of the disease. A good bronchoscopy particularly for lesions in the middle and upper one-third will give adequate information regarding invasion of the tracheobronchial tree. In experienced hands, bronchoscopic findings will give as much information about the state of trachea and bronchus as a CT scan.

A routine ultrasound of the abdomen is the next logical step; however, in today's high technology era, a CT or a PET/CT scan is more often the next investigation (Figs 4.5A to C). This is particularly useful to exclude distant metastasis in a locally advanced cancer. Metastasis in the liver and the lungs are frequent in an advanced esophageal cancer and the importance of these investigations cannot be understated as it can often radically change the therapeutic approach.

BIBLIOGRAPHY

1. Cancer of the Esophagus—DeVita, Hellman and Rosenberg's Principle and Practice of Oncology 10th edition.
2. Carcinoma of the Esophagus—Contemporary issues in cancer imaging—Sheila C. Rankin. 2008.
3. Practical Clinical Oncology—Praful Desai. 2014.

5

Diagnostic Endoscopy in Esophageal Cancer
(Viewing, Micro Viewing and Staging)

Samir Parikh, Anuj Parikh

Esophageal cancer (EC) is the eighth common highly virulent malignancy worldwide with an increasing incidence and a high, one and five year mortality.[1] It comprises 4% of newly diagnosed cancers per year with yearly incidence comparable to yearly cancer related mortality.[2] Squamous cell carcinoma (SCC) and adenocarcinoma (EAC) account for over 95% of all esophageal malignant tumors. Though the incidence of SCC is static, the incidence of EAC arising on the background of Barrett's esophagus (BE) is increasing.[3] SCC involves upper third in 30%, mid third 50% and lower third in 20% without involvement of the cardia. About 95% of EAC occur in mid and lower third with majority involving the cardia.

Most patients present with progressive dysphagia of short duration often accompanied by an average weight loss of 10 kg. Dysphagia occurs with reduction in the esophageal luminal diameter to <13 mm and is often a sign of unresectable tumor. Hoarseness of voice due to invasion of recurrent laryngeal nerve and Horner's syndrome due to invasion of sympathetic trunk in cervical esophageal cancer also suggest inoperability. Early diagnosis, accurate staging and protocol-based therapy by an expert team can reduce mortality and associated morbidity. Flexible video-endoscopy is an important tool to directly visualize the tumor and achieve a histological confirmation.[4] Endoscopy has largely replaced barium swallow as it is more sensitive and specific in the diagnosis of esophageal cancer (Fig. 5.1).[5]

Endoscopy is useful for:
a. Initial evaluation (visualize tumor and biopsy).
b. Staging (EUS, laparoscopy and biopsy).

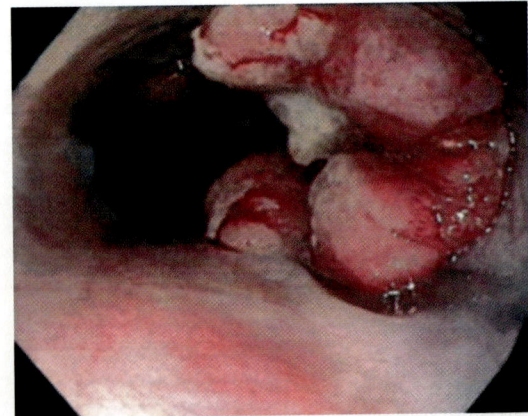

Fig. 5.1: Polypoidal, ulcerated mid esophageal tumor of 4 cm length with no luminal compromise or tracheo-esophageal fistula

c. Post-treatment evaluation (endoscopy, EUS and biopsy).

d. Detection of superficial esophageal cancer (newer endoscopic methods and biopsy).

e. Surveillance of high-risk population.

Initial Evaluation

Viewing Tumor

Initial endoscopy with white light high end video-endoscope aims to directly visualize various aspects of the tumor: morphology (polypoidal vs stricturous), length (<5 cm, >5 cm), location (upper, mid, lower third), distance from the cricopharynx and cardia, extension in stomach, luminal compromise, presence of hiatus hernia and BE, synchronous lesions in the esophagus or cricopharynx, associated tracheoesophageal fistula, extrinsic compression, change of esophageal axis and previous surgeries.

Esophageal cancers at cardia must be classified as per Siewert's classification: type I—predominantly in the esophagus, type II—equally distributed in the esophagus and stomach and type III—predominantly in the stomach (Fig. 5.2).[6] Like a protocol-based

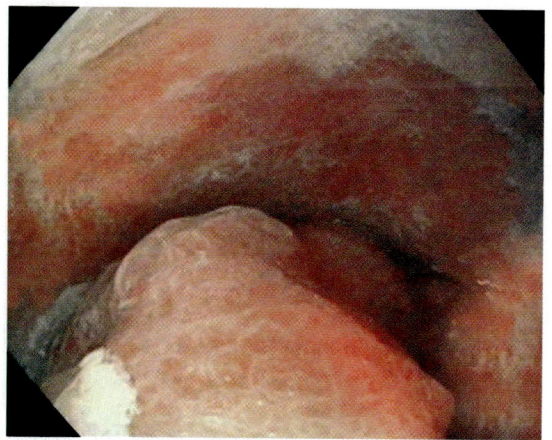

Fig. 5.2: Esophageal adenocarcinoma reaching cardia, Siewert type I

CT evaluation a trained gastrointestinal endoscopist must detail all the above aspects and preferably record and print them. Though an endoscopic view of a polypoidal ulcerated mass is suggestive of cancer, a histological confirmation is a must.

Biopsy

Endoscopic biopsy performed under direct vision reduces sampling error and gives accurate diagnosis, cell of origin and degree of tumor differentiation. Multiple biopsies (>7) have a sensitivity of about 98%.[7] Recently available Jumbo biopsy forceps (larger cups, central spike) allow sufficient material for routine histology, special stains and molecular biology studies. Biopsies must be performed from ulcer edges rather than slough (necrotic tissue). Obtained tissue must be placed on a filter paper for its proper orientation to the pathologist. For small doubtful lesions or post-therapy, biopsies are performed in a well method to achieve submucosal tissue. For a stricturous tumor, dilation (up to 11 mm) is performed to achieve biopsy material and reduce sampling error. Alternately a brush cytology may be performed before and after dilation along with routine biopsies to improve diagnostic yield.[8, 9]

Staging

The American Joint Committee of Cancer (AJCC) suggested staging classification of esophageal cancer based on primary tumor (T), lymph node (N) and distant organ metastasis (M) (Table 5.1).[10, 11] It is used for guiding therapy, assessing resectability, assessing prognosis, response to therapy and survival.[12] Newer modifications in staging includes location, pathological subtypes and response to neoadjuvant therapy.[12–17] Multiple modalities including CT, PET-CT, EUS, laparoscopy are used to accurately stage the disease.

Table 5.1	TNM staging AJCC, UICC 2017

Primary tumors (T), SCC and EAC	
T-Category	**T Criteria**
T_x	Tumor cannot be assessed
T_0	No evidence of primary tumor
T_{is}	High grade dysplasia (malignant cells confined to epithelium of the basement membrane)
T_1	Tumor invades the lamina propria, muscularis mucosa or submucosa
T_{1a}	Tumor invades the lamina propria or muscularis mucosa
T_{1b}	Tumor invades the submucosa
T_2	Tumor invades the muscularis propria
T_3	Tumor invades the adventitia
T_4	Tumor invades adjacent structures
T_{4a}	Tumor invades the pleura, pericardium, azygous vein, diaphragm or peritoneum
T_{4b}	Tumor invades other adjacent structures such as the aorta, vertebral body or airway

Regional lymph nodes (N), SCC and EAC	
N-Category	**N Criteria**
N_x	Regional lymph nodes cannot be assessed
N_0	No regional lymph node metastasis
N_1	Metastasis in one or two regional lymph nodes
N_2	Metastasis in three to six regional lymph nodes
N_3	Metastasis in seven or more lymph nodes

Distant metastasis (M), SCC and EAC	
M-Category	**M criteria**
M_0	No distant metastasis
M_1	Distant metastasis

Histological grade (G) SCC and EAC	
G	**G definition**
G_x	Grade cannot be assessed
G_1	Well-differentiated
G_2	Moderately differentiated
G_3	Poorly differentiated, undifferentiated

Location (L) SCC	
Location category	**Location criteria**
X	Location unknown
Upper	Cervical esophagus to lower border of azygous vein
Middle	Lower border of azygous vein to lower border of inferior pulmonary vein
Lower	Lower border of inferior pulmonary vein to stomach including gastroesophageal junction

Location is defined by epicenter of the tumor
Location plays a role in the stage grouping of esophageal SCC

Contd...

Prognostic stage groups, SCC (cTNM)

cT	cN	M	Group
T_{iS}	N_0	M_0	0
T_1	N_0–N_1	M_0	I
T_2	N_0–N_1	M_0	II
T_3	N_0	M_0	II
T_3	N_1	M_0	III
T_{1-3}	N_2	M_0	III
T_4	N_{0-2}	M_0	IV A
Any T	N_3	M_0	IV A
Any T	Any N	M_1	IV B

Pathological stage, SCC (pTNM)

pT	pN	M	Location	Stage
T_{iS}	N_0	M_0	Any	0
T_{1a}	N_0	M_0	Any	I A
T_{1b}	N_0	M_0	Any	I B
T_2	N_0	M_0	Any	II A
T_3	N_0	M_0	Lower	II A
T_3	N_0	M_0	Upper/middle	II B
T_3	N_0	M_0	Location X	II B
T_1	N_1	M_0	Any	II B
T_1	N_2	M_0	Any	III A
T_2	N_1	M_0	Any	III A
T_2	N_2	M_0	Any	III B
T_3	N_{1-2}	M_0	Any	III B
T_{4a}	N_{0-1}	M_0	Any	III B
T_{4a}	N_2	M_0	Any	IV A
T_{4b}	N_{0-2}	M_0	Any	IV A
Any T	N_3	M_0	Any	IV A
Any T	Any N	M_1	Any	IV B

Postneoadjuvant therapy, SCC (ypTNM)

ypT	ypN	M	Stage
T_{0-2}	N_0	M_0	I
T_3	N_0	M_0	II
T_{0-2}	N_1	M_0	III A
T_3	N_1	M_0	III B
T_{0-3}	N_2	M_0	III B
T_{4a}	N_0	M_0	III B
T_{4b}	N_{1-2}	M_0	IV A
T_{4a}	N_x	M_0	IV A
T_{4b}	N_{0-2}	M_0	IV A
Any T	N_3	M_0	IV A
Any T	Any N	M_1	IV B

Contd...

Prognostic stage, EAC (cTNM)			
cT	**cN**	**M**	**Stage**
T_{iS}	N_0	M_0	0
T_1	N_0	M_0	I A
T_1	N_1	M_0	II A
T_2	N_0	M_0	II B
T_2	N_1	M_0	III
T_3	N_{0-1}	M_0	III
T_{4a}	N_{0-1}	M_0	III
T_{1-4a}	N_2	M_0	IV A
T_{4b}	N_{0-2}	M_0	IV A
Any T	N_3	M_0	IV A
Any T	Any N	M_1	IV B

Pathological stage, EAC (pTNM)				
pT	**pN**	**M**	**G**	**Stage**
T_{iS}	N_0	M_0	NA	0
T_{1a}	N_0	M_0	G_1	I A
T_{1a}	N_0	M_0	G_x	I A
T_{1a}	N_0	M_0	G_2	I B
T_{1b}	N_0	M_0	G_{1-2}	I B
T_{1b}	N_0	M_0	G_x	I B
T_1	N_0	M_0	G_3	I C
T_2	N_0	M_0	G_{1-2}	I C
T_2	N_0	M_0	G_3	II A
T_2	N_0	M_0	G_x	II A
T_1	N_1	M_0	Any	II B
T_3	N_0	M_0	Any	II B
T_1	N_2	M_0	Any	II B
T_2	N_1	M_0	Any	III A
T_2	N_2	M_0	Any	III A
T_3	N_{1-2}	M_0	Any	III B
T_{4a}	N_{0-1}	M_0	Any	III B
T_{4a}	N_2	M_0	Any	III B
T_{4b}	N_{0-2}	M_0	Any	IV A
Any T	N_3	M_0	Any	IV A
Any T	Any N	M_1	Any	IV B

Contd...

Postneoadjuvant therapy, EAC (ypTNM)			
ypT	ypN	M	Stage
T_{0-2}	N_0	M_0	I
T_3	N_0	M_0	II
T_{0-2}	N_1	M_0	III A
T_3	N_1	M_0	III B
T_{0-3}	N_2	M_0	III B
T_{4a}	N_0	M_0	III B
T_{4a}	N_{1-2}	M_0	IV A
T_{4a}	N_x	M_0	IV A
T_{4b}	N_{0-2}	M_0	IV A
Any T	N_3	M_0	IV A
Any T	Any N	M_1	IV B

(TNM: tumor, node, metastasis; AJCC: American Joint Committee on Cancer; UICC: Union for International Cancer Control)

Role of Endoscopic Ultrasound (EUS)

T Stage

EUS allows distinct visualization of all layers of the esophagus. The depth of tumor invasion can be identified by hypoechoic disruption of esophageal layers. EUS is reliable, useful, cost-effective and the most accurate method to assess loco-regional staging. Its sensitivity for T stage varies from 81–92% and specificity from 94–97%.[18] It is more reliable for tumors in stage T4 than stage T1 (Fig. 5.3). In patients with stricture EUS may underestimate T stage.[19] A dilation up to 14–16 mm to allow standard EUS scope to traverse the stricture, carries a minor risk of perforation.[20–21] High frequency miniprobes (15–20 MHz) and wire guided echoendoscopes are useful in such cases.[22] Miniprobes can accurately differentiate T_{1a} from T_{1b} allowing the former to undergo endoscopic mucosal resection.[23] EUS miniprobes at present are expensive, have limited life, undergo rapid image deterioration, need water infusion in esophagus increasing the risk of aspiration and are poor for nodal detection as it has poor depth of penetration (about 3 cm).[24]

N Stage

Esophageal cancer has higher incidence of nodal disease with an incidence of 60% in T_2 and 80% in T_3/T_4 tumors.[2] Increasing number of nodes carry poorer outcome.[25] Nodal involvement does not prevent surgical resection but reduces cure rates,[25–27] suggesting a need for neoadjuvant chemotherapy.[28]

In the past involvement of coeliac node was considered a sign of unresectability which has now changed. EUS is more sensitive and specific compared to CT scan in detecting malignant nodes.[29] On EUS a malignant node has width >10 mm, round shape, smooth border and are hypoechoic.[30,31] If all 4 features are present the sensitivity of EUS is 80–100% in detecting malignant nodes.[31] Of all the features, size >10 mm and hypoechoic appearance are considered more specific. As all the 4 features are present in only one-third of patients, EUS guided FNA of the node is required when in doubt.[32] While performing EUS guided FNA, care must be taken not to traverse esophageal tumor. EUS guided FNA is the most cost-effective method to assess nodal stage compared to CT-PET and laparoscopy with distinct survival advantage.[33,34] A high volume center (>50 staging procedures/year),[35] a well-trained EUS operator (>75 staging procedures under supervision)[36] may yield best results on accurately staging T and N stage of esophageal cancer.

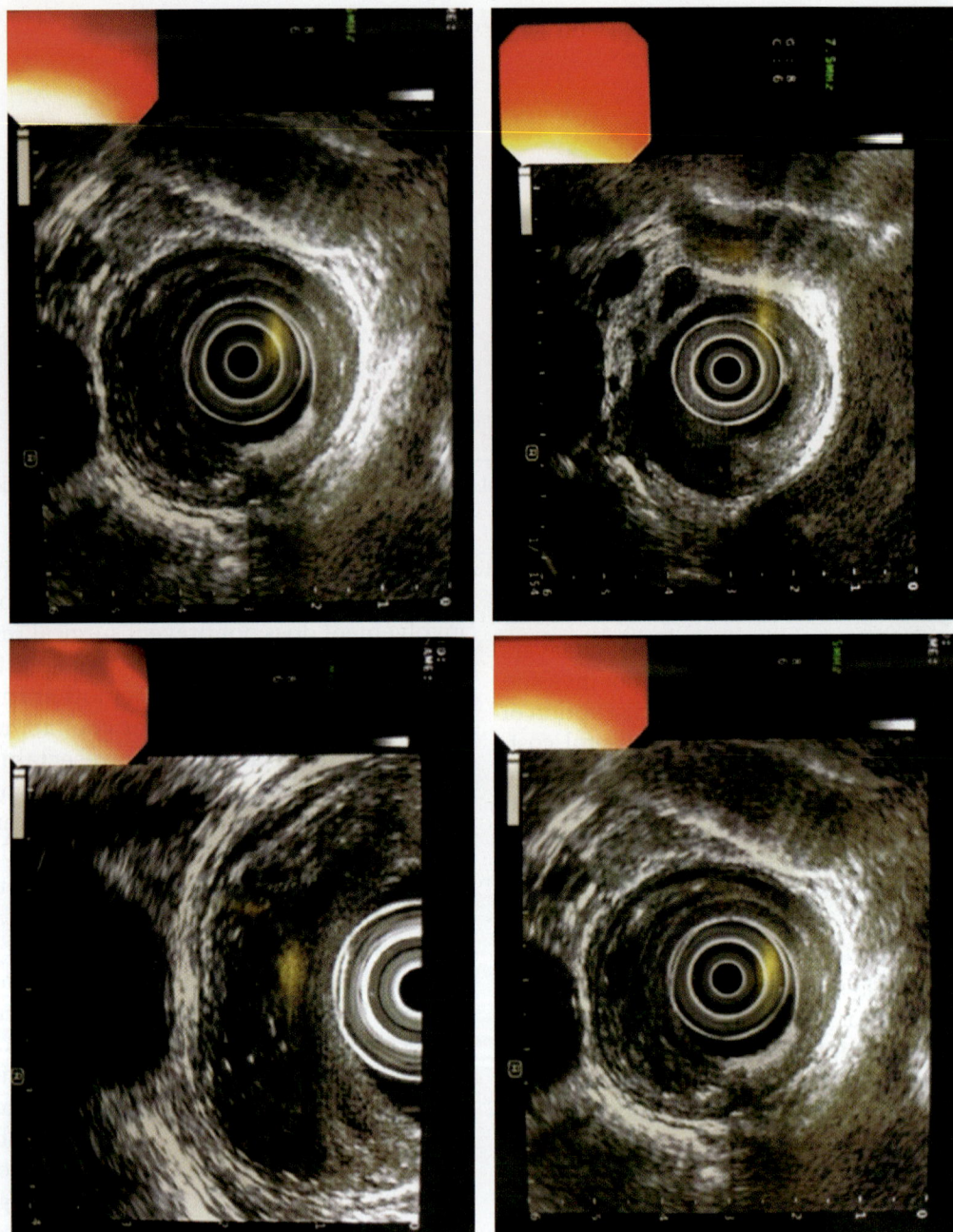

Fig. 5.3: EUS showing tumor extending to adventitia, locally abutting the left pleura with a small periesophageal node

Bronchoscopy and Laryngoscopy

Cervical esophageal cancers above the level of carina often need bronchoscopy with brush cytology in a preoperative evaluation when tumor is locally advanced.[37] Bronchoscopy is more reliable than CT in identifying airway invasion.[38] For SCC affecting cervical esophagus, a laryngoscopic evaluation is recommended to rule out local involvement or a synchronous lesion. Patients experiencing cough or stridor during diagnostic endoscopy warrants bronchoscopy to identify airway invasion or tracheoesophageal fistula.

Laparoscopy

Laparoscopy is performed in a few centers for patients with T_3/T_4 resectable tumors, Siewert II or III EAC or mild ascites where peritoneal deposits cannot be ruled out.[39–41] Its sensitivity to identify celiac lymph node is comparable to that of EUS. Laparoscopic ultrasonography often helps detect deep seated liver metastasis. Laparoscopy allows viewing of omentum, the liver surface, obtain a biopsy and a peritoneal lavage for cytology. However, its routine use for operable EAC on PET-CT is controversial.

Thoracoscopy and Mediastinoscopy

Thoracoscopy from right hemithorax allows visualization of thoracic esophagus and peri-esophageal nodes. When performed from left hemithorax it allows visualization of lower esophagus, aortopulmonary and peri-esophageal nodes. Its diagnostic accuracy is 90% and its specificity is enhanced by its ability to perform nodal and pleural biopsies. Mediastinoscopy allows viewing of regional lymph nodes in the right and left paratracheal regions, along the main bronchi, aorto-pulmonary window and subcarinal region. Both thoracoscopy and mediastinoscopy are now rarely performed with the advent of EUS even in developing countries.

M Stage

EUS can detect liver metastasis in left lobe of size <1 cm and malignant ascites. However, CT thorax/abdomen with PET combined remains investigation of choice for detecting distant metastasis. CT scan has about 70% accuracy to establish resectability and about 60% accuracy to detect nodal metastasis (Fig. 5.4). It can identify metastatic deposits of size >1 cm. PET-CT is cost-effective to detect bone metastasis but is poor in detecting brain

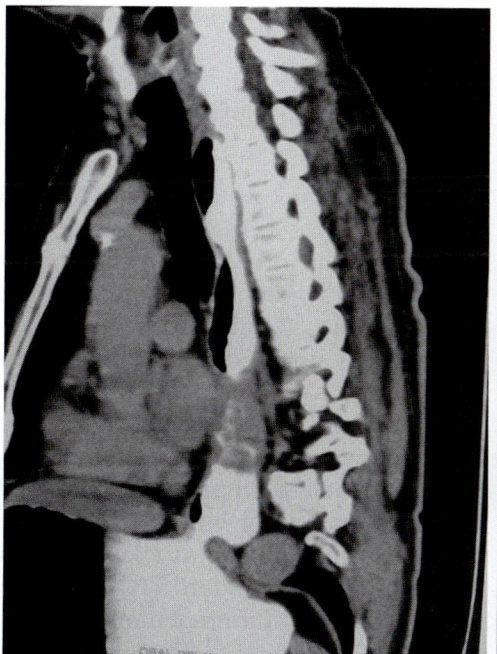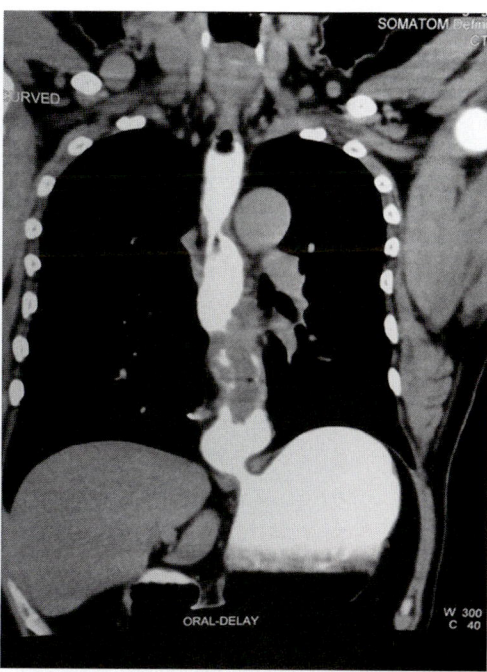

Fig. 5.4: CT scan showing polypoidal enhancing lower thoracic tumor with wall thickening, no nodes with hiatus hernia and tumor 3 cm above the cardia

lesions. At most centers after initial diagnosis of EC on endoscopic biopsy, CT scan of thorax/abdomen is performed to assess metastatic disease. If it is absent EUS is performed to assess loco-regional staging. A decision for resecting the tumor is most often taken after EUS evaluation.

POST-TREATMENT EVALUATION

Most centers perform barium swallow after a few months of successful tumor resection. If normal, endoscopy and CT scans are performed within the first year or when patient has symptomatic recurrence. Threshold to perform biopsy should be low and often multiple samples are required to detect early recurrence in an area of inflammation/fibrosis. Narrow band imaging (NBI) and chromoendoscopy's utility is not well evaluated in such a situation. A benign looking stricture must be dilated and biopsies with or without cytology should be performed. Mucosal irregularity on endoscopy post therapy must be biopsied (Fig. 5.5). EUS plays an important role in the evaluation of patients postchemoradiotherapy or post-chemotherapy. The sensitivity and specificity

of EUS in assessing T_1 stage is (23%, 95%), T_2 stage is (29%, 84%), T_3 stage is (81%, 42%), T_4 stage is (43%, 96%) and nodal stage is (69%, 52%) respectively.[42] Sensitivity was relatively high in T_3 disease and specificity in T_1, T_2 and T_4 stages.[42] Newer techniques did not contribute in enhancing the results.[43] EUS is unable to differentiate between post-treatment inflammation and fibrosis from tumor tissue.[44–48] Three dimensional EUS probes allow simultaneous radial and linear images to measure tumor volume and its relationship to surrounding structures. They are useful in restaging patients but only in expert hands. Tumor volume reduction of 50% in cross sectional area is a reasonable indicator of good response[48–50] and improved survival.[48,51] Patients with symptomatic recurrences may have normal endoscopy. EUS has a sensitivity of >92% and specificity of >96% in detecting loco-regional relapse.[52,53] Asymptomatic patients may be followed up every 9–12 months by endoscopy and imaging. For symptomatic patients even if endoscopy and imaging are negative EUS must be performed to diagnose early recurrence.[54]

DETECTION OF SUPERFICIAL ESOPHAGEAL CANCER

The incidence of superficial esophageal carcinoma (invading no deeper than the submucosa) is increasing in Asian countries especially where high-risk population screening is performed with endoscopy.[55] It is also increasingly detected in USA where patients with Barrett's esophagus are screened for the development of dysplasia. Esophageal lymphatic vessels within the submucosa allow tumor spread via lymphatics and hence detecting the tumor involvement of the submucosa is critical in defining available options of treatment.[56] The standard TNM classification is inadequate to differentiate nodal involvement of T_{1a} from T_{1b}.[11] The estimated risk of nodal metastasis from T_{1a} is 5% and that for T_{1b} is 16.6%.[57] Subclassification of early

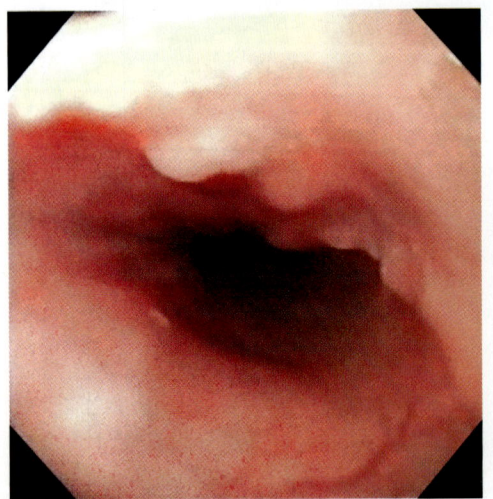

Fig. 5.5: Postneoadjuvant chemoradiotherapy white light imaging showing mucosal irregularity but no tumor on histology

esophageal cancer helps to determine treatment and assess prognosis (Fig. 5.6).[58,59] Comparison of subclassification and AJCC TNM classification is shown in Table 5.2.[59] The incidence of nodal involvement as per the depth of the tumor is shown in Table 5.3.[58-67] The rates of nodal metastasis for EAC and SCC are identical.[64] Endoscopic treatment is justifiable in M_1, M_2 and M_3 tumors without lymphovascular invasion, whereas all submucosal tumors and mucosal tumors with lymphovascular invasion should undergo surgery. Patients with non-flat tumors (Fig. 5.7) have a higher risk of nodal invasion compared to flat lesions (37 vs 17% respectively).[59] Size of lesion >2 cm and high-grade lesions are more commonly associated with nodal invasion.[57] Though EUS accurately differentiates T_{1a} from T_{1b} most centers prefer to perform endoscopic mucosal resection whenever feasible for mucosal tumors, check for lymphovascular invasion on biopsy and then decide on further need for surgery.

Table 5.2	Subclassification of early esophageal carcinoma	
Japanese Classification		**TNM (AJCC)**
Mucosal Tumors		
M_1	Limited to epithelial layer	T_{is}
M_2	Invades lamina propria	T_{1a}
M_3	Invades into muscularis mucosa	
Submucosal Tumors		
SM_1	Invades shallowest $1/3^{rd}$ of submucosa	
SM_2	Invades intermediate $1/3^{rd}$ of submucosa	T_{1b}
SM_3	Invades deepest $1/3^{rd}$ of submucosa	

SURVEILLANCE OF HIGH-RISK POPULATION

The etiological agents and association of both SCC and EAC are listed in Table 5.4. Like all cancers, esophageal cancer diagnosed at an early stage has better outcomes. The annual incidence of EAC has increased by sixfold in the USA.[68] Most EAC occurs on the

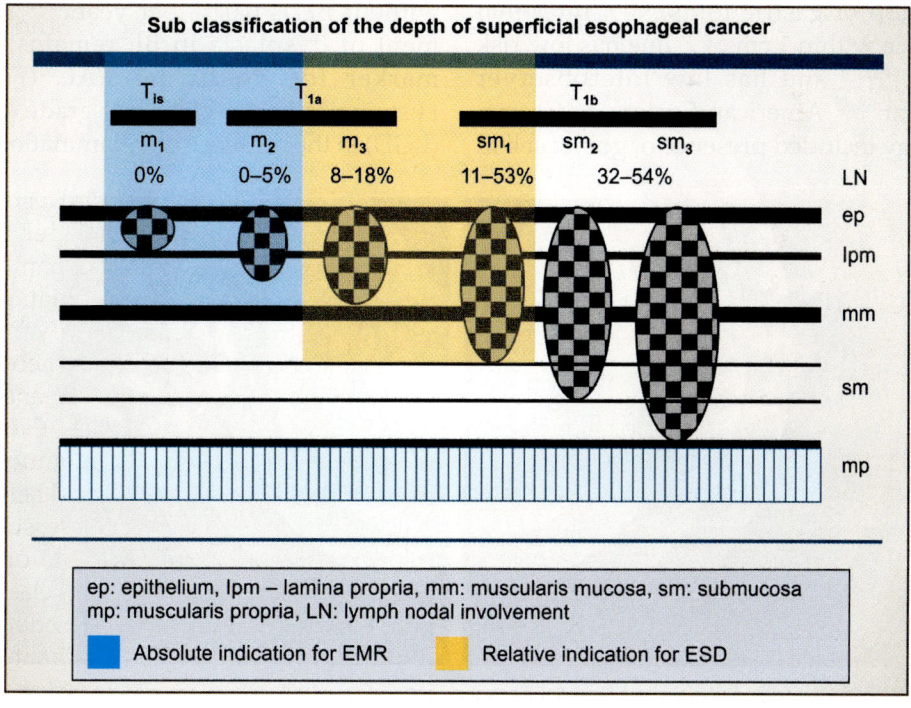

Fig. 5.6: Superficial esophageal cancer

Table 5.3 Incidence of lymph node involvement in superficial esophageal cancer according to the depth of its invasion

Author/Year	Histology	N	Lymph node in mucosal lesion			Lymph node in submucosal lesion		
			M_1	M_2	M_3	SM_1	SM_2	SM_3
Endo M[58] 2000	SCC	236	0	0	8	11	30	61
Fujita H[60] 2001	SCC	150	0	0	4	25	22	40
Westerterp M[62] 2005	EAC	120	0	0	4	0	26	67
Shimada H[59] 2006	SCC	160	0	0	6	32	31	42
Ancona E[64] 2011	EAC	31	0	0	0	8	29	54
	SCC	67						
Holschar A[66] 2011	EAC	121	0	0	0	13	19	56
	SCC	50						
Yamashina T[67] 2013	SCC	402	0.4*	0.4*	9	8	36	NR

LN: lymph node; SCC: Squamous cell cancer; EAC: Esophageal adenocarcinoma
* M_1/M_2 combined

background of Barrett's esophagus. BE is a metaplastic change in the esophageal mucosa from squamous cell to a specialized columnar lined mucosa. Endoscopically BE is identified by its salmon color and is situated 1 cm proximal to the squamocolumnar junction (Z-line, top of gastric folds).[69–72] Intestinal metaplasia within 1 cm of Z line has low risk for EAC,[73, 74] and has low interobserver agreement.[68,75] American Society of Gastro-enterology included presence of goblet cell in defining metaplasia of BE whereas British Society of Gastroenterology defined BE as a mere presence of columnar lined epithelium. Long segment of BE (>3 cm) (Fig. 5.8) has a higher risk of EAC. The annual incidence of EAC with BE is 0.38% per year whereas without BE is 0.07% per year.[68,76] Development of dysplasia in BE remains the best marker for predicting EAC (Fig. 5.9). Histologically detecting low grade dysplasia (LGD) in the presence of inflammation is often

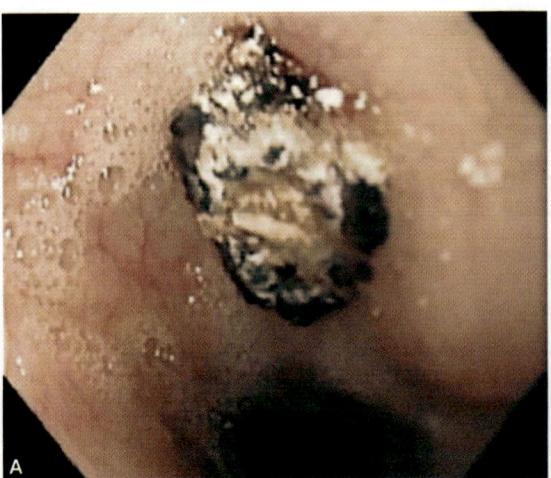
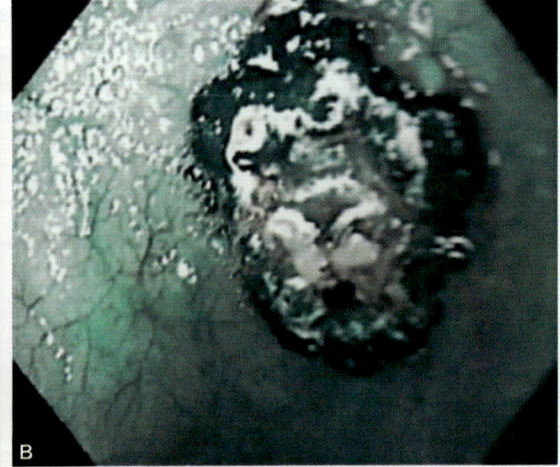

Fig. 5.7: (A) White light imaging of elevated superficial esophageal cancer of 2.5 × 2 cm size in mid esophagus. (B) Narrow Band Imaging (NBI)

Table 5.4	Etiological agents and high-risk factors	
Squamous cell carcinoma		
Etiological agents		**High-risk association**
1. Human papilloma Virus 2. Diet: Low in vitamin A, C, riboflavin, excess of nitrates and nitrosamine, contamination by aflatoxin 3. Smoking and alcohol		1. Head and neck cancer 2. Achalasia cardia 3. Corrosive injury 4. Zenker's diverticulum 5. Esophageal web 6. Tylosis
Adenocarcinoma		
1. Gastroesophageal reflux 2. Obesity, visceral obesity 3. Tobacco 4. Eradication of *H. Pylori* from gastric corpus 5. Western diet		Barrett's esophagus

difficult. Most studies use confirmation of dysplasia by two experienced pathologists. The risk of progression from LGD to high grade dysplasia (HGD) ranges from 0.5 to 13.4% per patient year and from HGD to invasive EAC is 0.6% per patient year (Fig. 5.10).[69] Once BE is identified on endoscopy four-quadrant biopsies must be performed every 2 cm to detect dysplasia. Timing of follow-up endoscopy with biopsies is suggested in Flowchart 5.1.[69,77,78] All patients with BE with/without dysplasia will receive proton pump inhibitors (PPI) for life.

Postendoscopic ablation therapy biopsies have to be performed in a well fashion to identify buried BE.

SCC is endemic in northern China, South Africa, Iran, Russia and India. Data for surveillance of SCC are scanty. In patients with achalasia cardia and corrosive injury, surveillance endoscopy should be performed within first 15 years, though no data is available for follow-up evaluation.[77] Surveillance endoscopy for other premalignant conditions for SCC like esophageal web is not standardized.

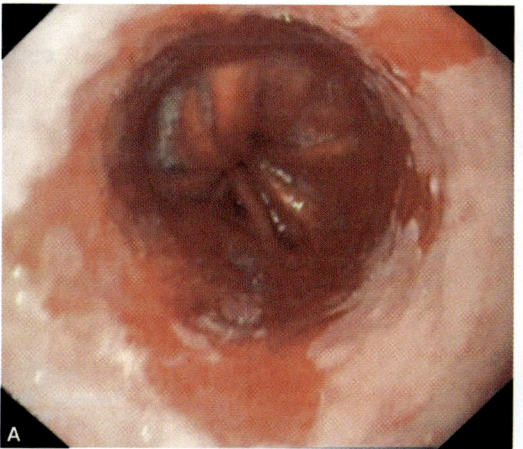 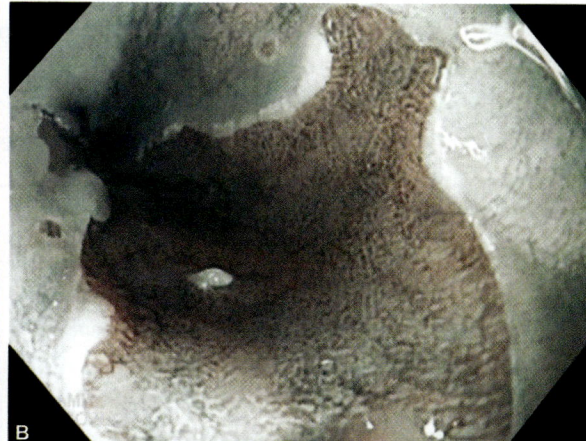

Fig. 5.8: (A) White light endoscopy showing long segment of Barrett's esophagus. (B) NBI showing long segment Barrett's esophagus with normal IPCL and regular mucosal surface (C2M4 by Prague criteria)

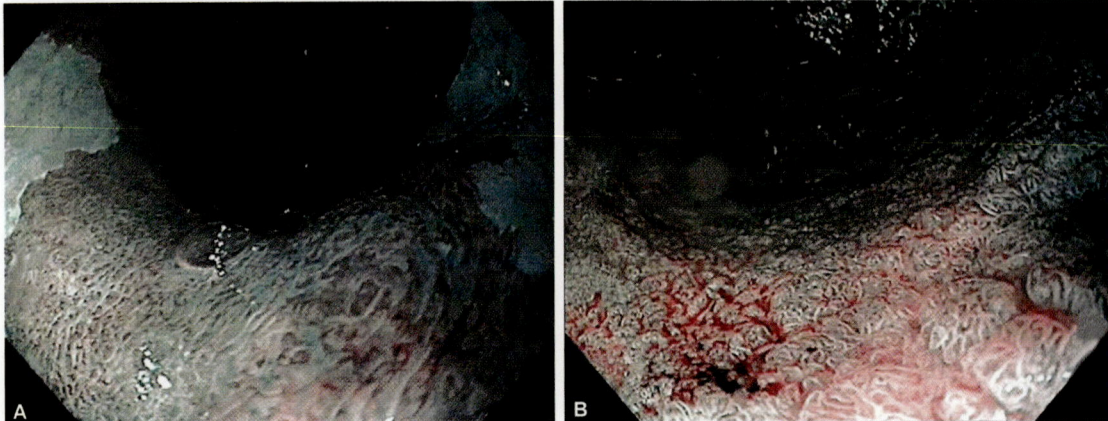

Fig. 5.9: (A) NBI showing disturbed intrapapillary capillary loop with mild irregularity suggesting dysplasia on underlying Barrett's esophagus. (B) NBI showing disturbed IPCL with mucosal irregularity suggesting HGD

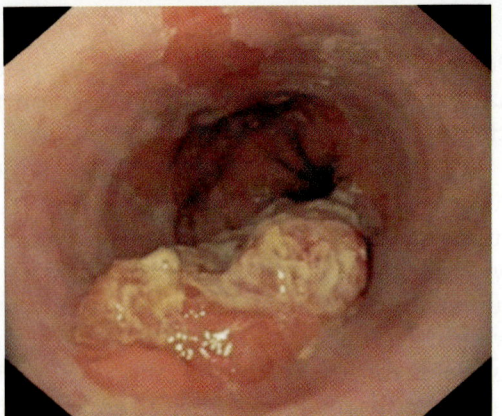

Fig. 5.10: Long segment Barrett's esophagus with a 3 × 2 cm well-differentiated adenocarcinoma detected on surveillance

Newer Endoscopic Techniques

Endoscopic advances have occurred to identify subtle changes in the esophageal mucosa to allow targeted biopsy to detect dysplasia, early cancer which was difficult to diagnose with standard white light video-endoscopes. They include chromoendoscopy, narrow band imaging, magnification endo-scopy, confocal endomicroscopy, optical coherence tomography, autofluorescence imaging, elastic scattered spectroscopy and wireless capsule endoscopy to name a few. Innovations in the field of endoscopy have allowed viewing of dysplastic cells (virtual histology). Most of the technology is

Flowchart 5.1: Follow-up endoscopy for Barrett's esophagus

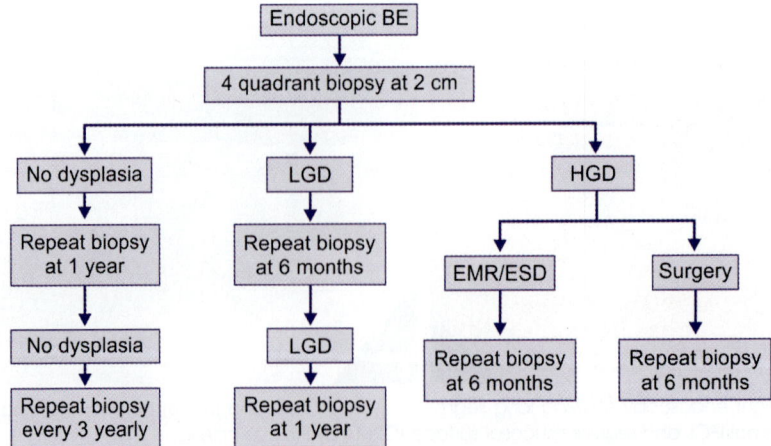

expensive, has a learning curve, increase endoscopic viewing time and needs validation before its regular use is recommended especially in the developing countries like India.

Chromoendoscopy

It includes spraying of dye on mucosa to improve tissue localization, characterization and allow targeted biopsies.[79] Dyes used can be classified as absorptive, contrast or reactive stains. Staining effects are transient, the technique is simple, quick, inexpensive and safe.

Lugol's Iodine

Lugol's iodine (LI) contains potassium iodide which has high affinity for glycogen in non-keratinized squamous epithelium. It stains normal squamous cell black or dark brown. It is used in concentration of 1–3%, about 30 ml is sprayed over esophageal mucosa after administering glucagon. Majority of inflamed, dysplastic, cancer containing mucosa and BE remain unstained to allow targeted biopsy.[80–84] It helps identify synchronous lesions, boundaries of abnormal tissue allowing complete evaluation.[82,83] Sensitivity of LI to detect early SCC ranges from 46–96%.[81,82] It can occasionally produce mild chest discomfort and lead to allergic reactions.

Methylene Blue (MB)

MB is taken up by goblet absorptive cells in BE.[85] Technique involves spraying of 10% N-acetylcysteine to remove the mucus on the epithelium. MB 0.5% is then sprayed over BE and washed away after 2–3 minutes. Unlike LI with MB stained mucosa is biopsied to detect BE. Heterogenous uptake may suggest dysplasia within BE. The sensitivity of MB to detect BE is high[86] but its sensitivity to detect dysplasia within BE is low.[86] Though it is cost effective to use MB it has several disadvantages: time consuming, possible induction of genetic damage, longer learning curve as it is a multi-step technique.

Indigo Carmine (IC)

IC is a contrast enhancing agent which pools in cervices between epithelial cells and helps identification of mucosal irregularity. Dye is diluted to 0.1–5% and sprayed on the mucosa. It is used only occasionally with magnification endoscopy for the detection of BE.[87]

Narrow Band Imaging (NBI)

NBI uses special red-green-blue filters to enhance visualization of superficial mucosal texture and vasculature with short wave length light. Currently available NBI scopes allow use of this technique by change of an electronic switch. NBI has several advantages over chromoendoscopy: no requirement of dye, easy to use, quick inspection of entire mucosa, viewing of intrapapillary capillary loop and short learning curve.

It is however expensive to use. Initial classification used three mucosal patterns (ridged/villous, circular and irregular/distorted) and two vascular patterns (normal and abnormal).[88] Ridge/villous pattern has sensitivity of 94% to detect BE whereas irregular/distorted pattern has sensitivity of 100% to detect HGD.[88] The overall sensitivity and specificity of NBI to detect BE was 95 and 65% respectively.[89] Its sensitivity and specificity to detect HGD was 96 and 94% respectively.[90] NBI compatible scopes are now available in most teaching centers.

Magnification Endoscopy (ME)

ME allows an image to be magnified from 1.5X to 150X. A cap is applied to the tip of the scope, an area of abnormality is identified, and a rotatory dial is used to zoom in. It not only allows detection of early esophageal cancer but also helps detect the depth of the tumor invasion (virtual histology).[90] Currently, its cost, longer time, long learning curve, interobserver variability and unavailability of uniform classification limits its use in day to day practice.

Confocal Endomicroscopy (CE)

CE allows optical biopsies from an area in focus using focal laser illumination. Its sensitivity and specificity in detecting BE is 98% and 94% respectively and associated cancer is 92% and 99% respectively.[91] Limited data is available on this technique.

Optical Coherence Tomography (OCT)

OCT uses light waves for cross sectional subsurface imaging. Catheter probes are introduced from biopsy channel to create radial/linear images of mucosal glands, crypts and villi. Disruption of various layers (epithelium, muscularis propria) can help diagnose BE, HGD and intramucosal cancer.[92,93] Spectral OCT is now evaluated to improve the contrast of the images.[94]

Autofluorescence Imaging (AFI)

AFI involves stimulation of endogenous molecules (fluorophores) by ultraviolet light. Light emitted by normal tissue is non-homogenous and appears green whereas neoplastic lesion emits pink or magenta color. To reduce false positive detection of dysplasia with AFI most studies have used NBI with AFI.[95]

Advances in optical imaging, excellence in engineering and higher understanding of molecular biology has allowed endoscopist to view, biopsy, predict outcomes and offer stage-based therapy to reduce morbidity and mortality of esophageal cancer. We have reached the beginning of the end as far as endoscopic diagnosis of esophageal cancer is concerned. In future, we should be looking at cost-effectiveness rather than cost, be able to offer technological advances to our patients, derive uniform methods of diagnosis and classification. Our understanding of how to evaluate patients with neoadjuvant chemo-radiotherapy need to improve. Recording, notifying and large scale screening will need team work, funds and manpower to succeed.

REFERENCES

1. Blot W, Devesa SS, Kneller RW, et al. Rising incidence of adenocarcinoma of the esophagus and gastric cardia. JAMA 1991;165:1287–9.
2. Newnham A, Quinn MJ, Babb P, et al. Trends in esophageal and gastric cancer: incidence, mortality and survival in England and Wales. Aliment Pharmacol Ther 2003;17:655–64.
3. Thrift AP. The epidemic of esophageal carcinoma - where are we now? Cancer Epidemiol 2016;41:88.
4. Lightdale CJ. Esophageal cancer. American College of Gastroenterology. Am J Gastroenterol 1999;94:20–9.
5. Doley CP, Larson AW, Stac NH, et al. Double contrast barium meal and upper gastrointestinal endoscopy. A comparative study. Ann Intern Med 1984;101:538–45.
6. Siewert J, Stein HJ. Classification of adenocarcinoma of the esophago-gastric junction. Br J Surg 1998;85:1457–9.
7. Graham DY, Schwartz JT, Cain GD, et al. Prospective evaluation of biopsy of esophageal and gastric carcinoma. Gastroenterology 1982; 82:228–31.
8. Kobayashi S, Kasugai T. Brushing cytology for the diagnosis of gastric cancer involving the cardia or the lower esophagus. Acta Cytol 1978; 22:155–7.
9. Zargar SA et al. Prospective comparison of the value of brushing before and after biopsy in the endoscopic diagnosis of gastroesophageal malignancy. Acta Cytol 1991;35:549–52.
10. Ajani JA, In H, Sano T, et al. Stomach. In AJCC cancer staging manual, 8th Amin MB (Ed). AJCC Chicago 2017;20–3.
11. Rice TW, Kelsen D, Blackstore EH, et al. Esophagus and esophago-gastric junction. In AJCC cancer staging manual 8th Amin MB (Ed) AJCC 2018.
12. Rice TW, Apperson-Hansen C, Di Paola LM, et al. Worldwide esophageal cancer collaboration: clinical staging data. Dis Esophagus 2016:29;707.
13. Rice TW, Lerut TE, Oringer MB, et al. Worldwide esophageal cancer collaboration: neoadjuvant pathological staging data. Dis Esophagus 2016: 29: 715.
14. Rice TW, Chen LQ, Hofstetter WL, et al. Worldwide esophageal cancer collaboration: Pathological staging data. Dis Esophagus 2016; 29:724.

15. Rice TW, Ishwaran H, Kelsen DP, et al. Recommendation for neoadjuvant pathological staging (ypTNM) of cancer of the esophagus and esophago-gastric junction for the 8th Edition AJCC/UICC staging manuals. Dis esophagus 2016;29:906.

16. Rice TW, Ishwaran H, Blackstone EH, et al. Recommendation for clinical staging (cTNM) of cancer of the esophagus and esophago-gastric junction for the 8th edition AJCC/UICC staging manuals. Dis esophagus 2016;29:913.

17. Rice TW, Ishwaran H, Hofstetter WL, et al. Recommendation for pathological staging (pTNM) of cancer of the esophagus and esophago-gastric junction for the 8th edition AJCC/UICC staging manuals. Dis Esophagus 2016;29:897.

18. Puli SR, Reddy JB, Bechfold ML, et al. Staging accuracy of esophageal cancer by endoscopic ultrasound: a metanalysis and systemic review: World J Gastroenterol 2018;14:1479.

19. Van Dam J, et al. High grade malignant stricture is predictive of esophageal tumor stage. Risk of endosonographic evaluation. Cancer 1993;71:2910–17.

20. Wallace MB, et al. Dilation of malignant esophageal stenosis to allow EUS guided fine needle aspiration: safety and effect on patient management. Gastrointest Endosc 2000;51:309–13.

21. Kallimanis GE, et al. Endoscopic ultrasound for staging esophageal cancer with or without dilation is clinically important and safe. Gastrointest Endosc 1995;41:540–6.

22. Mallary S, Van Dam J. Increased rate of complete EUS staging of patients with esophageal cancer using the nonoptical wire guided echoendoscope. Gastrointest Endosc 1999;50:53–7.

23. Murata Y, et al. Preoperative staging of superficial esophageal carcinoma: comparison of ultrasound probe and standard endoscopic ultrasonography. Gastrointest Endosc 1996;44:388–93.

24. Menzel J, Domschke W. Gastrointestinal miniprobe sonography: the current status. Am J Gastroenterol 2000;95:605–16.

25. Pfau P, Ginsberg GG, Lew RJ, et al. EUS predictors of long term survival in esophageal carcinoma. Gastrointest Endosc 2001;53:463–9.

26. Roder J, Busch R, Stein HJ, et al. Ratio of invaded to removed lymph nodes as a predicator of survival in squamous cell carcinoma of the esophagus. Br J Surg 1994;81:410–3.

27. Natsugoe S, Yoshinaka H, Shimada M, et al. Number of lymph node metastasis determined by presurgical ultrasound and endoscopic ultrasound is related to prognosis in patients with esophageal carcinoma. Ann Surg 2001;234:613–8.

28. Killinger W, Rice TW, Adelstein DJ, et al. Stage II esophageal carcinoma: the significance of T and N. J Thorac Cardiovasc Surg 1996;111:935–40.

29. Bolet JF, et al. Preoperative staging of esophageal cancer: comparison of endoscopic US and dynamic CT. Radiology 1991;181:419–25.

30. Catalano M, Sivak MV Jr, Rice T, et al. Endosonography features predictive of lymph node metastasis. Gastrointest Endosc 1994;40:442–6.

31. Bhutani M, Hawes RH, Hoffman BJ. A comparison of accuracy of echo features during endoscopic ultrasound (EUS) and EUS guided fine needle aspiration for diagnosis of malignant lymph node invasion. Gastrointest Endosc 1997;45:474–9.

32. Vazquez-Sequeiros E, et al. Impact of EUS guided fine needle aspiration on lymph node staging in patients with esophageal carcinoma. Gastrointest Endosc 2001;53:751–7.

33. Harewood G, Kumar KS. Assessment of clinical impact of endoscopic ultrasound on esophageal cancer. J Gastroenterol Hepatol 2004;19:433–9.

34. Wallace M, Netter PJ, Earle C, et al. An analysis of multiple staging management strategies for carcinoma of the esophagus computed tomography, endoscopic ultrasound, positron emission tomography and thoracoscopy/laparoscopy. Ann Thorac Surg 2002;74:1026–32.

35. Van Vilet EPM, Eijkemans MJC, Poley JW, et al. Staging of esophageal carcinoma in a low volume EUS center compared with reported results from high volume centers. Gastrointest Endosc 2006;63:938–47.

36. Schlick T, Heintz A, Junginger T. The examiners learning effect and its influence on the quality of endoscopic ultrasonography in carcinomas of the esophagus and gastric cardia. Surg Endosc 1999;13:894–8.

37. National comprehensive cancer network (NCCN). NCCN Clinical practice guideline in oncology 2018.

38. Riedel M, Hauck RW, Stein HJ, et al. Preoperative bronchoscopic assessment of airway invasion by esophageal cancer a prospective study. Chest 1998;13:687.

39. Kaushik N, Khalid A, Brody D, et al. Endoscopic ultrasound compared with laparoscopy for staging esophageal cancer. Ann Thorac Surg 2007;83:2000.

40. Yau KK, Siu WT, Cheung HY, et al. Immediate preoperative laparoscopic staging for squamous cell carcinoma of the esophagus. Surg Endosc 2006;20:307.

41. Bryan RT, Cruickshank NR, Needham SJ, et al. Laparoscopic peritoneal lavage in staging gastric and esophageal cancer. Eur J Surg Oncol 2001; 27:291.

42. Sun F, Chen T, Han J, et al. Staging accuracy of endoscopic ultrasound for esophageal cancer after neoadjuvant chemotherapy: a meta-analysis and systemic review. Dis Esophagus 2015;26:757.

43. Cerfolio R, Bryant AS, Bohja, et al. The accuracy of endoscopic ultrasonography with fine needle aspiration, integrated positron emission tomography with computed tomography and computed tomography in restaging patients with esophageal cancer after neoadjuvant chemo-radiotherapy. J Thorac Cardivasc Surg 2005;129:1232–41.

44. Kalha I, Kaw M, Fukamis N, et al. The accuracy of endoscopic ultrasound for restaging esophageal carcinoma after chemoradiation therapy. Cancer 2004;101:940–7.

45. Zuccaro G, Rice TW, Goldblum J, et al. Endoscopic ultrasound cannot determine sutability for esophagectomy after aggressive chemoradiotherapy for esophageal cancer. Am J Gastroenterol 1999;94:906–12.

46. Beseth B, Bedford R, Isacoff WH, et al. Endoscopic ultrasound does not accurately assess pathological stage of esophageal cancer after neoadjuvant chemoradiotherapy. Am Surg 2000;66:827–31.

47. Bowrey D, Clark GW, Roberts SA, et al. Serial endoscopic ultrasound in the assessment of response to chemoradiotherapy for carcinoma of the esophagus. J Gastrointest Surg 1999;3: 462–7.

48. Hirata N, Kawamoto K, Ueyama T, et al. Using endosonography to assess the effect of neoadjuvant therapy in patients with advanced esophageal cancer. AJR Am J Roetgenol 1997; 169:485–91.

49. Isenberg G, Chak A, Canto MI, et al. Endoscopic ultrasound in restaging esophageal cancer after neoadjuvant chemoradiation. Gastrointest Endosc 1998;48:158–63.

50. Willis J, Cooper GS, Isenberg G, et al. Correlation of EUS measurement with pathological assessment of neoadjuvant therapy response in esophageal carcinoma. Gastrointest Endosc 2002; 55:555–61.

51. Chak A, Canto MI, Cooper GS, et al. Endosonographic assessment of multimodality therapy predicts survival of esophageal carcinoma patients. Cancer 2000;88:1788–95.

52. Catalano MF, Sivak MV Jr, Rice TW, et al. Postoperative screening for anastomotic recurrence of esophageal carcinoma by endoscopy ultrasonography. Gastrointest Endosc 1995;42:540.

53. Fockens P, Manshanden CG, Van Lansohot JJ, et al. Prospective study on the value of endosonographic follow up after surgery for esophageal carcinoma. Gastrointest Endosc 1997; 46:487.

54. Muller C, Kahler G, Scheele J. Endosonographic examination of gastrointestinal anastomosis with suspected locoregional tumor recurrence. Surg Endosc 2000;14:45.

55. Tachibana M, Hirahara N, Kinugasa S, et al. Clinicopathologic features of superficial esophageal cancer: results of consecutive 100 patients. Ann Surg Oncol 2008;15:104.

56. Barbour AP, Jones M, Brown I, et al. Risk stratification of early esophageal adenocarcinoma: analysis of lymphatic spread and prognostic factors. Ann Surg Oncol 2010;17: 2494.

57. Merkow RP, Bilimoria KY, Keswani RN, et al. Treatment trends, risk of lymph node metastasis and outcomes for localized esophageal cancer. J Natl Cancer Inst 2014;106.

58. Endo M, Yoshino K, Kawano T, et al. Clinicopathological analysis of lymph node metastasis in surgically resected superficial cancer of the thoracic esophagus. Dis Esophagus 2000;13:125.

59. Shimada H, Nabeya Y, Matsubara H, et al. Prediction of lymph node status in patients with superficial esophageal carcinoma: analysis of 160 surgically resected cancers. Am J Surg 2006;191: 250.

60. Fujita H, Sueyoshi S, Yamana H, et al. Optimum treatment strategy for superficial esophageal cancer: endoscopic mucosal resection versus radical esophagectomy. World J Surg 2001;25: 424.

61. Liu L, Hofsletter WL, Rashid A, et al. Significance of the depth of tumor invasion and lymph node metastasis in superficial invasive (T1) esophageal adenocarcinoma. Am J Surg Pathol 2005;29:1079.

62. Westerterp M, Koppert LB, Buskens CJ, et al. Outcome of surgical treatment for early adenocarcinoma of the esophagus or gastro-esophageal junction. Virchow's Arch 2005;446:497.

63. Araki K, Ohno S, Egashira A, et al. Pathological features of superficial esophageal squamous cell carcinoma with lymph node and distant metastasis. Cancer 2002;94:570.

64. Ancona E, Rampado S, Cassaro M, et al. Prediction of lymph node status in superficial esophageal carcinoma. Ann Surg Oncol 2008;15:3278.

65. Sepesi B, Watson JJ, Zhou D, et al. Are endoscopic therapies appropriate for superficial submucosal esophageal adenocarcinoma: An analysis of esophagectomy specimens. J Am Coll Surg 2010;210:418.

66. Holscher AH, Bollschweiter E, Schroder W, et al. Prognostic impact of upper, middle and lower third mucosal or submucosal infiltration in early esophageal cancer. Ann Surg 2011;254:802.

67. Yamashina T, Ishihara R, Nagai K, et al. Long-term outcome and metastatic risk after endoscopic resection of superficial esophageal squamous cell carcinoma. Am J Gastroenterol 2013;108:544.

68. Hur C, Miller M, Kong CY, et al. Trends in esophageal adenocarcinoma incidence and mortality. Cancer 2013;119(6):1149–58.

69. Spechler SJ, Sharma P, et al. American Gastro-enterological Association Medical position statement on the management of Barrett's eso-phagus. Gastroenterology 2011; 140(3):1084–91.

70. ASGE standards of practice committee. Evans JA, Early DS, Fulcami N, et al. The role of endoscopy in Barrett's esophagus and other premalignant conditions of the esophagus. Gastrointest Endos 2012;76(6):1087–94.

71. Shaheen NJ, Falk GW, Iyer PG, et al. American College of Gasteroenterology. ACG Clinical guideline: diagnosis and management of Barrett's esophagus. Am J Gastroenterol 2016; 111(1):30–50.

72. Fitzgerald RC, Pietrom DI, Ragunath K, et al. British Society of Gastroenterology guidelines on the diagnosis and management of Barrett's esophagus. Gut 2014;63(1):7–42.

73. Jung KW, Talley NJ, Romero Y, et al. Epidemio-logy and natural history of intestinal metaplasia of the gastroesophageal junction and Barrett's esophagus a population-based study. Am J Gastroenterol 2011;106(8):1447–55.

74. Thota PN, Veenalaganti P, Veenalaganti S, et al. Low risk of high-grade dysplasia or esophageal adenocarcinoma among patients with Barrett's esophagus less than 1 cm (irregular Z line) within 5 years of index endoscopy. Gastroentero-logy 2016.

75. Sharma P, Dent J, Armstrong D, et al. The development and validation of an endoscopic grading system for Barrett's esophagus: the Prague C & M criteria. Gastroenterology 2006; 131(5):1392–9.

76. Bhat S, Coleman HG, Yousef F, et al. Risk of malignant progression in Barrett's esophagus patients: results from a large population-based study. J Natl Cancer Inst 2011;103(13):1049–57.

77. Hirota WK, et al. ASGE guideline: the role of endoscopy in the surveillance of premalignant conditions of the upper GI tract. Gastrointest Endosc 2006;63:570–80.

78. Wang KK, Sampling RE. Updated guideline 2008 for the diagnosis, surveillance and therapy of Barrett's esophagus. Am J Gastroenterol 2008; 103:788–97.

79. Fennerty MP. Tissue staining. Gastrointest Endosc Clin N Am 1994;4:297.

80. Yokoyama A, Ohmori T, Makuuchi H, et al. Successful screening of early esophageal cancer in alcoholics using endoscopy and mucosa iodine staining. Cancer 1995;76:919–21.

81. Dawsey S, Fleischer DE, Wang CQ, et al. Mucosal iodine staining improves endoscopic visuali-zation of squamous dysplasia and squamous cell carcinoma of the esophagus in Linxian, China. Cancer 1998;83:220–31.

82. Fagundes R, de Barros SGS, Putten ACK, et al. Occult dysplasia is disclosed by Lugol's chromo-endoscopy in alcoholics in high risk for squamous cell carcinoma of the esophagus. Endoscopy 1999;31:281–5.

83. Meyer V, Burtin P, Bour B, et al. Endoscopic detection of early esophageal cancer in a high-risk population: does Lugol's staining improve video-endoscopy? Gastrointest Endosc 1997;45:480–4.

84. Carr-Locke D, Alchaws FH, Branch MS, et al. Technology assessment status evaluation: endo-scopic tissue staining and tattooing. Gastrointest Endosc 1996;43:652–6.

85. Kowklakis GS, et al. Methylene blue chromo-endoscopy for the detection of Barrett's esophagus in a Greek Cohort. Endoscopy 2003; 35:383–7.

86. Ngamruengphong S, Sharma VK, Das A. Diagnostic yield of methylene blue chromoendoscopy for detecting specialized intestinal metaplasia and dysplasia in Barrett's esophagus: a metanalysis. Gastrointest Endosc 2009;69:1021–8.

87. Sharma P, Weston AP, Topalovski M, et al. Magnification chromoendoscopy for the detection of intestinal metaplasia and dysplasia in Barrett's esophagus. Gut 2003;52:24–7.

88. Sharma P, Bansal A, Mathur S, et al. The utility of novel narrow band imaging endoscopy system in patients with Barrett's esophagus. Gastrointest Endos 2006;64:167.

89. Mannath J, Subramanian V, Hawkey CJ, et al. Narrow band imaging for characterization of high-grade dysplasia and specialized intestinal metaplasia in Barrett's esophagus: a metanalysis. Endoscopy 2010;42:351.

90. Kumagai Y, Inone H, Nagai K, et al. Magnifying endoscopy, stereoscopic microscopy and the microvascular architecture of superficial esophageal carcinoma. Endoscopy 2002;34:269–375.

91. Kiesslich R, Dahlmann AM, Vieth M, et al. *In vivo* histology of Barrett's esophagus and associated neoplasias by confocal laser endomicroscopy. Gastrointest endosc 2005;61:AB101.

92. Poneros J, Brand S, Bouma BE, et al. Diagnosis of specialized intestinal metaplasia by optical coherence tomography. Gastroenterology 2001; 120:7–12.

93. Evans JA, Poneros JM, Bouma BE, et al. Optical coherence tomography to identify intramucosal carcinoma and high-grade dysplasia in Barrett's esophagus. Clin Gastroenterol Hepatol 2006;4: 38–43.

94. Li X, Boppart SA, J Van Dam, et al. Optical coherence tomography: advanced technology for the endoscopic imaging of Barrett's esophagus. 2000;32:921–30.

95. Kara M, Peters FP, Fockens P, et al. Endoscopic video-autofluorescence imaging followed by narrow band imaging for detecting early neoplasia in Barrett's esophagus. Gastrointest Endosc 2006;64:176–85.

6

Pathology of Esophageal Tumors

Sarabjeet Kaur Arneja

Histological classification of esophageal tumors:[1]

EPITHELIAL TUMORS

Squamous Cell Carcinoma

Esophageal squamous cell carcinoma is predominantly located in the middle and the lower third of the esophagus, approximately 10–15% are located in the upper third of esophagus. The gross appearance (Fig. 6.1) varies from exophytic, fungating to ulcerative, plaque like infiltrative lesion. It is composed of neoplastic squamous epithelium that penetrates through the epithelial basement membrane and infiltrates the lamina propria or deeper tissue layers (Fig. 6.2). The precursor lesion of esophageal squamous cell carcinoma is thought to be intraepithelial neoplasia (dysplasia and carcinoma *in situ*). It is frequently seen adjacent to invasive squamous cell carcinoma in esophagectomy specimens (Fig. 6.3).

Variants of Squamous Cell Carcinoma

Verrucous carcinoma: On gross examination, its appearance is that of exophytic, warty tumor, microscopically it is composed of

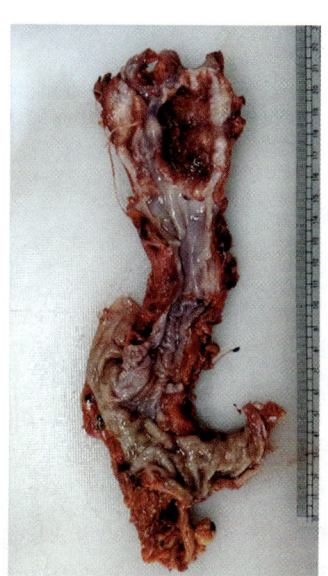

Fig. 6.1: Gross Appearance. Ulcerative, infiltrative lesion involving upper esophagus

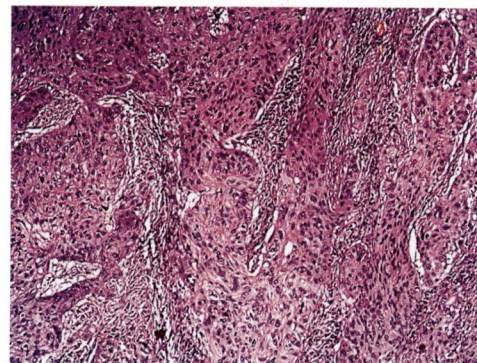

Fig. 6.2: Squamous cell carcinoma, moderately differentiated. Invasive nests of neoplastic epithelium showing evident squamous differentiation

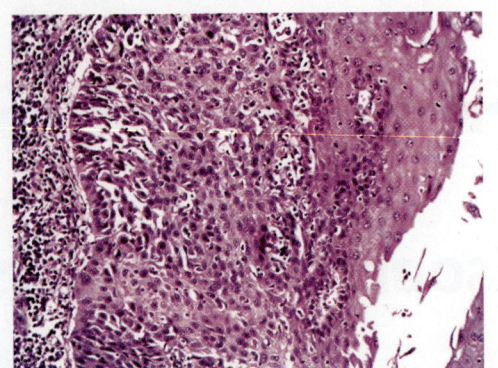

Fig. 6.3: Intraepithelial neoplasia. High grade dysplasia/carcinoma *in situ*. Cellular atypia is marked and is seen involving full thickness of the epithelium

well-differentiated keratinizing squamous epithelium with minimal cytological atypia, forming broad pushing island of neoplastic epithelium rather than infiltrating margins.

Spindle cell carcinoma: Squamous cell carcinoma with a spindle (sarcomatoid) cell component. Immunohistochemically the sarcomatoid spindle cells show evidence of epithelial differentiation.

Basaloid squamous cell carcinoma: This rare variant shows a solid growth pattern composed of closely packed cells with scant basophilic cytoplasm hyperchromatic nuclei and central comedo-type necrosis.

Grading of Squamous Carcinoma

Grade 1: Well-differentiated tumors show a high proportion of large, differentiated, keratinocyte like squamous cells and a low proportion of small basal-type cells located at the periphery of the cancer cell nests.

Grade 2: Moderately differentiated, the most common type, show differentiation between the well and poorly differentiated types.

Grade 3: Poorly differentiated, consists predominantly of basal-type cells.

Adenocarcinoma

A malignant epithelial tumor of the esophagus showing glandular differentiation. It arises predominantly from Barrett's mucosa that involves the lower third of the esophagus. On gross examination tumors are flat, ulcerated or polypoid, exophytic, fungating appearance. Microscopically majority are tubular and/or papillary (Fig. 6.4) in appearance a few tumors are of the diffuse type that show rare, insignificant glandular formations (Fig. 6.5), and sometimes signet ring cells.

Grading of Adenocarcinoma

Grade 1: Well-differentiated (>95% of tumor composed of glands).

Grade 2: Moderately differentiated (50–95% of tumor composed of glands).

Grade 3: Poorly differentiated (<50% of tumor composed of glands).

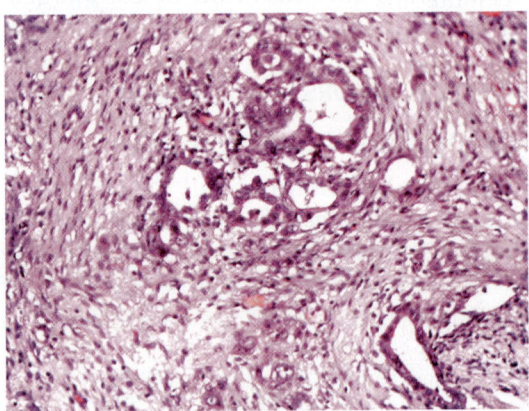

Fig. 6.4: Adenocarcinoma, well-differentiated. Tumor is composed of neoplastic glandular epithelium forming well-formed tubular glands

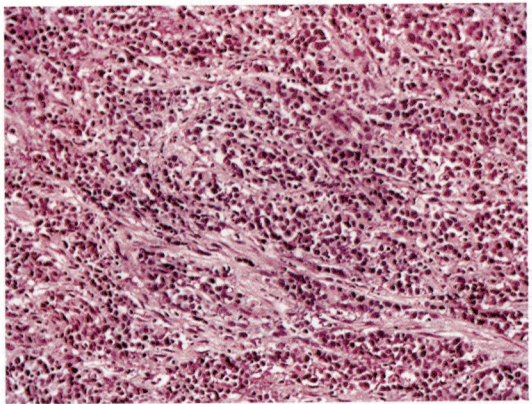

Fig. 6.5: Adenocarcinoma, poorly differentiated. Glandular differentiation is completely absent in this tumor

Neuroendocrine Tumors

Neuroendocrine tumors of the esophagus are rare tumors, and include well-differentiated neuroendocrine tumors (carcinoid tumors) and poorly differentiated endocrine carcinoma (small cell carcinoma) (Fig. 6.6).

WHO classification of the digestive NETs is applied to grade the tumors. WHO Grade 1 tumors have <2 mitoses per 10 HPF or Ki67 labeling index <3%, while WHO Grade 2 tumors have 2 to 20 mitoses per 10 HPF or Ki-67 labeling index 3–20%, and rare WHO grade 3 well-differentiated tumors have >20 mitoses per 10 HPF or Ki67 labeling index >20%.

NONEPITHELIAL TUMORS

- Leiomyoma and its malignant counterpart, leiomyosarcoma
- Gastrointestinal stromal tumor (GIST).

Leiomyoma and its malignant counterpart, Leiomyosarcoma: These are tumors of smooth muscle origin. They are composed of spindle cells that show smooth muscle differentiation evidenced by eosinophilic, fibrillary cytoplasm. Cellularity is low to moderate, mitotic activity is insignificant in benign tumors. On immunohistochemistry cells express desmin and smooth muscle actin, and are negative for CD34 and CD117 (C- KIT).

Gastrointestinal stromal tumor: Esophageal GISTs are identical to their counterparts elsewhere in gastrointestinal tract. Tumors are characterized by their positivity for KIT and CD34, variable reactivity for smooth muscle actin and negativity for desmin (Fig. 6.7).

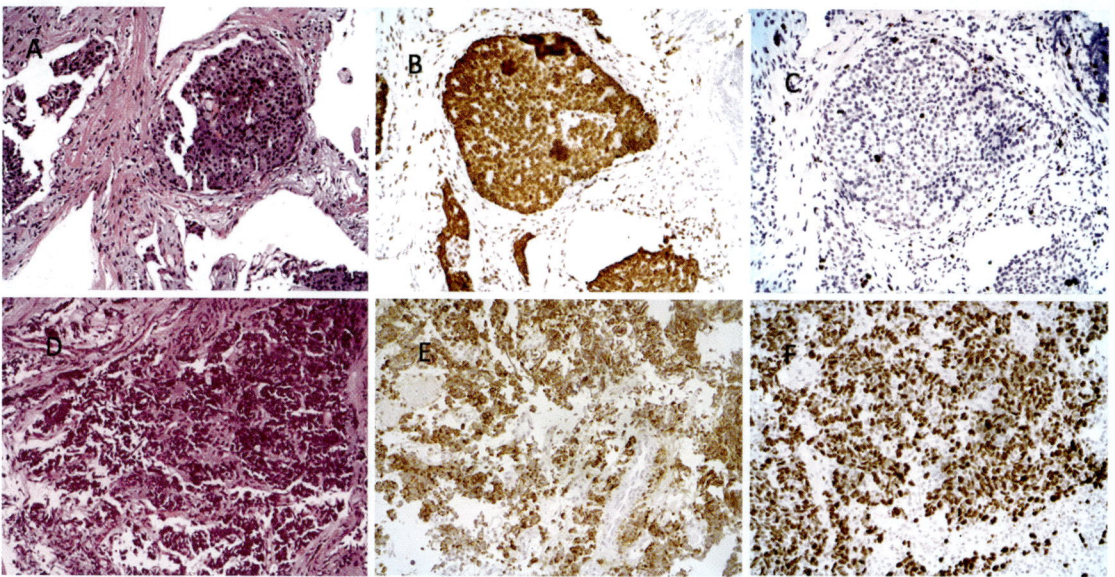

Fig. 6.6: Neuroendocrine tumor of esophagus. (A to C) Well-differentiated neuroendocrine tumor Grade 1. (A) H&E, organized nests of monotonous cells. (B) Strong cytoplasmic positivity for neuroendocrine marker, chromogranin. (C) MIB-1(Ki67) labelling index is approximately 2%. (D to F) Poorly differentiated small cell neuroendocrine carcinoma. (D) H&E, nuclear crowding and molding with indistinct cytoplasm. (E) Chromogranin is positive, evidently with lesser intensity as compared to well-differentiated neuroendocrine carcinoma. (F) MIB-1(Ki67) labelling index is high, approximately 60–70%

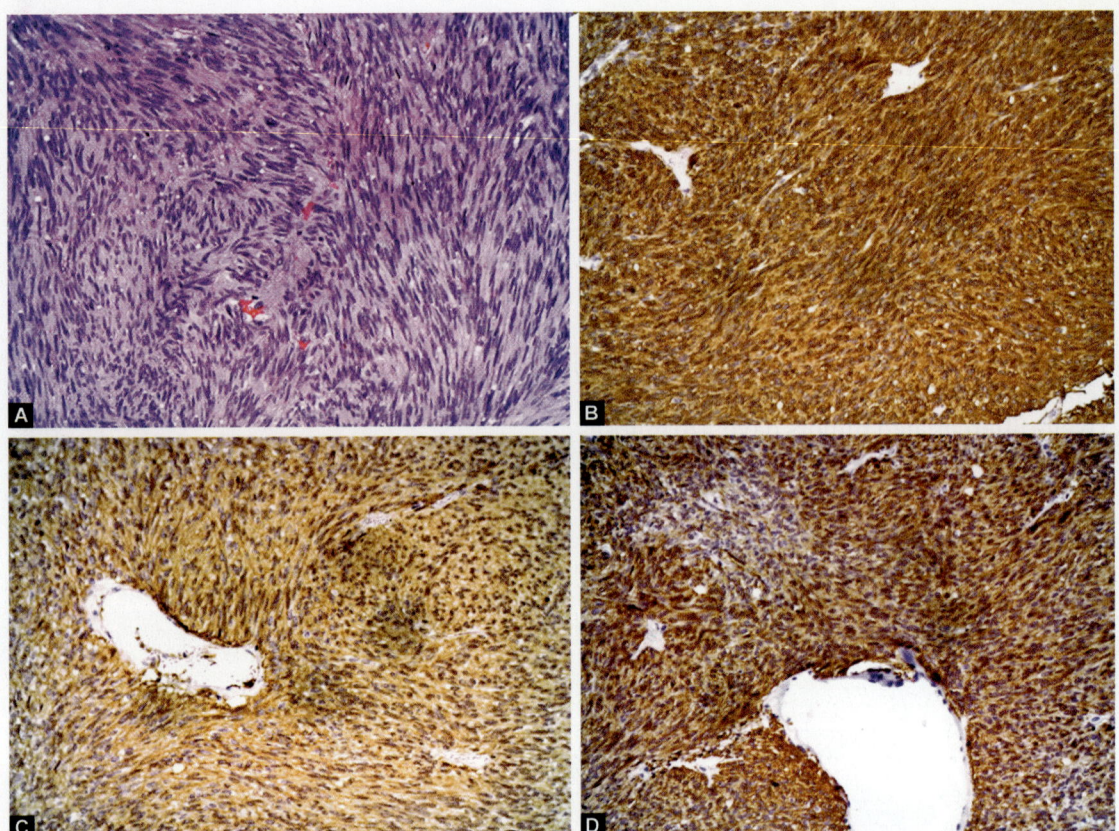

Fig. 6.7: Gastrointestinal Stromal Tumor (GIST) of esophagus. (A) H&E, Tumor is composed of spindle cells. (B to D) Immuno-histochemistry for CD117 (c-Kit), CD34 and DOG-1 respectively. Strong cytoplasmic positivity for all the three markers, characteristic of GIST

BIBLIOGRAPHY

WHO classification of tumours of the digestive system. 4th Edition, Volume 3 http://publications.iarc.fr/

7

Imaging in Esophageal Cancer

Anirudh Kohli

Imaging plays an important role in staging of esophageal cancer (EC). Computed tomography (CT) complements endoscopy and endoscopic ultrasound (EUS) in staging of esophageal cancer. Though CT scan and magnetic resonance imaging (MRI) are inferior to EUS in identifying tumor invasion of the esophageal wall, they play an important role in estimating local spread, nodal involvement, distant metastasis, response to chemoradiotherapy and tumor recurrence. Current treatment of esophageal cancer is based on the stage of the disease. It is therefore, mandatory to accurately stage every patient as per TNM classification maintained by the American Joint Committee on Cancer (AJCC) and the Union for International Cancer Control (UICC) (Fig. 7.1).

The esophagus has distinct anatomical features which is conducive to rapid spread: The absence of a serosa, rich and diffuse lymphatic plexus with a bidirectional flow and the only organ to traverse three anatomical regions (the neck, the thorax and the abdomen). Therefore, a tumor can easily spread to the adjacent pericardium or aortic adventitia and can metastasize to cervical or celiac nodes. The four anatomical regions of the esophagus are cervical: from the cricoid cartilage to the thoracic inlet; upper thoracic: from the thoracic inlet to the carina; mid thoracic: from the carina to the diaphragm and lower thoracic/abdominal: from the diaphragm to the gastroesophageal junction (Fig. 7.2).

To determine the level of the tumor, the upper edge of the tumor should be considered and not the epicenter where it has the largest volume. There may be confusion about tumors which occur at the esophagogastric junction and extend into the esophagus and stomach as to whether they are esophageal or stomach cancers. Any tumor in the distal esophagus with its center within the distal 5 cm of the esophagus and proximal 5 cm of stomach is considered to be an esophageal carcinoma. A tumor in the proximal 5 cm of the stomach but no esophageal extension is considered a stomach cancer. This is important, so that the appropriate staging system can be applied, depending on its origin, whether from the esophagus or stomach.

Barium Swallow

A barium swallow is the first imaging investigation for the evaluation of dysphagia. An ideal barium technique is a double contrast swallow. An early esophageal cancer appears as a small protruded lesion which may be plaque like with central ulceration or as a small sessile polyp with lobulated contours.

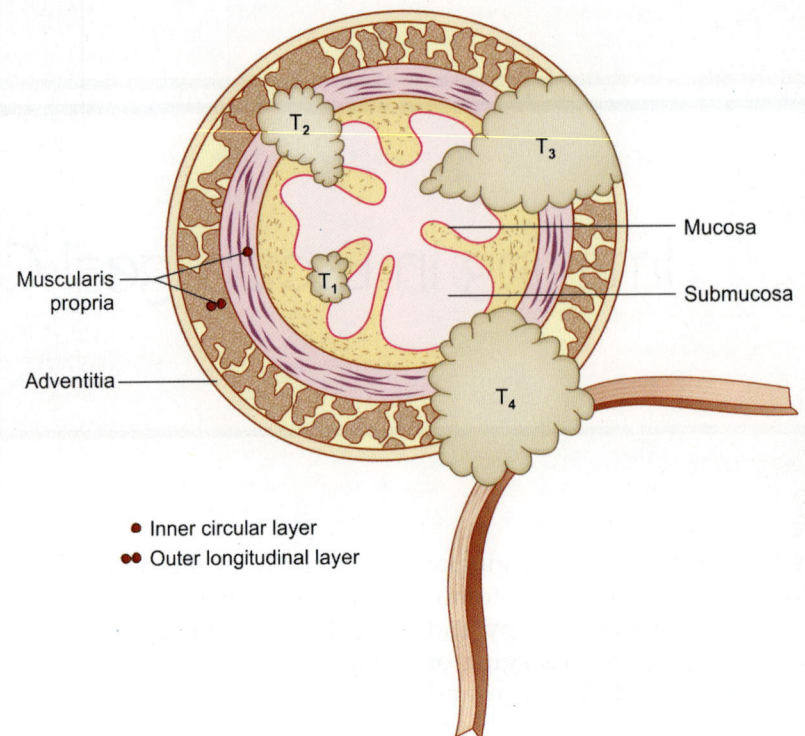

Muscularis
propria

Adventitia

Mucosa

Submucosa

● Inner circular layer
●● Outer longitudinal layer

Fig. 7.1: Esophageal wall showing four layers—mucosa, submucosa, muscularis propria and adventitia; T_1: Invasion up to the submucosa; T_2: Invasion of the muscularis propria; T_3: Invasion of the adventitia; T_4: Invasion of adjacent structures

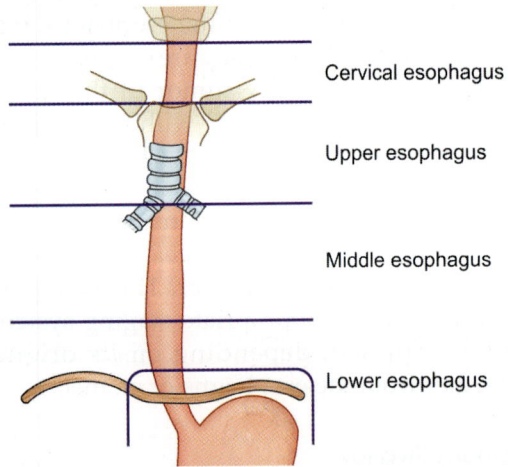

Cervical esophagus

Upper esophagus

Middle esophagus

Lower esophagus

Fig. 7.2: The four anatomical regions of the esophagus

Advanced esophageal cancer presents as an infiltrating irregular narrowing which constricts the lumen with well-defined proximal and distal margins. They may also present as a polypoidal lobulated intraluminal mass with surface irregularity representing erosions or as ulcerative lesions where there is a large outpouching of the barium column, representing a deep ulcer (Fig. 7.3). Occasionally it can identify a tracheoesophageal fistula. Esophagoscopy has largely replaced barium studies as it allows tissue diagnosis. Most centers use barium swallow post-deployment of self-expandable metal stents for palliation of advanced esophageal cancer to assess position and expansion of the stent, as endoscopic viewing in early stage may lead to its migration (Fig. 7.4).

Computed Tomography

On a CT scan EC appears as an esophageal wall thickening or as an intraluminal mass (Fig. 7.5). The normal esophageal wall is not more than 3 mm thick in a distended state. A wall thickness of 5 mm or greater is considered abnormal especially in a clinical setting.[1] The wall thickening may be

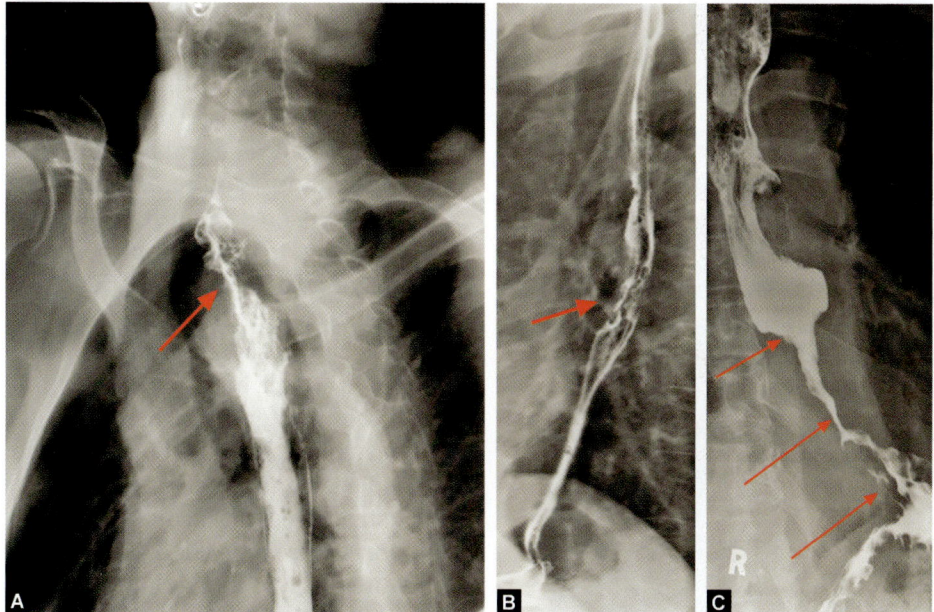

Figs 7.3A to C: Barium studies demonstrating esophageal cancer in the cervicothoracic, mid thoracic with mucosal irregularity and distal thoracic esophagus with apple core appearance with shouldering and stricture

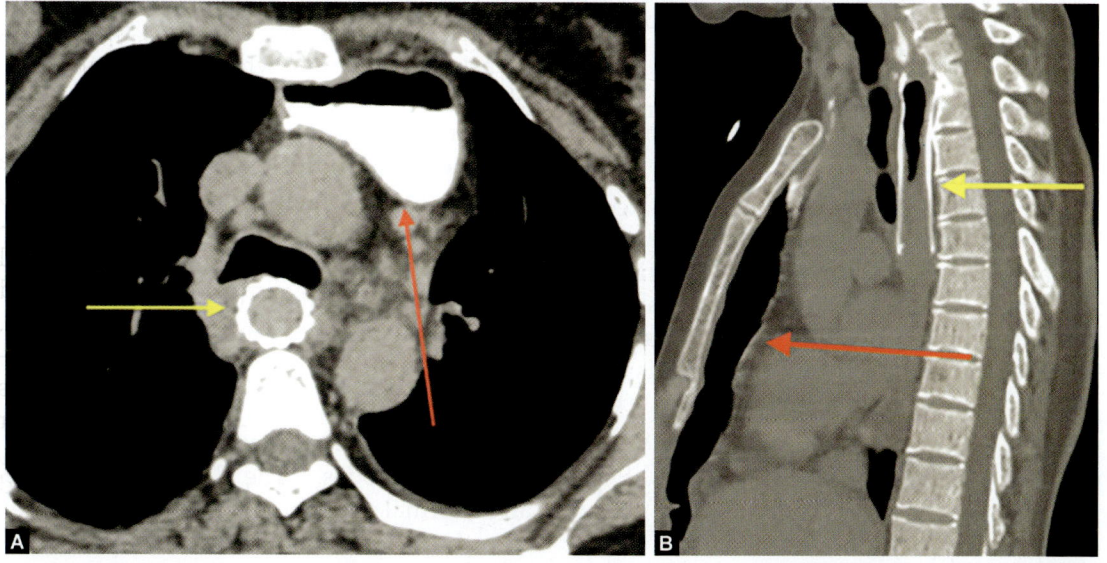

Fig. 7.4: (A) Plain axial CT study demonstrates a stent *in situ* in the esophagus. The stent (yellow arrow) is occluded by the intraluminal tumor extension. A pull through surgery using colon (red arrow) has been performed as evidenced by the oral positive contrast in the anterior mediastinum. (B) Sagittal CT image demonstrates a stent *in situ* in the esophagus with evidence of tumor occluding the lumen (yellow arrow). Pull through colon is seen in the anterior mediastinum (red arrow)

concentric or asymmetric, which is best delineated by a thin contrast.[2] There may be a mild or marked esophageal dilatation proximal to the lesion. The neoplasm may also be seen as an intraluminal mass lesion coated by the contrast media. Additional signs such as local infiltration into adjacent structures may be seen. In advanced esophageal cancer

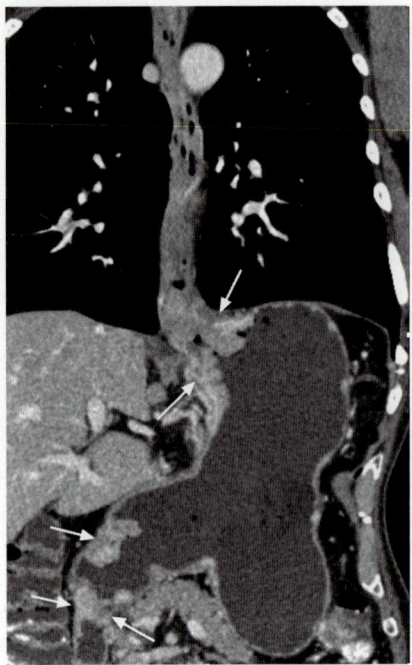

Fig. 7.5: Coronal CT image demonstrates an ill-defined soft tissue mass lesion involving the distal esophagus as well as fundus of the stomach, representing a primary esophageal neoplasm

infiltration of the tumor can occur into the trachea, producing a tracheoesophageal fistula, which results in extension of the contrast into the tracheobronchial tree. Recent studies have suggested that a triple phase dynamic CT may allow tumor identification in the late arterial phase even in the absence of wall thickening.[3] CT scan accurately assesses tumor bulk, a width >3 cm is associated with a higher incidence of extra-esophageal spread, an advanced stage and poor prognosis.[4] Axial CT imaging often overestimates the length of the tumor and is unreliable for detecting the length of stomach involvement.[5]

Tumor Staging

The CT scan is the most widely used modality to determine the T staging. It has limitations in determining the exact depth of tumor infiltration of the esophageal wall as it is unable to differentiate between $T_1/T_2/T_3$

lesions. This is an important requirement when considering the use of neoadjuvant chemotherapy and radiation therapy. Endoscopic ultrasound has a much higher accuracy than a CT scan. The real benefit of CT scan is in determining T_4 disease.[6] Since the esophagus lacks a serosa and it is attached to the neighboring structures by loose adventitia, there is no real anatomic barrier to the spread of disease into the mediastinum. Spread can occur easily into the neck, thyroid, larynx, trachea, bronchi, lung, pericardium, aorta and diaphragm. There may be loss of fat planes between the lesion and the adjacent structures or displacement/indentation of other mediastinal structures. Aortic invasion is suggested if there is more than 90° contact with the aorta or obliteration of triangular fat space between the esophageal tumor, aorta and spine[7, 8] (Figs 7.6 and 7.7). Aortic invasion is best viewed in the prone position. Other signs seen are tracheal displacement, indentation of posterior tracheal wall (Fig. 7.8). Pericardial invasion is suspected when there is loss of fat plane with the pericardium. Other signs of pericardial invasion are pericardial thickening, pericardial effusion or indentation of the heart by the esophageal mass.[9, 10] A caveat to be remembered is, it may be difficult to delineate the normal fat planes in severely underweight patients or those who have undergone chemo/radiotherapy.

Nodal Staging

A bulky tumor may interfere with evaluation of regional nodes.[10] The CT scan criteria for an abnormal adenopathy is based on the size. Intrathoracic and abdominal lymph nodes greater than 1 cm and supraclavicular lymph nodes more than 5 mm in short axis are considered to be metastatic.[11] Nodes smaller than 1 cm in short axis diameter, smooth well-defined borders, uniform homogeneous attenuation and a central fatty hilum are considered as normal. Occasionally, normal sized lymph nodes may contain metastatic

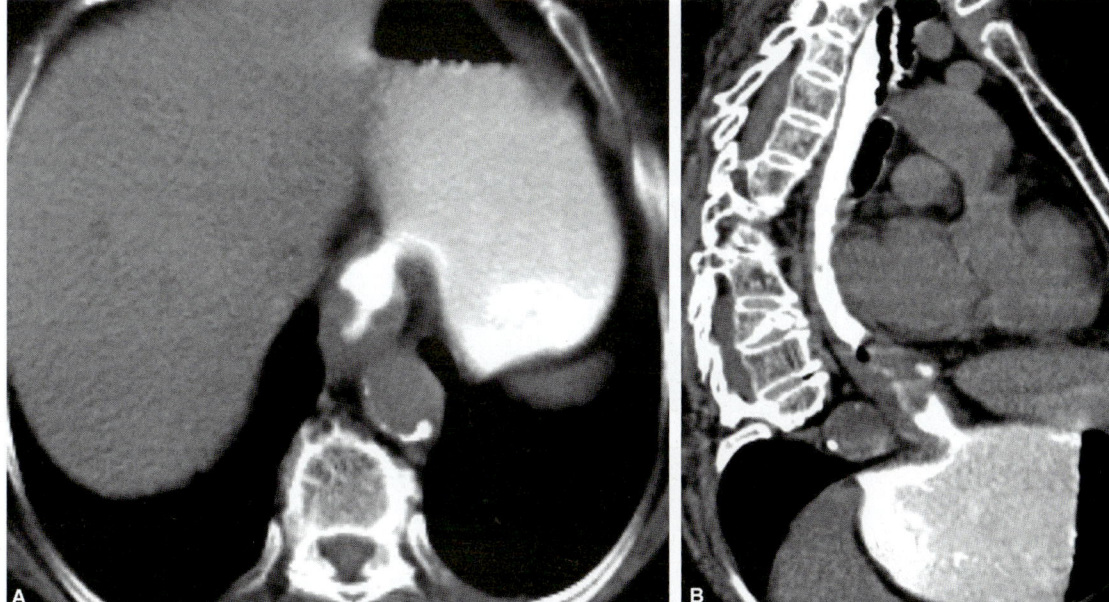

Figs 7.6A and B: Axial and sagittal CT images demonstrate a mass lesion involving the distal esophagus and gastroesophageal junction representing a primary esophageal neoplasm. The contact surface with aorta is less than 90°, therefore, not indicative of aortic invasion.

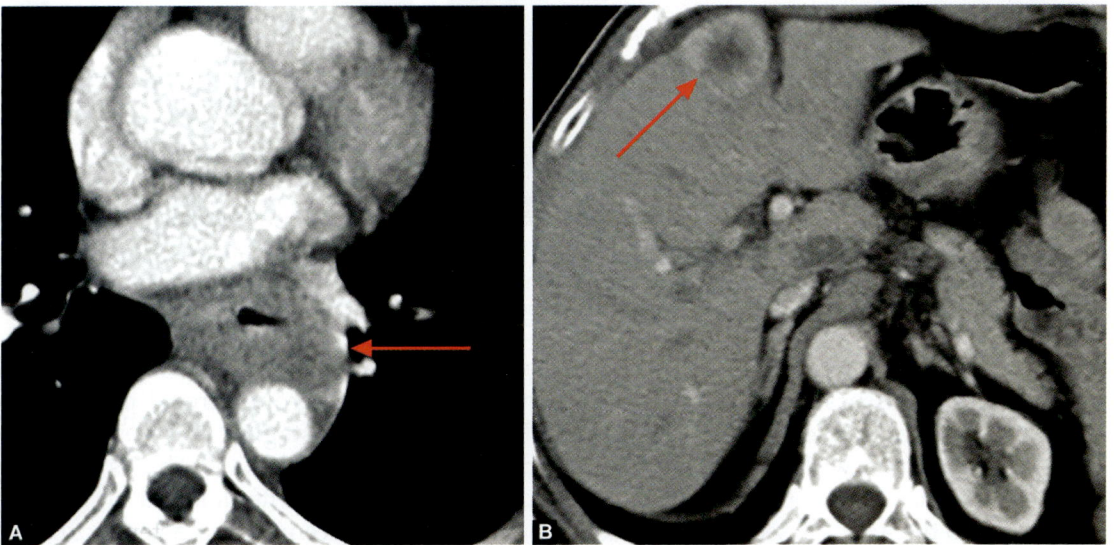

Fig. 7.7: (A) Axial CT image demonstrates a mass lesion involving the distal esophagus with aortic invasion as there is more than 90° contact in relation to the aorta. (B) Axial CT image demonstrates a focal hepatic lesion most likely representing a metastatic deposit

foci and CT scan cannot differentiate these which can lead to understaging.[12] Likewise, benign/reactive adenopathy larger than 1 cm may be falsely classified as positive.

Metastatic Staging

Distant metastasis may occur due to hematogenous spread to distant organs most commonly seen in the liver, lungs, bone,

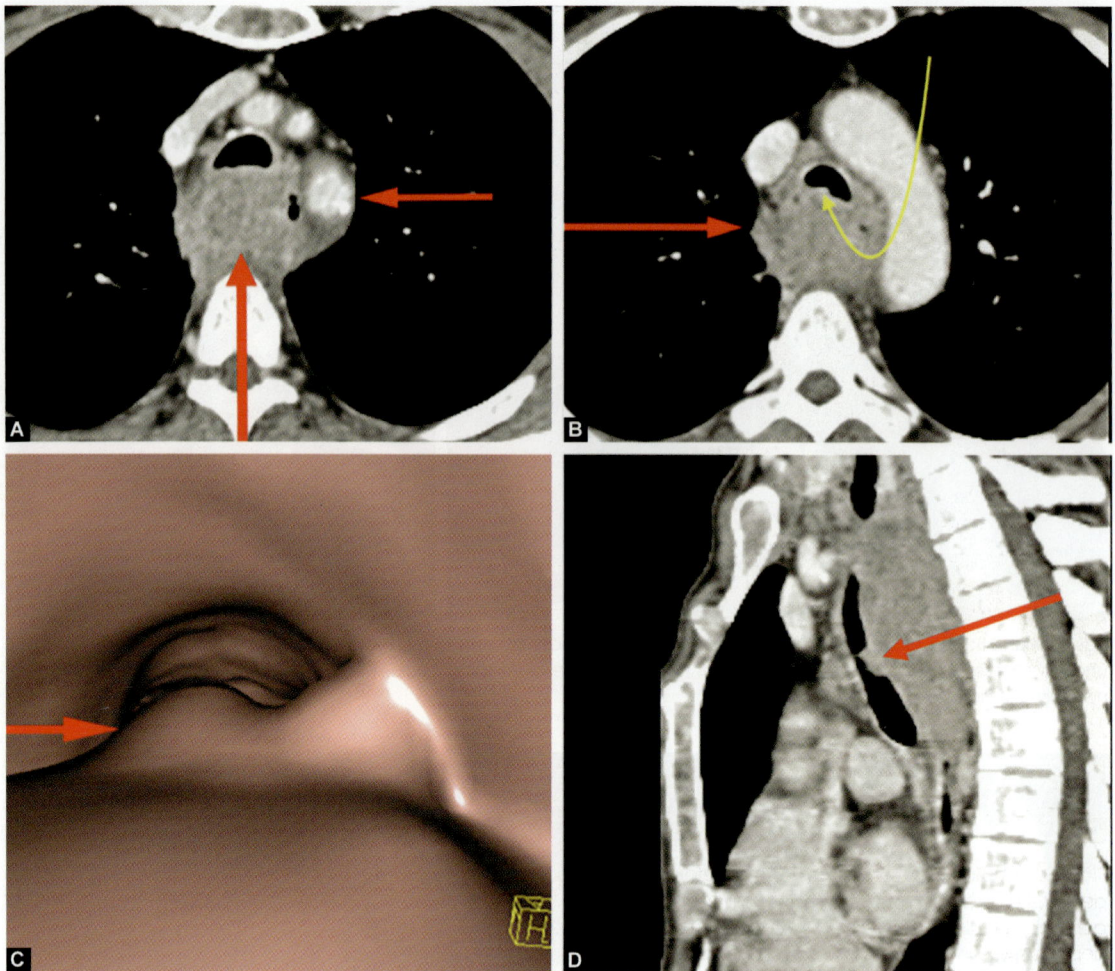

Fig. 7.8: (A and B) Axial CT images demonstrate a mass lesion involving the proximal thoracic esophagus displacing the trachea anteriorly with encasement of left subclavian artery. (C and D) Virtual endoscopy and sagittal CT images demonstrate extension of the lesion into the trachea representing tracheal invasion

adrenal glands and rarely in the brain or the peritoneum. To assess metastasis patients should have a contrast enhanced CT of the chest and abdomen with a dedicated liver technique to visualize hepatic metastasis.[13] Metastases to the liver are seen as focal well-circumscribed mass lesions in the liver. They are hypoechoic on sonography and hypo-dense on portal venous phase imaging on CT scan. Distant metastases to the lungs are seen as pulmonary nodules on chest X-ray or CT scan (Fig. 7.9). Distant metastases to adrenal gland are seen as focal enlargement of the adrenal gland. As benign adrenal adenomas are common it is important to differentiate adrenal adenoma from adrenal metastases. There may be upstaging of disease if this differentiation is not done. This is possible using a number of criteria based on the HU values and enhancement characteristics of the lesion on CT scan. Chemical shift MRI scan is also useful to help in differentiation.

Postoperative Imaging

Intraoperative complications, like recurrent laryngeal nerve injury may occur due to dissection in the neck when the trachea and thyroid are retracted or during intrathoracic

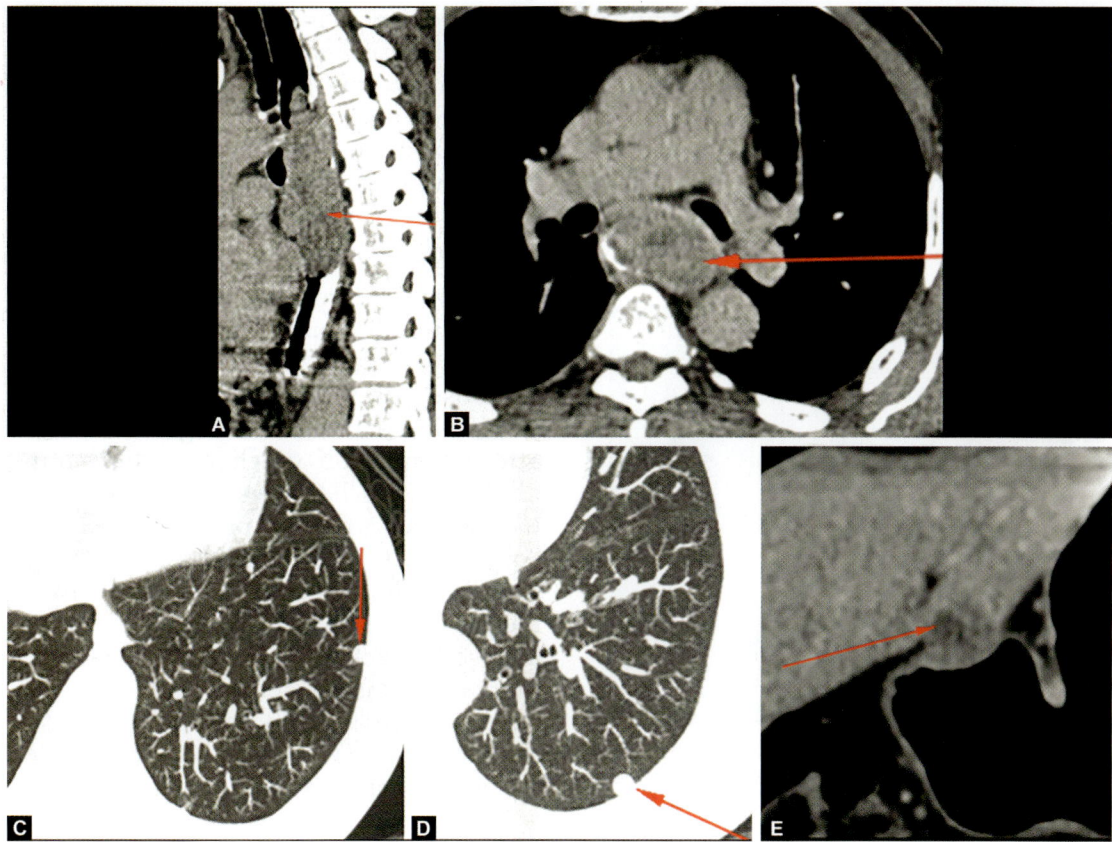

Fig. 7.9: (A) Sagittal CT image demonstrates a lobulated mass lesion involving mid-esophagus. (B) Axial CT image demonstrates a mass lesion at subcarinal level causing displacement of the left main bronchus. However, no bronchial or aortic invasion noted. (C and D) Axial CT images demonstrate pulmonary nodules most likely representing metastatic deposits. (E) Axial CT image demonstrates a focal hepatic lesion representing metastatic deposit

mobilization of the esophagus with lymph node dissection. Injury to the recurrent laryngeal nerve impairs the ability of the patient to cough in the postoperative period leading to the possibility of aspiration pneumonia. Other intraoperative complications are tracheobronchial injury essentially involving membranous portion of the airway. This leads to fistula formation with consequent empyema, recurrent pneumonia and respiratory compromise. This may require stent placement or a surgical repair.

CT imaging is useful to identify postoperative complications, which are common in such major surgical procedures. Pulmonary and pleural complications such as atelectasis, aspiration pneumonia, pleural effusion and empyema can be seen on imaging. Esophagus related complications such as anastomotic leak, chylothorax, delayed emptying of the stomach, herniation of abdominal viscera through the hiatus and reflux esophagitis can also be identified.

Anastomotic leak may occur early or late. Early anastomotic leaks (2–3 days) occur due to technical failure. Late anastomotic leaks occur after 3–4 days due to ischemia of the pulled up gastric stump or below the anastomotic level. Clinically anastomotic leaks present as an increasing or persistent pleural drainage, pus in the drainage tube, fever or sepsis. On imaging there may be an increasing hydropneumothorax, new air fluid levels or a persistent pneumonia. Contrast studies using water soluble contrast under fluoroscopy or CT scan will demonstrate the leak, its exact site and extent of the leak (Figs 7.10 and 7.11). There may be esophagopleural, esophagobronchial or esophagocutaneous fistulas. Subclinical leaks usually heal without treatment and are followed up by serial imaging.

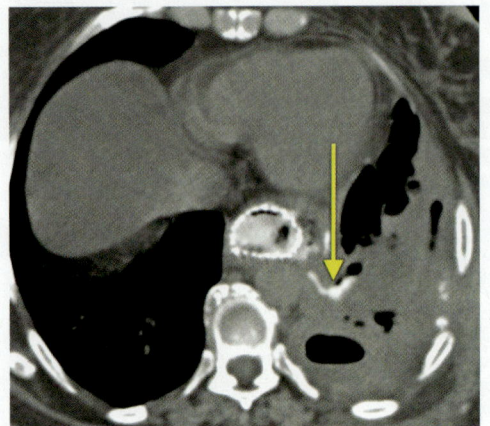

Fig. 7.10: Axial CT study demonstrates a stent *in situ* in the esophagus, oral contrast is seen in the stent lumen. There is extravasation of the orally administered contrast from the stent lumen into the left pleural space

Delayed emptying of stomach may occur. This will be seen as a large air fluid level in the mediastinum. This sign is a good indicator of delayed emptying. A contrast study can be performed and the stomach emptying can be evaluated.

Postneoadjuvant Therapy

CT scan/PET scan (Positron Emission Tomography) may be done after three to four cycles of chemotherapy, to assess the therapy response and to essentially identify nonresponding patients. Imaging is also useful after completion of chemoradiotherapy to identify which tumors have responded to therapy. This is a useful prognostic indicator. Another utility is to detect new distant metastases during the interval period between the start and end of therapy. CT accurately assesses reduction of the tumor volume. A partial response is defined as reduction in volume by 50% with no new lesions on two examinations 4 weeks apart.[14] A reduction in tumor volume by more than 50% on CT scan performed 2 weeks after neoadjuvant

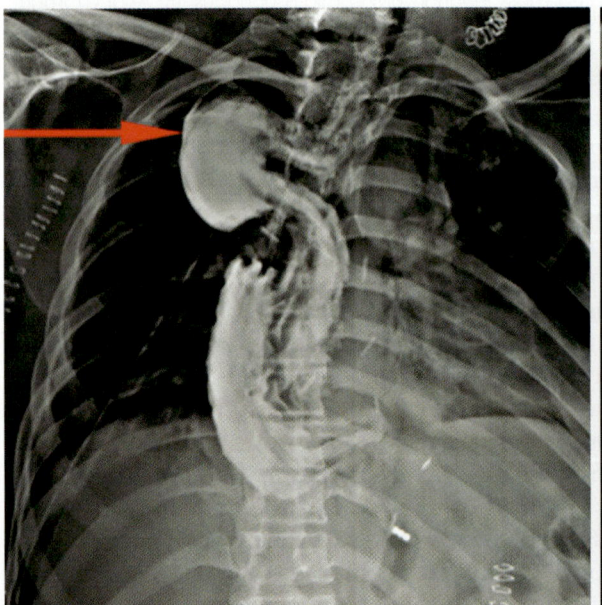

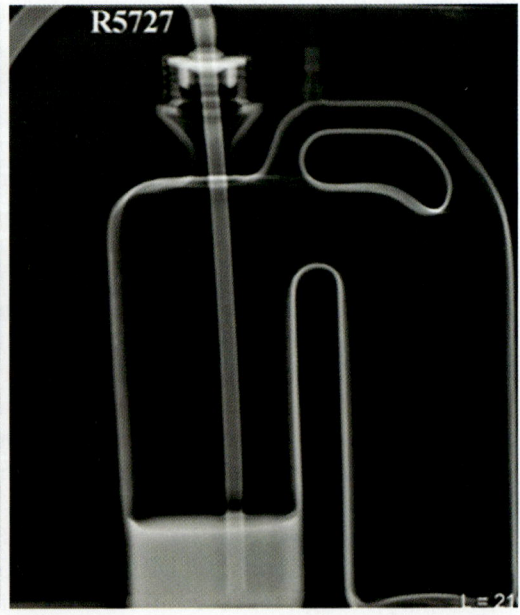

Fig. 7.11: (A) Oral contrast swallow following a pull through surgery demonstrates large extravasation of orally administered contrast in the upper thoracic region. (B) There is evidence of the contrast seen in the drainage bottle

chemotherapy can predict histopathological response with high sensitivity but low specificity.[15] However results of volume reduction must be validated by pathological response.[16] F-fluoro-2deoxy-D-glucose (FDG PET) is the modality of choice for demonstrating a quantitative decrease in FDG uptake, decrease in tumor and size of metastasis, post-therapy. A good response on FDG PET correlates closely with improved patient survival. CT scan is not an ideal imaging modality to assess the therapeutic response as it fails to differentiate between T_1–T_3 tumors. CT scan also has limitation in differentiating residual tumor from post-therapy changes such as inflammation and scar tissue. Endoscopic ultrasound examination also may not be able to differentiate between the residual tumor and post-therapy changes.

Post Definitive Treatment

CT scan is not routinely performed after definitive therapy for esophageal cancer. However, if patient has any symptom or sign suspicious for recurrence a CT chest and abdomen must be performed. Most recurrences occur in the abdominal nodes.[17] In the absence of any surgical complications an early CT (within 3 months) should be avoided after surgery as postoperative soft tissue thickening, pleural effusion and mediastinal fat infiltration may simulate early recurrence.[17, 18]

Magnetic Resonance Imaging

CT scan and MRI are comparable in staging esophageal cancers. Most centers prefer to use CT scan over MRI as it is less expensive, less time consuming and easily available.

Positron Emission Tomography

Positron emission tomography (PET) is now increasingly used in esophageal cancer in assessing response to therapy and predicting survival.[18] F-fluoro-2-deoxy-D-glucose (FDG) is commonly used isotope during PET as tumor cells have an increased uptake and delayed clearance allowing its differentiation from normal tissue. After 40 minutes of intravenous administration of 300–400 MBq of FDG, its uptake by tumor cells can be identified. Higher tumor to background activity may be seen on delayed images at 60 minutes. The spatial resolution of most FDG-PET system is 5–8 mm. At higher concentrations of FDG even lesions <1 cm can be detected.

Fusion of multidetector CT and PET scanner in PET/CT is now available in India. PET/CT is better than PET in identifying metastatic disease thus reducing unnecessary surgeries in patients with esophageal cancer.[19–21]

Tumor Staging

Both squamous cell carcinoma (SCC) and adenocarcinoma (EAC) cells take up FDG.[22] PET scan can identify primary tumor in about 80% with sensitivity of 40% for T_1 and 100% for T_4 tumors.[23,24] Its sensitivity is <25% for adenocarcinoma at gastroesophageal junction, signet ring and mucin secreting tumors.[25–29] Combining PET/CT yields very little to the diagnosis of T stage above EUS and hence it is rarely performed.[21]

Nodal Staging

Five years survival of node negative patient is about 4–5 times better than node positive patients.[30] Patients with more than 4 to 5 nodes and large size nodes have worst outcomes.[31–33] FDG PET was more sensitive to CT in identifying the nodes but with variable specificity.[34, 35] PET/CT has higher sensitivity, specificity and accuracy compared to PET in nodal staging of esophageal cancer. Currently EUS with fine needle cytology/biopsy is considered as the most accurate and specific method to diagnose nodal involvement irrespective of nodal size.[36]

Metastatic Staging

FDG PET is superior to CT in identifying non-regional nodal involvement, metastasis in the liver and bones.[37,38] PET/CT combined improves anatomical localization, reduces false positive rate and alters patient management when compared to PET alone.[39,40] PET/CT combined is most ideal for detecting occult metastasis. CT + EUS with fine needle aspiration cytology (FNAC) is inexpensive and offers more quality adjusted life years.[41] PET/CT combined with EUS/FNAC is an ideal option but at a much higher cost in staging esophageal cancer.[41] Currently, most surgeons would perform FDG-PET prior to attempting curative surgery in order to identify and exclude occult metastases.[42]

Treatment and Prognosis

PET is extremely useful in planning radiotherapy treatment for accuracy in length of tumor and identifying non-regional nodes.[43] FDG-PET may be used as an independent predictor of survival.[44] Higher SUV max was associated with poorer outcome in few studies.[45,46]

Response Assessment

Use of neoadjuvant therapy improves not only resection rates but also survival. Patients with complete histological response have a 3 year survival of >60%.[47] Identifying reduction of SUV suggests good response to treatment. Post-treatment SUV reduction by >10 suggests a good response. Patients who have increase in SUV post-treatment, need an alternative form of therapy. SUV reduction postchemotherapy is often associated with a pathological response, reduction in recurrence and improved survival.[48–50] However, results following radiotherapy are unreliable as radiotherapy induces marked inflammation which itself changes the SUV. FDG-PET is a useful guide though not always perfect in assessing outcomes of patients undergoing neoadjuvant therapy. Protocol based studies, larger numbers and standardization of PET evaluation is a must to improve care and cure in patients with esophageal cancer (Fig. 7.12).

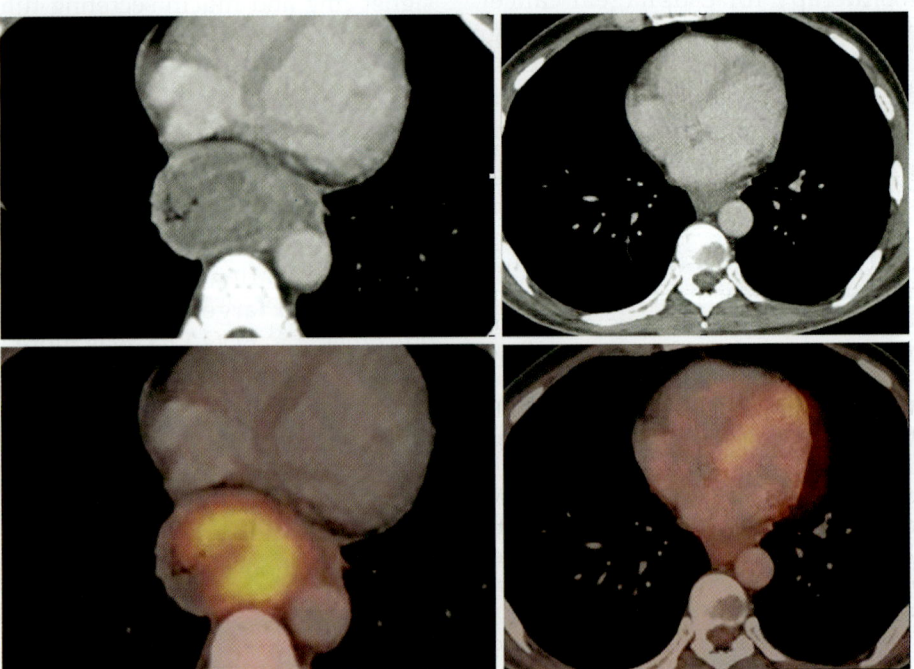

Fig. 7.12: 51-year-old male with a mass lesion in the distal thoracic esophagus indicative of a primary esophageal neoplasm. PET-CT done two months apart. CT and PET images demonstrate near complete resolution of the primary esophageal malignancy indicating response to the treatment

CONCLUSION

In esophageal carcinoma accurate preoperative staging and assessment is essential to determine appropriate therapy. Similarly, following neoadjuvant therapy an accurate assessment of therapeutic response is the key to deciding further management. Endoscopic ultrasound is the ideal modality to determine the depth of invasion and presence of regional lymph nodes. It can also be used as a guide to sample adjacent adenopathy to determine if the adenopathy is benign or malignant. CT scan is very useful for determining extent of tumor, adjacent organ invasion as well as presence of distant metastases, essentially for determining operability. PET CT scan is very useful in detecting metastatic local adenopathy, distant metastases as well as in follow-up after therapy to determine therapeutic response as well as recurrence of the disease.

REFERENCES

1. Halber MD, Daffner RH. Thompson WM. CT of the esophagus: I. Normal appearance. AJR Am J Roentgenol 1979;133:1047–50.
2. Rise TW. Clinical staging of esophageal carcinoma. CT, EUS and PET. Chest Surg Clin N Am 2000;10:471–85.
3. Umeoka S, Koyama T, Togashi K, et al. Esophageal cancer: Evaluation with triple-phase dynamic CT-initial experience. Radiology 2006;239:777–83.
4. Lefor AT, Merino MM, Steinberg SM, et al. Computerized tomographic prediction of extraluminal spread and prognostic implications of lesion width in esophageal carcinoma. Cancer 1988;62:1287–92.
5. Quint LE, Glazer GM, Orringer MB, Gross BH. Esophageal carcinoma: CT findings. Radiology 1985;155:171–5.
6. Coulomb M, Lebas JF, Sarrazin R, Geindre M. [Oesophageal cancer extension. Diagnostic contribution and effects on therapy of computed tomography. Report on 40 cases (author's trans.)]. J Radiol 1981;62:475–87.
7. Picus D, Balfe DM, Koehler RE, Roper CL, Owen JW. Computed tomography in the staging of esophageal carcinoma. Radiology 1983;146:433–8.
8. Takashima S, Takeuchi N, Shiozaki H, et al. Carcinoma of the esophagus: CT vs MR imaging in determining resectability. AJR Am J Roentgenol 1991;156:297–302.
9. Saunders HS, Wolfman NT, Ott DJ. Esophageal cancer. Radiologic staging. Radiol Clin North Am 1997;35:281–94.
10. Kumbasar B. Carcinoma of the esophagus: radiologic diagnosis and staging. Eur J Radiol 2002;42:170–80.
11. Balfe DM, Mauro MA, Koehler RE, et al. Gastrohepatic ligament: normal and pathologic CT anatomy. Radiology 1984;150:485–90.
12. Schroder W, Baldus SE, Monig SP, et al. Lymph node staging of esophageal squamous cell carcinoma in patients with and without neoadjuvant radiochemotherapy: histomorphologic analysis. World J Surg 2002;26:584–7.
13. Gollub MJ, Lefkowitz R, Moskowitz CS, et al. Pelvic CT in patients with esophageal cancer. AJR Am J Roentgenol 2005;184:487–90.
14. Miller AB, Hoogstraten B, Staquet M, Winkler A. Reporting results of cancer treatment. Cancer 1981;47:207–14.
15. Beer AJ, Wieder HA, Lordick F, et al. Adenocarcinomas of esophagogastric junction: multidetector row CT to evaluate early response to neoadjuvant chemotherapy. Radiology 2006;239:472–80.
16. Griffith JF, Chan AC, Chow LT, et al. Assessing chemotherapy response of squamous cell oesophageal carcinoma with spiral CT. Br J Radiol 1999;72:678–84.
17. Carlisle JG, Quint LE, Francis IR, et al. Recurrent esophageal carcinoma: CT evaluation after esophagectomy. Radiology 1993;189:271–5.
18. Becker CD, Barbier PA, Terrier F, Porcellini B. Patterns of recurrence of esophageal carcinoma after transhiatal esophagectomy and gastric interposition. AJR Am J Roentgenol 1987;148:273–7.
19. Rampin L, Nani C, Fanti S, et al. Value of PET-CT fusion imaging in avoiding potential pitfalls in the interpretation of 18 F-FDG accumulation in the distal oesophagus. Eur J Nucl Med Mol Imaging 2005;32:990–2.
20. Muden RF, Macapiniac HA, Erasmus JJ. Esophageal cancer: the role of integrated CT-PET in initial staging and response assessment after preoperative therapy. J Thorac Imaging 2006;21:137–45.
21. Bar-Shalom R, Guralnik L, Tsalic M, et al. The additional value of PET/CT over PET in FDG imaging of oesphageal cancer. Eur J Nucl Med Mol Imaging 2005;32:918–24.

22. Kim K, Park SJ, Kim BT, Lee KS, Shim YM. Evaluation of lymph node metastases in squamous cell carcinoma of the esophagus with positron emission tomography. Ann Thorac Surg 2001;71:290–4.

23. Kato H, Miyazaki T, Nakajima M, et al. The incremental effect of positron emission tomography on diagnostic accuracy in the initial staging of esophageal carcinoma. Cancer 2005;103:148–56.

24. Yoon YC, Lee KS, Shim YM, et al. Metastasis to regional lymph nodes in patients with esophageal squamous cell carcinoma: CT vs FDG PET for presurgical detection-prospective study. Radiology 2003;227:764–70.

25. Flamen P, Lerut T, Haustermans K, Van Cutsem E, Mortelmans L. Position of positron emission tomography and other imaging diagnostic modalities in esophageal cancer. Q J Nucl Med Mol Imaging 2004;48:96–108.

26. Rasanen JV, Sihvo EI, Knuuti MJ, et al. Prospective analysis of accuracy of positron emission tomography, computed tomography and endoscopic ultrasonography in staging of adenocarcinoma of the esophagus and esophago-gastric junction. Ann Surg Oncol 2003;10:954–60.

27. Stahl A, Ott K, Weber WA, et al. FDG PET imaging of locally advanced gastric carcinomas: correlation with endoscopic and histopathological findings. Eur J Nucl Med Mol Imaging 2003;30:288–95.

28. Kawamura T, Kusakabe T, Sugino T, et al. Expression of glucose transporter-1 in human gastric carcinoma: Association with tumor aggressiveness, metastases and patient survival. Cancer 2001;92:634–41.

29. Takita KH, Myazaki T, Nakajima M, et al. Correlation of 18-F-fluorodeoxyglucose (FDG) accumulation with glucose transporter (Glut-1) expression in esophageal squamous cell carcinoma. Anticancer Res 2003;23:3263–72.

30. Lerut T, Coosemans W, Decker G, et al. Cancer of the esophagus and gastro-esophageal junction: Potentially curative therapies. Surg Oncol 2001;10:113–22.

31. Eloubeidi MA, Desmond R, Arguedas MR, Reed CE, Wilcox CM. Prognostic factors for the survival of patients with esophageal carcinoma in the US: the importance of tumor length and lymph node status. Cancer 2002;95:1434–43.

32. Rizk N, Venkatraman E, Park B, et al. The prognostic importance of the number of involved lymph nodes in esophageal cancer: implications for revisions of the American Joint Committee of Cancer staging system. J Thorac Cardiovasc Surg 2006;132:1374–81.

33. Komori T, Doki Y, Kabuto T, et al. Prognostic significance of the size of cancer nests in metastatic lymph nodes in human esophageal cancers. J Surg Oncol 2003;82:19–27.

34. Kole AC, Plukker JT, Niewag OE, Vaalburg W. Positron emission tomography for staging of esophageal and gastroesophageal malignancy. Br J Cancer 1998;78:521–7.

35. Kneist W, Schreckenberger M, Bartenstein P, et al. Positron emission tomography for staging esophageal carcinoma: Does it lead to a different therapeutic approach? World J Surg 2003;27:1105–12.

36. Vazquez-Siqueiros E. Nodal status: number or site of nodes? How to improve accuracy? Is FNA always necessary? Junctional tumors-what's N and what's M? Endoscopy 2006;38:54–8.

37. Kinkel K, Ly Y, Both M, et al. Detection of hepatic metastases from cancers of the gastrointestinal tract by using non-invasive imaging methods (US, CT, MR Imaging, PET): A meta-analysis. Radiology 2002;224:748–56.

38. Kaato H, Miyazaki T, Nakajima M, et al. Comparison between whole-body positron emission tomography and bone scintigraphy in evaluating bony metastases of esophageal carcinomas. Anticancer Res 2005;25:4439–44.

39. Stahl A, Stollfus J, Ott K, et al. FDG PET and CT in locally advanced adenocarcinoma of the distal esophagus. Nuklearmedizin 2005;44:249–55.

40. Jadvar H, Henderson RH, Conti PS. 2-Deoxy-2-[F-18] fluoro-D-glucose-positron emission tomography/computed tomography imaging evaluation of esophageal carcinoma. Mol Imaging Biol 2006;8:193–200.

41. Wallace MB, Nietert PJ, Earle C, et al. An analysis of multiple staging management strategies for carcinoma of the esophagus: Computed tomography, endoscopic ultrasound, positron emission tomography and thoracoscopy/laparoscopy. Ann Thorac Surg 2002;74:1026–32.

42. Imdahl A, Hentschel M, Kleimaier M. et al. Impact of FDG-PET for staging of oesophageal cancer. Langenbecks Arch Surg 2004;389:283–8.

43. Leong T, Everitt C, Yuen K, et al. A Prospective study to evaluate the impact of FDG-PET or CT-based radiotherapy treatment planning for oesophageal cancer. Radiother Oncol 2006;78:254–61.

44. Choi JY, Jang HJ, Shim M, et al. 18F-FDG PET in patients with esophageal squamous cell

carcinoma undergoing curative surgery: prognostic implications. J Nucl Med 2004;45:1843–50.

45. Cerfolio RJ, Bryant AS. Maximum standardized uptake values on positron emission tomography of esophageal cancer predicts stage, tumour biology and survival. Ann Thorac Surg 2006;82:391–5.

46. Rizk N, Downey RJ, Akhurst T, et al. Preoperative 18-F-fluorodeoxyglucose positron emission tomography standardized uptake values predict survival after esophageal adenocarcinoma resection. Ann Thorac Surg 2006;81: 1076–81.

47. Geh JI, Crellin AM, Glynne-Jones R. Preoperative (neoadjuvant) chemoradiotherapy in oesophageal cancer. Br J Surg 2001;88:338–56.

48. Ott K, Weber WA, Lordick F, et al. Metabolic imaging predicts response, survival and recurrence in adenocarcinomas of the esophagogastric junction. J Clin Oncol 2006; 24: 4692–8.

49. Wieder HA, Beer AJ, Lordick F, et al. Comparison of changes in tumour metabolic activity and tumour size during chemotherapy of adenocarcinomas of the esophagogastric junction. J Nucl Med 2005;46:2029–34.

50. Wieder HA, Brucher BLDM, Zimmermann F, et al. Time course of tumour metabolic activity during chemoradiotherapy of esophageal squamous cell carcinoma and response to treatment. J Clin Oncol 2004;22:900–8.

8

Treatment Decisions

Praful Desai, Ratna Parikh

Pretherapy investigations and work up will give a reasonably precise idea of the clinical stage of the disease and will help in deciding whether the patient should be treated either with a curative or a palliative intent. This decision is vital as restoration of normal swallowing is the primary objective in most patients of esophageal cancer. Subjecting a patient with an incurable advanced cancer to major invasive surgery is a poor medical decision.

The Curative Group

All patients below the age of 70 years with a reasonably acceptable nutritional status, an albumin level of not less than 3 gm%, a normal hematologic and systemic status and a clinical stage not beyond T_3N_1 as determined by pretherapy assessment should be treated with a curative intent. For such a major surgical procedure, an acceptable cardiovascular, pulmonary and hepatorenal status are mandatory and of great significance for a smooth postoperative recovery. Patient's hematologic status could be subnormal for undertaking such a major surgical procedure as esophagectomy; however, this can be usually improved to a near normal status. Once a decision has been made to treat a patient with a curative intent, the treatment generally recommended is surgery, if feasible.

The type and extent of this major and difficult surgery needs to be discussed with the patient and the relatives, particularly as complications may develop in the postoperative phase. Rarely, chemoradiotherapy has to be primarily considered based on predictive criteria of a likely good response to avoid such a major surgery in selected cases. Presence of more than five metastatic nodes does convey a guarded prognosis;[1] however, presence of positive nodes when dissected and removed is often compatible with a long-term control, survival and occasional cures. Attempts must therefore be made to approach this group with a curative intent and appropriate management should be considered like surgery per primum or after chemoradiotherapy. This may achieve a good control for a reasonable period of time.

The Palliative Group

Patients with a subnormal or a below par hematologic and nutritional status or those with advanced disease are best managed with a non-surgical alternative with chemoradiotherapy. If this is not feasible only supportive therapy with nutrition management (gastrostomy/jejunostomy/stent placement) should be considered. Control with chemoradiotherapy is often possible in this group and often moderate to a reasonably good

68

response is possible to achieve. Palliative care with a reasonably normal swallowing for weeks or months is possible and known. It is very satisfying to treat and witness this improvement in a patient who presents with severe dysphagia, unable even to take liquids. At all times during treatment a good supportive therapy with intravenous fluids, proteins, vitamins and minerals are of importance. The diagnosis of esophageal cancer is generally delayed. An advanced tumor classified larger than T_3N_1 and those with severe back pain, often due to skeletal metastasis in the spine should be treated with a palliative intent with a view to ensure normal swallowing, if feasible. In this group, disease in the mediastinum, bronchial infiltration, adherence often to the aortic adventitia and around the inferior pulmonary vein is likely. Current imaging technology along with attention to clinical symptoms mentioned above will help to avoid unnecessary explorations in this group of patients.

These patients, as mentioned above, are more appropriately managed with chemo-radiotherapy or stents (Figs 8.1 and 8.2) as indicated. Indications for palliative resections include, a reasonably good general condition and absence of distant metastases. A small metastatic node in the supraclavicular or axillary region does not negate a palliative resection, which offers the best symptomatic relief for the major problem of dysphagia.

SURGICAL APPROACHES

Preoperative Induction Therapy

The main cause of poor survival rates in esophageal cancer is advanced disease, delayed clinical presentation and diagnosis, leading to local and systemic disease recurrence. The objective of preoperative induction chemotherapy is for down-staging the disease to facilitate surgical resection, improve local control, relief of dysphagia in responding patients and control of or possible eradication of micro-metastatic disease.

Localized (Loco-regional) Esophageal Cancer

Though surgical excision remains the therapy of choice in this clinical setting, a number of trials have indicated a better disease free

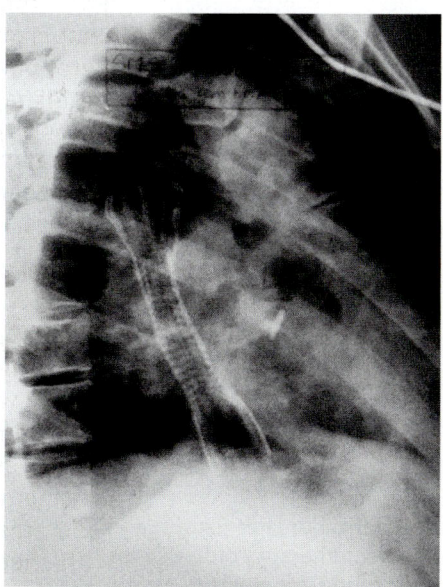

Fig. 8.1: Stent *in situ* for an inoperable strictured lesion

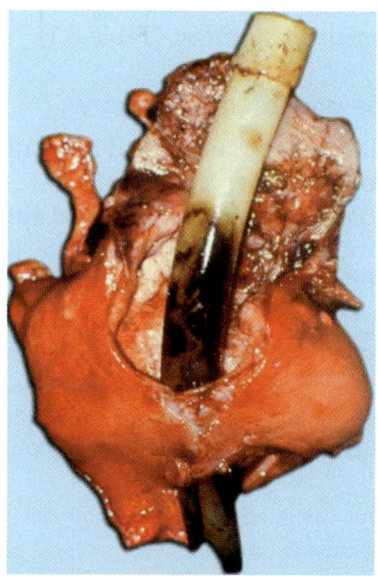

Fig. 8.2: Resected specimen of the esophagus with an *in situ* stent. A proper assessment of resectability of the lesion is mandatory before stenting. Complications due to stents are not uncommon

5 years survival by combining neoadjuvant chemo-radiotherapy (3 cycles cisplastin/5 fluorouracil/paclitaxel and 45Gy radiation therapy)[2,3] followed by a surgical resection, three to four weeks later. This is not universally accepted as neoadjuvant chemoradiotherapy can produce postoperative complications including cardiopulmonary and anastomotic healing issues; particularly so if, preoperative radical chemoradiotherapy has been used. Combination therapy is indicated if the lesion, though resectable, is locoregionally advanced. Surgical results of lesions of the supra-aortic region and thoracic inlet are unsatisfactory and are better treated by definitive chemo-radiotherapy, with surgery only as a salvage option. Indeed, any lesion with a length greater than 6 cm is best managed by neoadjuvant chemoradiotherapy. It is then assessed for a surgical resection or definitive chemoradiotherapy, if the response is satisfactory with a significant regression of the lesion and complete relief of dysphagia. The debate about the types of surgical procedures and the views regarding two or three field nodal dissection will continue; however, certain surgical principles have remained steadfast (Table 8.1).

The Type and Extent of Surgery

Experiences of the author and his team relate to the following procedures:

a. **Standard left thoracoabdominal approach:** for cancers of the cardioesophageal junction and infradiaphragmatic lesions.

b. **Standard Ivor-Lewis procedure (Transthoracic esophagectomy—TTE):** Abdominal mobilization of the stomach, a right thoracotomy and a middle or high right intrathoracic esophagogastrostomy, for supradiaphragmatic and low mid 1/3rd lesions with two field dissection.

c. **Total esophagectomy for middle and upper 1/3rd lesions:** (with three field dissection and cervical anastomosis)

d. **Transhiatal esophagectomy (THE)**

While personal experience and bias will remain with individual surgeons, the author and his team believe that sufficient data now exists, from personal series and the literature[4–6] to select a procedure based on the need of the patient which depends on the clinical setting and the general condition of the patient. Dogmas in clinical sciences should be avoided and the therapeutic procedure should be selected based on a given lesion, the condition of the patient, the choice and experience of the surgeon. Surgery for any cancer is a wide excisional surgery of the primary tumor and encompassing lymph nodes in the drainage area. While our biologic understanding of a tumor is steadily improving by far and large, the above adage is still true for most cancers that we treat surgically.

The unique anatomic location of the esophagus traversing three anatomic regions, the neck, the thorax and the abdomen, along with extremely rich lymphatic plexus particularly in the submucosa ensures that the lymphatic

Table 8.1	Standard Surgical approaches	
	Site of lesion	Surgical approaches
Adenocarcinoma squamous carcinoma	Cardioesophageal junction, lower esophagus, cardia	Left thoracoabdominal Ivor-Lewis/Tanner (TTE) Transhiatal esophagectomy (THE)
Squamous carcinoma adenocarcinoma (rare)	Middle one-third lesion	Three-stage total esophagectomy Transhiatal esophagectomy (THE)
Squamous carcinoma	Cervical, supra-aortic, thoracic inlet	Poor candidates for surgery chemotherapy/radiotherapy/ stenting, etc. are better options

TTE: Transthoracic esophagectomy; THE: Transhiatal esophagectomy

drainage is widespread. Total esophagectomy with extensive three field (abdomen, thorax and neck) lymph node dissection is the only way to encompass and remove the entire lymph drainage area. Much debate has raged about this procedure,[7-9] its morbidity and mortality in average hands and its inapplicability in all operable patients with esophageal cancer. Data is now available that in very early and advanced cancers such extensive surgery does not improve survival[4] but leads to significant morbidity. Obviously, therefore, every surgical procedure listed above has its indications in a given clinical setting. In surgery for cancer, "the bigger the better" does not necessarily hold true. The following procedures will suit the needs of most patients.

a. **A standard left thoracoabdominal approach** is suitable for cancers of the cardioesophageal junction and the infradiaphragmatic esophageal cancer. A total esophagectomy is not always necessary in these patients (Fig. 8.3). Besides the usual squamous cell cancer of the esophagus, this procedure can also be considered for a Barrett's adenocarcinoma of the lower

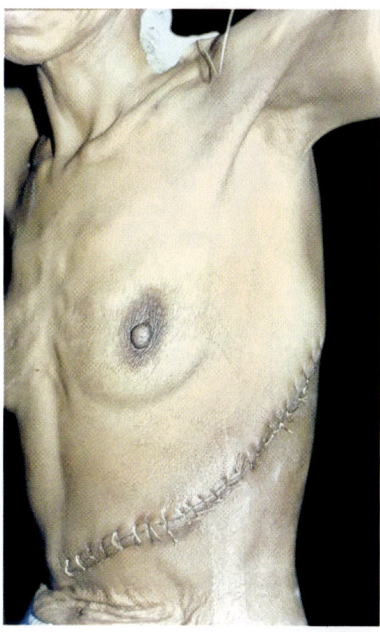

Fig. 8.3: Cachectic lady (due to disease) with an abdominothoracic incision after completion of esophageal resection

esophagus where the proximal limit of the disease will allow a good clearance of at least 4 to 5 cm of normal esophagus (Figs 8.4 and 8.5); if this is not feasible, an Ivor-Lewis procedure will become

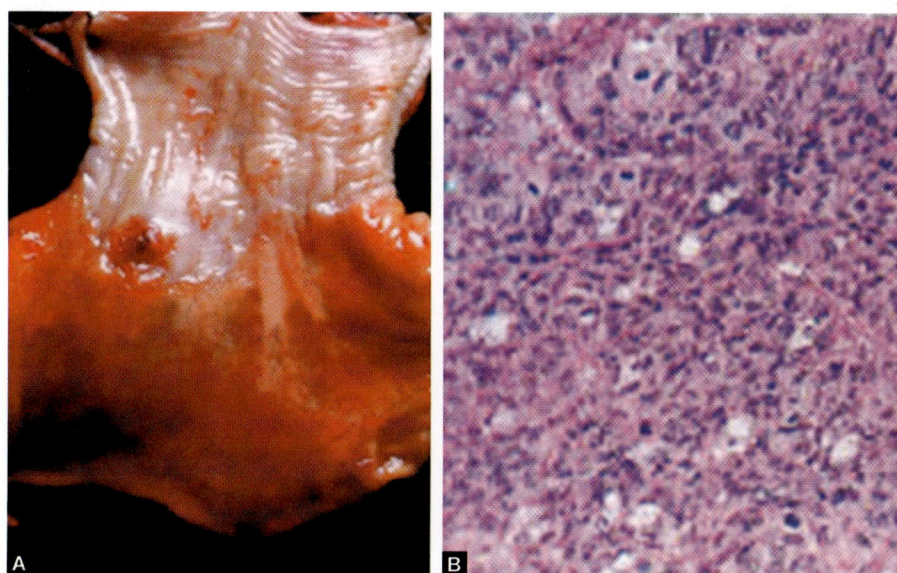

A   B

Fig. 8.4: (A) Early cardioesophageal lesion in the resected specimen via a left thoracoabdominal approach. Good proximal margin >5 cm. Margins shrink *in vitro*. (B) Histology of the same patient showing active tumor

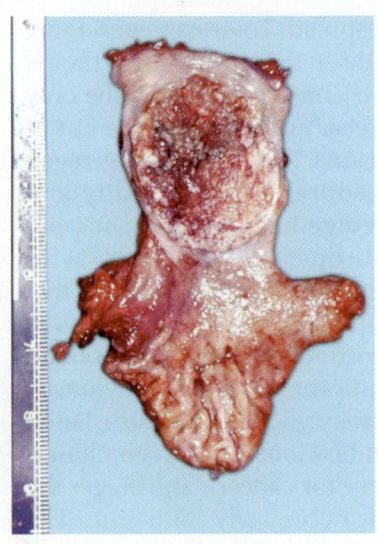

Fig. 8.5: (A) Resected specimen of a large proliferative growth with complete obstruction. (B) Resected specimen of a large ulceroproliferative growth in the lower esophagus

necessary. Nodal spread and metastasis from malignant lesions of the infra-diaphragmatic esophagus and those of the cardia generally drain towards the lesser curvature of the stomach, celiac and pancreatic region near its superior border and rarely to the retropancreatic space. In only 7% of patients the nodes are involved in a cephalad spread up to the inferior pulmonary vein. Involvement of subcarinal, mediastinal and paratracheal nodes is rare in lesions of the cardia or infra-diaphragmatic esophagus. The Fig. 8.6 shows the amount of area and nodal tissue

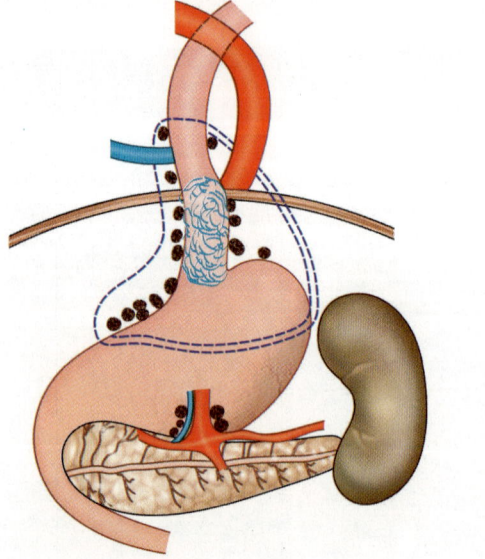

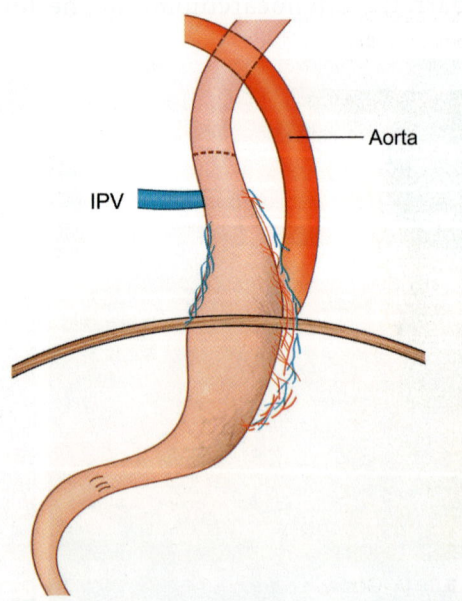

Fig. 8.6: Shows the extent of resection and nodal clearance for a lesion in the lower esophagus and cardia. The left esophagogastric anastomosis is well above the inferior pulmonary vein (IPV) about 3–4 cm below the aortic arch. Via left thoracoabdominal approach

that can be effectively excised by a standard left thoracoabdominal approach. Most metastatic failures here will occur in the liver, pancreatic and retropancreatic region. Akiyama[10] reports 13% involvement of cervical node metastasis in low esophageal cancers. It is possible that majority of such lower esophageal cancers may be advanced and where the nodal burden is high, retrograde lymphatic spread may travel to the neck. Majority of lesions in this region can have a satisfactory surgical clearance of lymph nodes and the procedure is extremely well-tolerated with the anastomosis well above the left pulmonary vein

giving a good proximal margin of 5 cm or more (Figs 8.7 and 8.8). With current methods of staging, pretherapy investigations and assessment the resectability rate for selected cases should be around 90%. Only in an occasional case the procedure needs to be abandoned because of an unexpected encounter with very advanced disease. This situation should be rare with appropriate preoperative clinical assessment and imaging studies as aforementioned (Table 8.2 and Graph 8.1).

b. **The Ivor-Lewis procedure:** Right sided middle or high intrathoracic esophagogastrostomy. This procedure has stood the

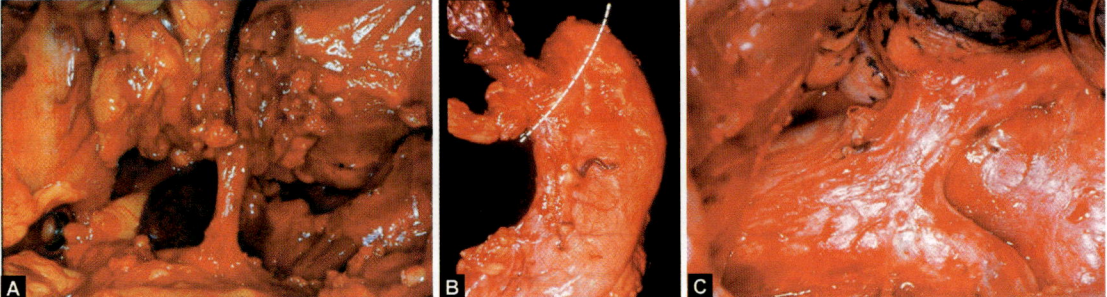

Fig. 8.7: (A) Celiac axis nodal clearance; the left gastric artery is cleared of nodes and fatty tissue and should be ligated at the upper border of the pancreas. (B) Clearance of nodes from lesser curvature of the stomach. (C) Subcarinal nodal clearance in the right chest, the right and left bronchus and subcarinal area is clearly visible (two field dissection)

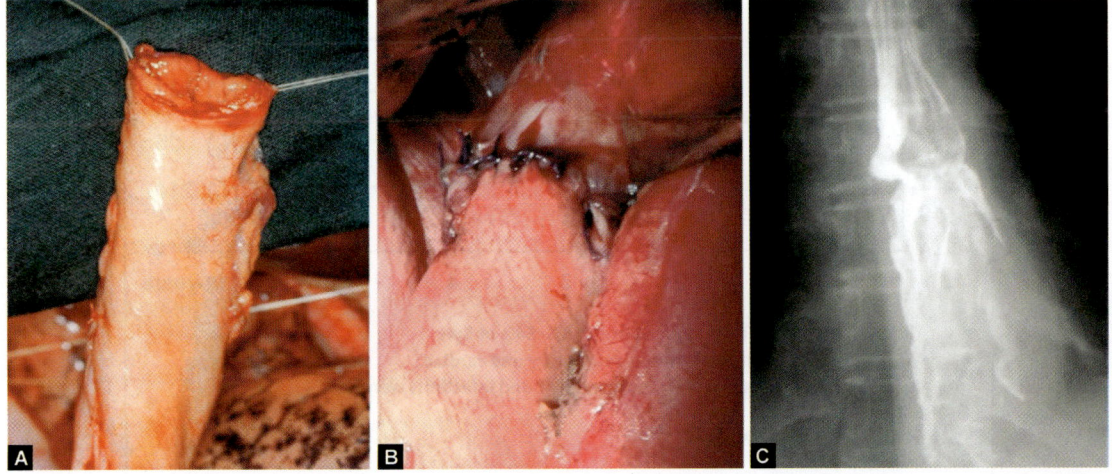

Fig. 8.8: (A) Gastric tube conduit prepared for the anastomosis. (B) Hand sewn left sided esophagogastric anastomosis for a lesion in the lower 1/3rd of the esophagus. Anastomosis just below the aortic arch. Descending thoracic aorta is clearly visible next to the stomach tube. (C) Contrast study 6 months later of the same patient showing a smooth passage with a wide anastomosis

Table 8.2	Left thoracoabdominal approach for cancers of the cardia, CO junction and lower esophagus		
N = 330		Sites	%
186 ⎰ 169 (SQ Ca) ⎱ 17 (Ad. Ca)		Lower esophagus	56
46 ⎧ 21 (SQ Ca) ⎨ 8 (Indeterm) ⎩ 17 (Ad. Ca)		Co junction	14
98 —— (Ad. Ca)		Fundus	30

test of time ever since it was described by Ivor-Lewis (Figs 8.9 to 8.12).[11] The only constant argument against it is the danger of an intrathoracic anastomotic leakage and likely fatality in the event of a major leak. With continuing improvement in surgical techniques and with increasing experience, anastomotic dehiscence rates have dropped below 5% and most of these are salvageable with early diagnosis and effective management. Most lesions of the lower 1/3rd

(below the inferior pulmonary vein) which extends into the middle segment can be effectively tackled with an Ivor-Lewis procedure. The stomach is mobilized in the abdomen with dissection of the regional nodes and through a separate right thoracotomy (5th intercostal space or rib resection) the lesion is mobilized encompassing the lymph nodes, the parietal pleura and the thoracic duct if needed. It is not a routine to excise the thoracic duct; however, in a stage III lesion and particularly in presence of para-esophageal nodes, excision of the thoracic duct is a good surgical practice. The lower end should be properly ligated; the tracheobronchial group of mediastinal nodal tissue up to the apex of the chest can be excised en-mass as a monobloc mass. No deliberate attempt is made to demonstrate the left recurrent nerve unless a packet of nodes are lying anterior to the tracheal wall.

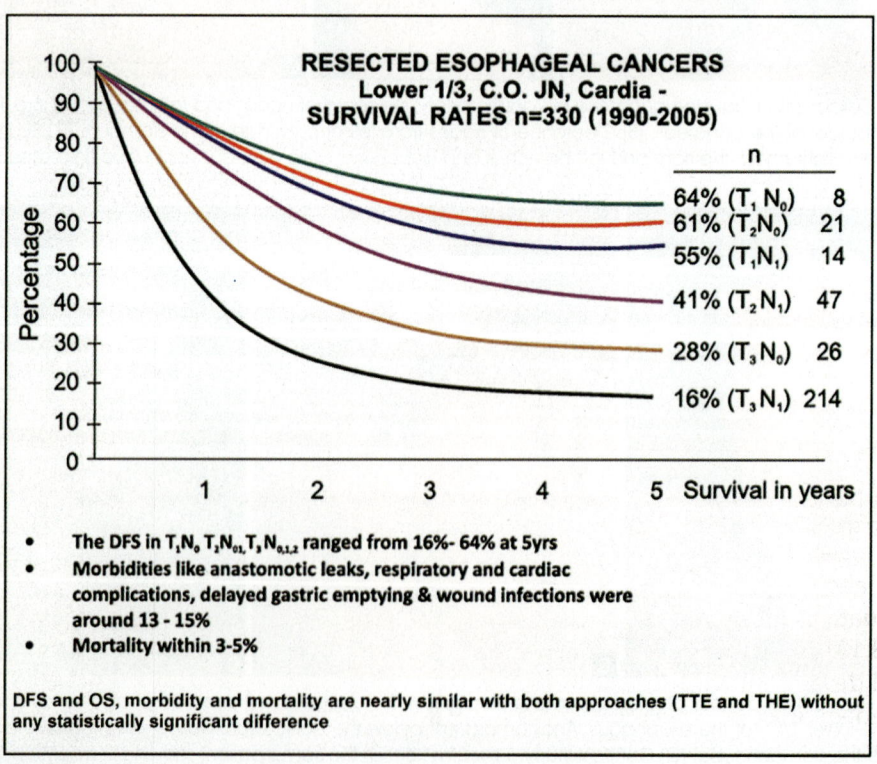

RESECTED ESOPHAGEAL CANCERS
Lower 1/3, C.O. JN, Cardia -
SURVIVAL RATES n=330 (1990-2005)

	n
64% (T_1N_0)	8
61% (T_2N_0)	21
55% (T_1N_1)	14
41% (T_2N_1)	47
28% (T_3N_0)	26
16% (T_3N_1)	214

- The DFS in T_1N_0 $T_2N_{0,1}$ $T_3N_{0,1,2}$ ranged from 16%- 64% at 5yrs
- Morbidities like anastomotic leaks, respiratory and cardiac complications, delayed gastric emptying & wound infections were around 13 - 15%
- Mortality within 3-5%

DFS and OS, morbidity and mortality are nearly similar with both approaches (TTE and THE) without any statistically significant difference

Graph 8.1: Desai et al. Personal series

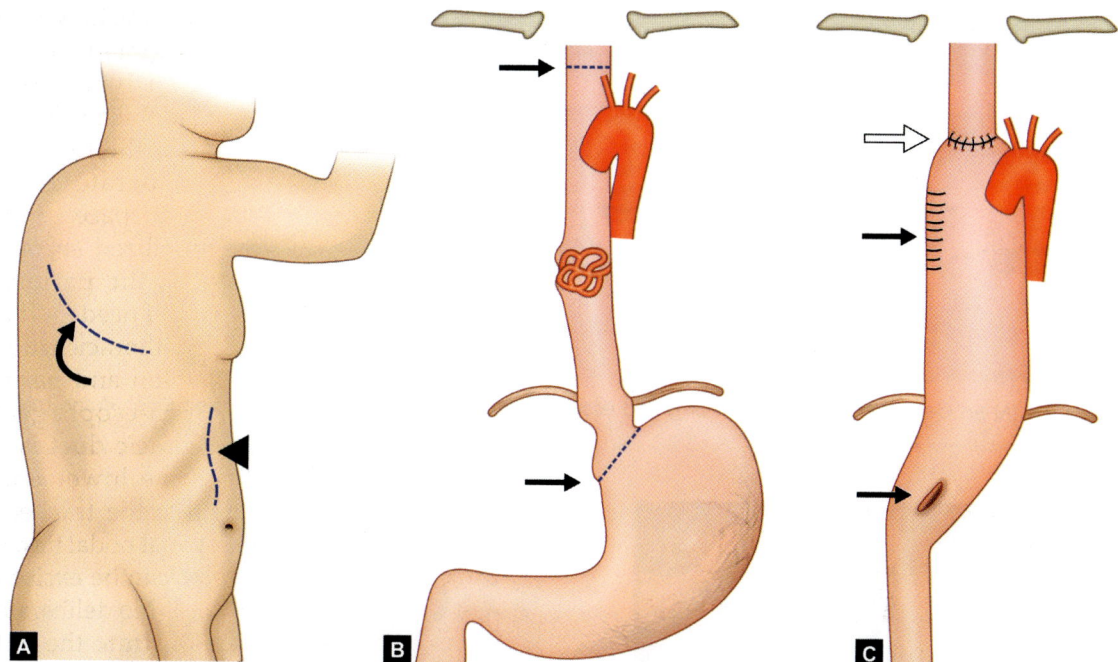

Fig. 8.9: Schematic diagram of Ivor-Lewis procedure: (A) Black arrows indicate surgical incisions for Ivor-Lewis. (B) Black arrows indicate line of transection. (C) White arrow indicates completed esophagogastric anastomosis, black arrows indicate suture or stapler line after transection of the stomach and pyloroplasty (author prefers a pyloromyotomy) respectively

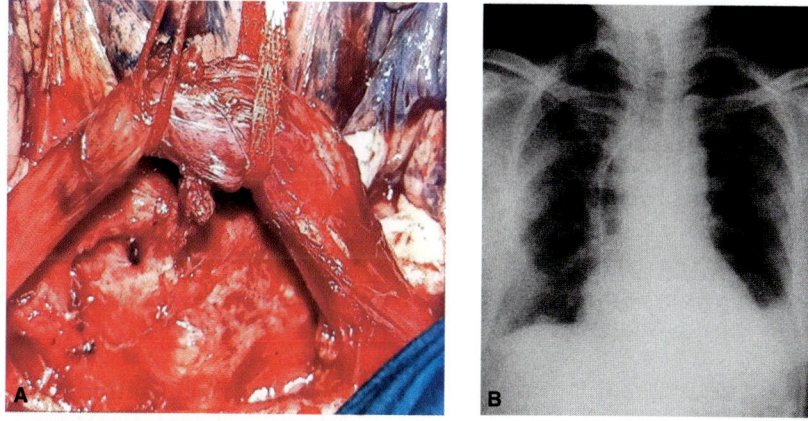

Fig. 8.10: (A) Dissected lesion in the mid esophagus hooked up with tapes in the right chest. (B) X-ray chest showing the stomach conduit lying snugly in the mediastinum with the anastomosis above the arch of aorta, high (Ivor-Lewis) in the right chest

We label the above procedure as "ARL" (Adequate Regional lymphadenectomy)[12] (Fig. 8.13) in contrast to the three field radical dissection. Nodal dissection of two field (adequate regional dissection— ARL) is an accepted standard. This includes (a) Celiac and left gastric, (b) Gastric lesser curvature, and (c) mediastinal and hilar region. Our analysis shows that ARL is effective in Stage I and II, but ineffective in increasing disease free survival in very late stages of the disease (Fig. 8.14, Graph 8.2 and 8.3).[12] Extensive three field radical dissection is not really needed as it does

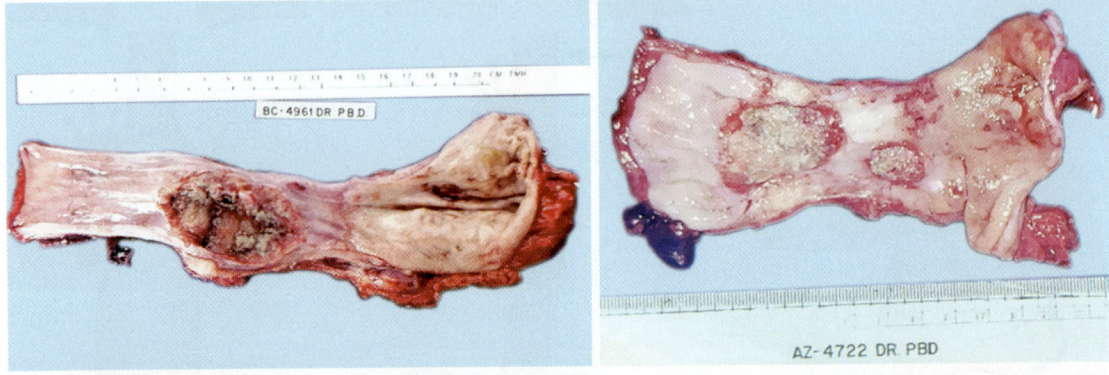

Fig. 8.11: (A) An ideal resection specimen of a mid esophageal cancer. (B) Multicentric ulcerated lesion in the mid-esophagus

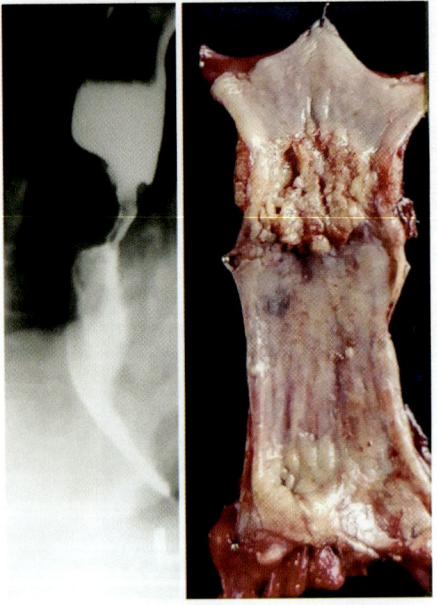

Fig. 8.12: Barium swallow showing a mid-esophageal lesion with the resected specimen

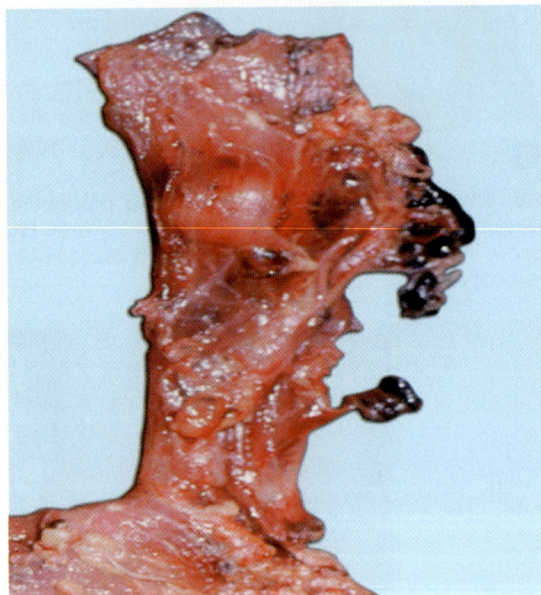

Fig. 8.13: Specimen of esophagectomy with two field lymph node dissection (Ivor-Lewis)

not impact on survival and is compatible with local complications due to radical dissection.

In a recent study[13] the presence of nodal metastasis was accurately reflected (with a concordance of 90%) by the feel of nodes.

Nodes which are soft to touch at surgery are generally devoid of metastasis and those which are firm or hard to feel is strongly indicative of the presence of metastasis.

If after mobilization of the lesion it is determined that a safe proximal margin is not available in the chest, it is easy to convert the procedure to a total esophagectomy and resort to a cervical anastomosis with the stomach pulled up in the neck through the posterior mediastinum, the shortest route to the neck. As always, at least 5 cm of normal esophagus proximal to the growth is a necessity and 7 cm would be an optimal margin. In a

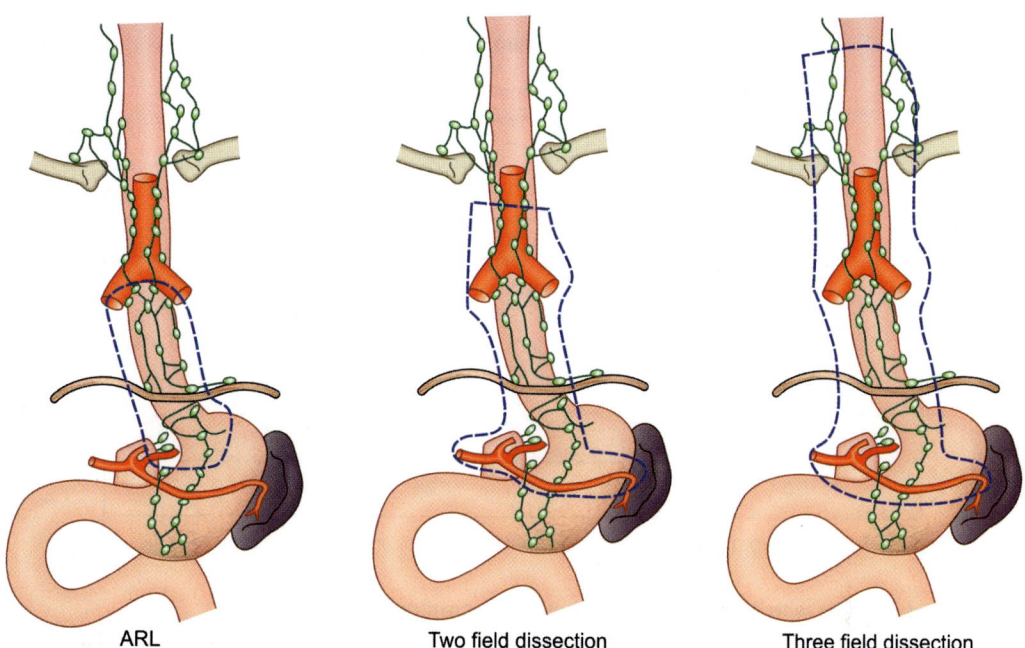

ARL   Two field dissection   Three field dissection

Fig. 8.14: ARL, two field and three field lymph node dissection

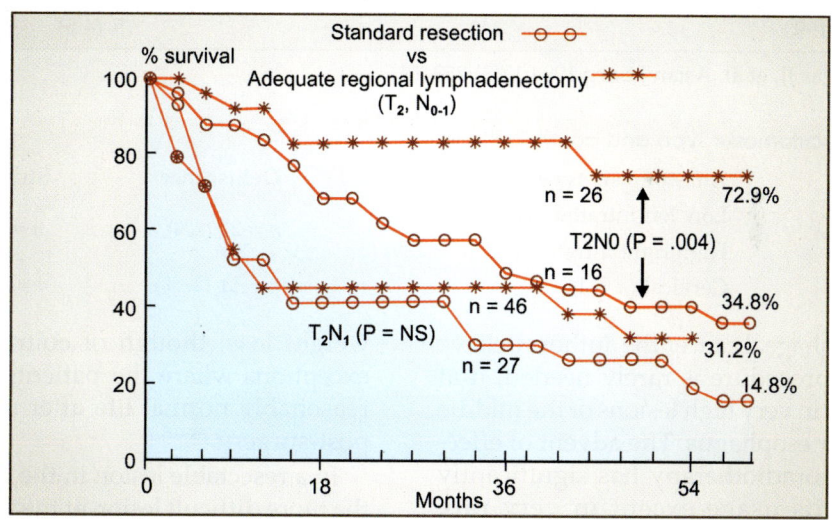

Graph 8.2: The standard resection versus adequate regional lymphadenectomy - ARL (T_2N_{0-1})

properly executed Ivor-Lewis procedure with ARL one can be radical in removing the nodes without inflicting any significant morbidity. Intrathoracic anastomosis heals well, is less prone to stricture and dehiscence rates are significantly less than cervical anastomosis. Tables 8.3A and B shows the overall data on esophageal resections over different periods of time, the type of anastomosis and dehiscence rates.

c. **Total esophagectomy for upper $1/3^{rd}$ and creeping mid $1/3^{rd}$ lesions:** Though a few surgeons still consider total esophagectomy (TE) for all localized middle and upper

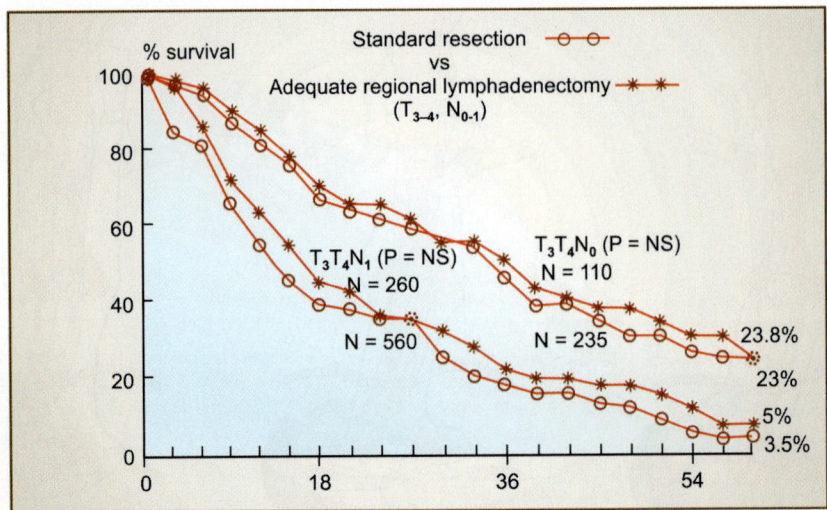

Graph 8.3: The standard resection versus adequate regional lymphadenectomy - ARL (T_{3-4}, N_{0-1})

Table 8.3A	Experiences with esophageal resections for cancer	
Period	**Total No. Resected**	**Postoperative 30 day mortality (%)**
1970–1985	1366	122 (9)
1986–1990	617	37 (6)
1991–1993	111	5 (4.5)

*Desai PB, Vyas JJ, et al. Asian J Surg 1994;17(3):253–61.

Table 8.3B	Anastomosis: Type and complications		
Period	**Anastomosis type**	**Dehiscence**	**Stenosis**
1986–1993 ($n = 728$)	Low left intrathoracic ($n = 445$)	$n = 27$ (4%)	$n = 96$ (14%)
	High right intrathoracic ($n = 239$)		
	Cervical ($n = 44$)	$n = 11$ (26%)	$n = 10$ (23%)

$1/3^{rd}$ esophageal cancer the authors believe that this procedure is rarely needed, if at all, except in very high lesions of the middle and upper esophagus. The advent of effective chemoradiotherapy has significantly reduced its usage except in very rare circumstances where chemoradiotherapy is contraindicated due to rare reasons of patient refusal or intolerance to chemotherapy. The morbidity and mortality of total esophagectomy is significantly higher and the quality of life issues are frequent in the form of anastomotic strictures, need for repeated dilatations, constant complaint of regurgitation, nausea, weight loss and inability to enjoy a normal meal, often with weight loss; though of course there are exceptions where the patients adjust to a reasonably normal life after a few weeks post-surgery.[14–16]

In a resectable lesion in the upper $1/3^{rd}$, the more difficult lesion at the thoracic inlet and the "creeping up" lesion of the middle $1/3^{rd}$, a total esophagectomy with a three field dissection becomes mandatory (Fig. 8.15). The initial steps are similar to the Ivor-Lewis procedure, but the dissection is extended into the neck keeping close to the esophagus. Damage to right and left recurrent laryngeal nerves is more likely and should be carefully avoided. Higher lesions do not metastasize frequently in

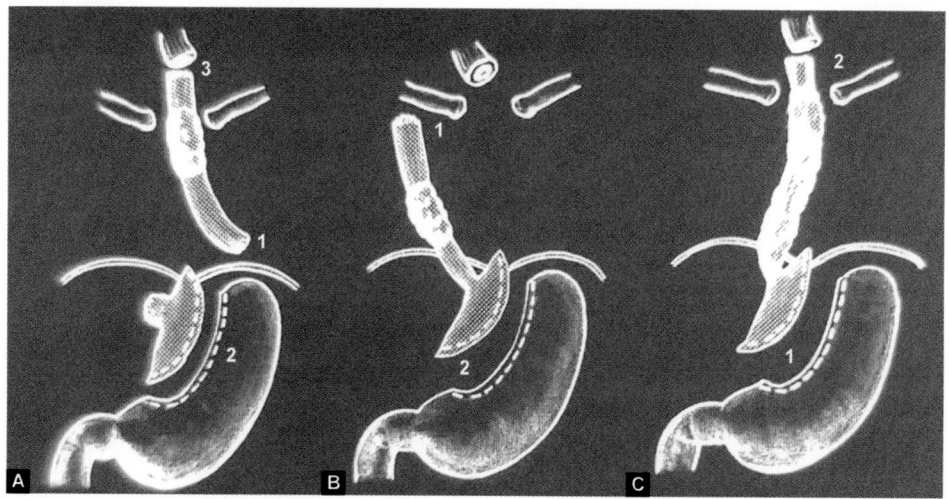

Figs 8.15A to C: Total esophagectomy for middle and upper 1/3rd lesions

the lower para esophageal region[11] and the abdominal and lower thoracic part of the dissection need not be very radical. The thorax is closed around a drain, patient is turned in the normal supine position and with the neck extended and face turned to the right side, with an incision along the lower 1/3rd of the left sternocleidomastoid, the mobilized lesion is removed by a gentle pull up and the anastomosis is created between the esophagus and the pulled-up stomach after ensuring its viability. The neck is drained. Any incidental nodes are dissected from the lower neck while doing a total esophagectomy.

d. **Transhiatal esophagectomy (THE):** It is worthwhile to know that THE evolved in 1980s, primarily to avoid the serious complication of an anastomotic disruption in the right or left chest. With increasing experience over the years the leakage rate is now less than 5% (even 2% in high volume hospitals and surgeons) and with aggressive management of an anastomostic disruption, most patients are salvaged from this dreaded complication. THE is feasible for any lesion in the entire thoracic esophagus and occasionally also for a cardia lesion; the procedure pre-supposes that there is less negative impact on the cardiovascular and pulmonary physiology.

Patients who are otherwise suboptimal in cardiopulmonary and nutritional status would better tolerate this procedure. In experienced hands the procedure is quick and expeditious; nonetheless, though an "extrathoracic" procedure, "intrathoracic" complications are frequent. Pneumothorax and intrathoracic bleeding sometimes require drainage and tracheal or bronchial tears are not unknown. The following criteria need to be fulfilled before THE can be considered.

CT scan and bronchoscopic assessment should confirm that the disease is not beyond the muscle wall, lest the lesion during blunt dissection and part of the tumor can tear or is left behind. Serious damage as mentioned above can occur. Lymph nodes are often left behind in this blind procedure which precludes chances of a cure. Similar results reported in THE and TTE[17] can be open to question as careful selection for THE may have more patients with N_0 node status and accurate pathologic staging will not be possible in patients undergoing THE. The procedure, however, has come to stay in the management of esophageal cancer and patients should be carefully selected and tackled only after adequate experience in transthoracic esophageal surgery.

LITERATURE REVIEW (Tables 8.4 to 8.6)

Table 8.4 Outcomes after transhiatal and transthoracic esophagectomy for cancer*

Outcome variables	Transthoracic (n = 643)	Transhiatal (n = 225)	p value
Thirty day mortality (%)	13.1	6.7	0.009
Hospital length of stay (days)	20.7	21.4	0.65
Need for anastomotic dilatation (%)	34.5	43.1	0.02
Overall survival (%) 5 years	22.7	30.5	0.02

*(Chang, et al. Ann Thorac Surg 2008;85:424–29. [Seer Database (1992–2002)]

Table 8.5 Transthoracic versus transhiatal esophagectomy for the treatment of esophageal cancer*

Total (n = 5905)	TTE (n = 3389)	THE (n = 2516)
Tumor characteristics	More often adopted for advanced stage ($T_{2,3}$–N_{0-1})	More often adopted for early stage ($T_{1,2}$–N_0)
Extent of lymphadenectomy	Better (8 or more lymph nodes were retrieved)	Lesser nodes retrieved
Length of operation	Took 85 m longer	Lesser time taken
Length of stay	More	Less by 4 days
Blood loss	—————— No difference ——————	
Postoperative complications	More respiratory complications, wound infections and early postoperative mortality	Anastomotic leaks, anastomotic strictures, RLN palsy higher
5 years survival	—————— No significant difference ——————	

*Boshier, Anderson, et al. Ann of surgery Dec 2011;Vol 254(6):894–904 [Meta analysis 1999–2001 (52 studies)]
Composite data-not confined to high vol. surgeons and institutions

Table 8.6 Extended resections will improve staging and improves loco-regional control. However, no reliable data confirming a survival benefit for these procedures*

	TTE	THE
Perioperative mortality	9.5%	6.3%
Perioperative complications	—————— No signif diff ——————	
Leaks	7.2%	13.6%
Anastomotic strictures	Less	More
RN palsy	None	Frequent (8–12%)
Pulmonary complications	18.7%	12.7%
5 years survival	26%	24%
(Various series)	23%	21.7%

*Data from 2 large meta-analysis. Rindani, et al. 5483 Pts, 44 series (1986–1996)

Transthoracic (TT) and Transhiatal (TH) Esophagectomy and Open/Minimally Invasive/Robotic Esophagectomy

Arguments and debates will continue over these issues as it has happened ever since TH approach and the minimally invasive surgery (MIS) began to be performed more frequently. It is now beyond any doubt, based on many well-studied randomized trials that the results are nearly equivalent in experienced hands, vis-à-vis node retrieval, complications and long-term results. There is also little doubt that every single case of resectable esophageal cancer need not undergo a total esophagectomy as lesions of the lower reaches of the esophagus and cardia can be easily and effectively handled by a subtotal esophagectomy (Ivor-Lewis or left thoracoabdominal approach). It may be of interest to note the very recent publication of Leuketich et al[18] of thousand MIS (with cervical anastomosis) in which there is now a shift towards a subtotal (Ivor-Lewis) type of esophagectomy with a right intrathoracic anastomosis. More importantly, it is the comfort zone of the operating surgeon, open or MIS or robotic, which is more important rather than any major differences in the procedures. Less pain, less complications and an early hospital discharge of 2 to 3 days are usually mentioned with MIS/robotic surgery. The overall complications, the node retrievals, the disease free survival (DFS) and overall survival (OS) are almost comparable. The learning curve for all three techniques is long and difficult. An experienced open surgeon can master the other techniques expeditiously; the reverse is probably not true.[19–21]

Few Points in Surgical Technique

Surgical technique has undergone modifications to achieve two main objectives in surgery for esophageal cancer.

1. To minimize and prevent anastomotic dehiscence which is the only major complication in established surgical procedures for curing esophageal cancer.
2. Removing lymph nodes en-mass with the primary tumor to get beyond the neoplastic spread to ensure a complete cancer operation as is feasible.

Two main factors to achieve the first objective is to ensure viable ends of the esophagus and the stomach (or colon or jejunum) for anastomosis, devoid of tension and using a 3–0 or 4–0 absorbable sutures to reduce stenosis at a later date. The anastomosis may be hand sewn or stapled, depending on ones' choice and experience as no significant differences are reported in the literature vis-à-vis breakdown, stenosis, etc. However,

occasional reports of increased stricture rates have been reported in stapled anastomosis.[22] If sound surgical principles are adhered to, no special tricks are necessary to prevent anastomotic disruptions. In most centers with experience in esophageal surgery the disruption rate is below 5% and most of these are salvageable.[5,22,23]

Lymph Node Dissection

Two field and three field lymph node dissections, mediastinal dissection and adequate regional lymphadenectomy all have their advocates with pros and cons;[24,25] however, this can be considered as a significant recent advance in surgery for esophageal cancer. There is a significant improvement in results reported by Japanese authors,[26] unfortunately such results are not reproducible at all centers; nonetheless, there is no doubt that within the realms of safety, lymph nodes ought to be removed, particularly, the tracheobronchial and paraesophageal group of nodes, to avoid later, morbidity of nodal infiltration into the bronchi, paralysis of recurrent laryngeal nerves and mediastinal pressure difficult to palliate later on (Flowchart 8.1 and Fig. 8.16).

Flowchart 8.1: Lymph node dissection

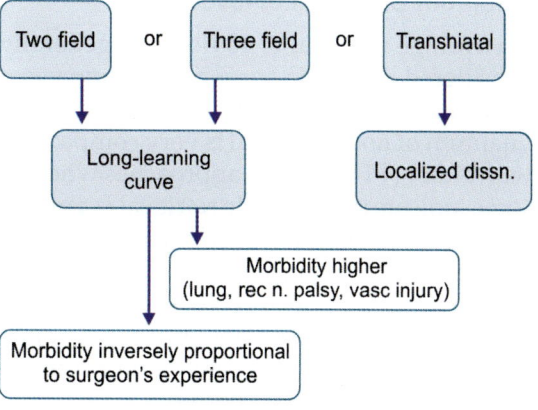

(Cited from John Bolton, Steve Tang - TT or TH Esophagectomy for Cancer. Does It Matter? S. Onc. Clin. N. Am 2002; 11:365–75)

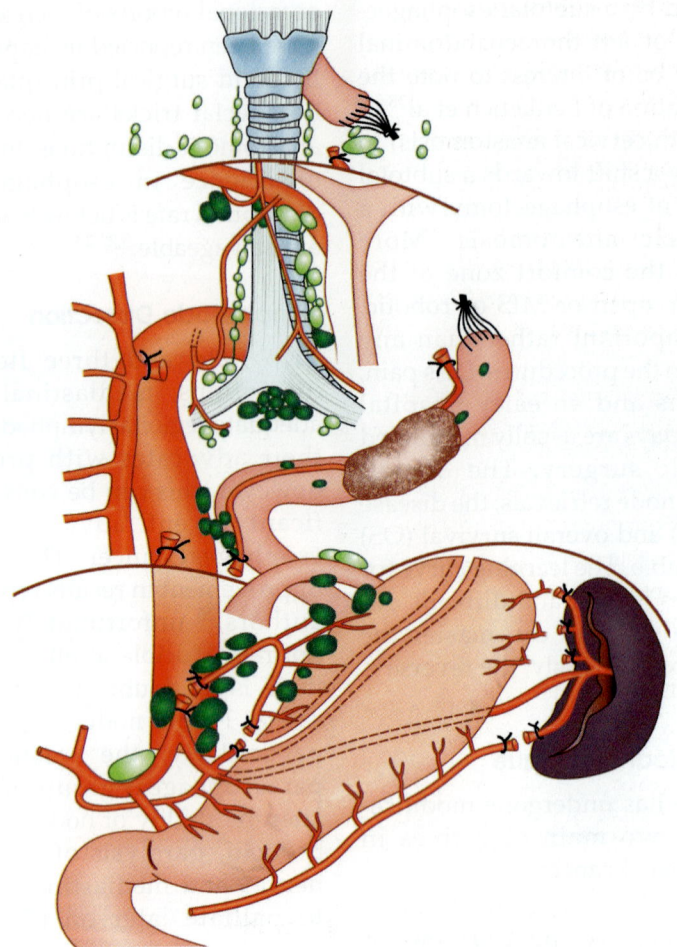

Fig. 8.16: Chaotic lymphatic drainage of the esophagus

Quantum of Node Retrieval

An average retrieval of 15 nodes is generally considered adequate surgery and conveys a good dissection. Recent reports indicate that quantum of node retrieval is very comparable with either (TTE or THE) approaches whereas some indicate that TT node retrieval is greater. This is indeed a theoretical debate and generally does not impact on ultimate control or cure rates. Clearance of 15 metastatic nodes or more, generally does not improve survival rates as prognosis is inversely proportional to the number of involved nodes.

Cornell university group studied 80 patients who underwent esophageal surgery with three field lymphadenectomy — overall 30 day mortality was 5%, with 31% of patients developing major postoperative complications including the need for reintubation in 16%, anastomotic leaks 11% and recurrent laryngeal nerve injury 9%, overall 5 year survival was 51%. Cervical node metastases were identified in 36% and 5 year survival with positive node was 25%.[27] Lerut et al[28] reported on 174 patients (squamous + adenocarcinoma), who underwent three field dissection, overall mortality was 58%, 5 years survival of stage III patients was 36.8%. The author suggest three field dissection may have a role in patients with squamous cell carcinoma but remains investigational for patients with adenocarcinoma. These results although impressive may also reflect both selection bias and stage migration. The Hulscher trial, employed an en bloc resection of the esophagus, compared to transhiatal esophagectomies, failed to improve outcome.[29] A small study by Nishihira et al[27] of 62 patients showed an improved but not statistically significant, survival advantage for extended lymphadenectomies (66.2% versus 48%; p = 0.19).

Extensive studies of multiple trials of two stage and three stage extended resections improved staging and may enhance loco-regional control; however, no reliable data of survival benefit is proven for these extensive procedures with associated complications. The authors believe a total esophagectomy is not always necessary or indicated for lesions of the lower esophagus, GE junction and fundus of the stomach.

Recent studies regarding the impact of high volume surgeon and high volume institutions, for very major surgeries like esophagectomy, pancreatectomy and liver resections, etc. have been studied extensively by many authors.[30,31] There is little doubt that the survival rates for such technically demanding procedures are better and complications and morbidities are lower with high volume surgeons working in a high volume tertiary institution. Centra-lization of such difficult surgical procedures, therefore needs to be seriously considered.

Tracheoesophageal (TE) Fistula

This is a potentially dangerous and lethal complication of locally advanced esophageal cancers. Very rarely in neglected cases patients may initially present with complaints of persistent cough (saliva aspiration) and obvious inability to swallow; fever, aspiration pneumonia and weight loss are constant features. Majority of tracheoesophageal (TE) fistulae occurs in the upper thoracic region or occasionally in the mid 1/3rd esophagus. Only

palliation is feasible with a short-term survival.

A. Expandable metal stents can occasionally block a small tracheoesophageal fistula temporarily; larger tracheoesophageal fistulae are difficult to palliate. If the patient's general condition is good and investigations reveal localized disease in a short segment, attempts can be made towards aggressive palliation by improving nutrition by:

   • A **feeding gastrostomy or jejunostomy** and re-evaluation after 3 to 4 weeks.

   • End cervical esophagostomy with closure of the distal end in the neck to prevent aspiration pneumonias and hectic fever.

B. Chemotherapy—2 to 3 cycles (cisplatin based) could be administered during this phase as occasionally in around 10% the fistula may close if there is disease response. Rarely, due to necrosis, fistula can worsen.

C. Radiation therapy is contraindicated in presence of a TE fistula due to the danger of worsening the fistula due to radiation necrosis.

D. If the general condition improves and in the event of a good response, attempts to do a colonic bypass (retrosternal) by a cervical esophagocolostomy and cologas-trostomy is a theoretical possibility. These are severe procedures and are compatible with morbidity and mortality. However, in very rare suitable clinical setting this procedure can be considered. No attempt should be made to do esophagectomy.

At the most palliation can last 6 to 8 months. Untreated, most patients will succumb in 2 to 3 months. A considered decision after a detailed discussion with the patient and relatives is imperative. Best supportive care is an alternative with poor outcomes in this very distressing complication of neglected esophageal cancer.

REFERENCES

1. Demeester Tom–Esophageal Cancer Current Controversies - Seminars in Surgical Oncology 1997;13:317–33.
2. Medical Research Council Esophageal working group. Surgical resection with or without preoperative chemotherapy in esophageal cancer. A randomized clinical trial. Lancet 2002;3(59):1727–33.
3. Lerut T, Moons J, et al. Multidisciplinary treatment of advanced carcinoma esophagus. S Clinics N Am 2008;17:485–502.
4. Desai PB, Vyas JJ, et al. Carcinoma of the Esophagus an Indian Experience. Asian J Surg 1994;17(3):253–61.
5. Lee R, Miller J. Esophagectomy for cancer. Surgical Clinics of North America 1997;77(5):1195.
6. Skinner DB, Little AB, et al. Selection of Operation for esophagus cancer based on staging. Ann Surgery 1986;204:391.
7. Isono K, Ochial T, et al. The treatment of lymph node metastasis from esophageal cancer by extensive lymphadenectomy. SPN J Surg 1990; 20:151–7.
8. Wu Y, Huang K. Chinese experience in the surgical treatment of cancer of the esophagus. Ann Surg 1979;190:360–5.
9. Akiyama H. Surgery for cancer of the esophagus. Current problems in Surgery 1980;17:53–120.
10. Akiyama H. Squamous cell cancer of the thoracic esophagus. Surgery for cancer of the esophagus P 117 Baltimore, Hongkong, London, Sydney William & Wilkins 1990.
11. Lewis I. The surgical treatment of cancer of the esophagus with special reference for growth in the middle third. British Journal of Surg 1946; 34:18–31.
12. Desai PB, Vyas JJ, et al. Adequate Regional Lymphadenectomy. Asian Journal Surg. 1994; 17(3):253–61.
13. Patil P, Badwe R, et al. Clinico Histologic relationship between nodal consistency and final histopathology. A study on dissected lymph nodes in esophageal cancer (In Press).
14. Andrew C Chang, Hong Ji, et al. Outcomes after transhiatal and transthoracic esophagectomy for Cancer. Ann Thorac Surg. 2008;85:424–9.
15. Piers R Boshier, Oliver Anderson, et al. Transthoracic Versus Transhiatal Esophagectomy for the treatment of Esophagogastric Cancer. Ann of Surg 2011;254(6);893–4.
16. Mark Orringer, Becky Marshall, et al. Two thousand Transhiatal esophagectomies Changing Trends, Lessons Learned. Ann of Surg 2007; 246(3);363–71.
17. Finley RJ, Inailet RI. The results of esophago-gastrostomy without thoracotomy for adeno-carcinoma of the esophago-gastric junction. Ann Surg 1989;210;535.
18. Leuketich, Pennathur, et al. Outcome after minimally invasive esophagectomy. Review 1000 patients.Ann Surgery 2007:246;363–72.
19. Rindani, et al. Data from meta-analysis 5483 patients 1986–1996.
20. Connors RC, Reuben B, et al. Journal of Am. College of surgeons 2007;205:6.
21. Brendon B, Stiles, et al. The annals of thoracic surgery 2011;92(2):49.
22. Fok M, Ah-Chong AK, et al. Comparison of a single layer continuous hand-sewn method and circular stapling in 580 esophageal anastomosis. Br J Surg 1991;580:342–5.
23. Mathison DB, et al. Thoracic Esophagectomy: A safe approach to cancer of the esophagus. Ann Th Surg 1988;45:137.
24. Desai PB, Deshpande RK, et al. Radical lymphy-adenectomy in esophagus cancer—does it improve survival? Dis Esophagus 1992;5:99–105.
25. Isono K, Sata H, et al. Results of nationwide study on the 3 field lymph node dissection of esophageal cancer. Oncology 1991;48:411–20.
26. Isono K, Ochia T, et al. The treatment of lymph node metastasis from esophageal cancer by extensive lymphadenectomy. Spn J Surg 1990; 20:151–7.
27. De Vita, Hellman and Rosenberg's Principles and Practice of Oncology 10th edition Vincent DeVita, et al. Cancer of the Esophagus 158.
28. Lerut TY, Nafteux P, Moons J, et al. Three field lymphadenectomy for carcinoma of the esophagus and gastro-esophageal junction in 174 R_0 resections: Impact on staging, disease-free survival and outcome: a plea for adaptation of TNM classification in upper-half esophageal carcinoma. Ann Surg 2004;240:962–72.
29. Omloo JM, Hulscher JB, et al. Extended transthoracic resection compared with limited transhiatal resection for adenocarcinoma of the mid/distal esophagus: five-year survival of randomized clinical trial. Ann Surg 2007;246: 992–1000.
30. Birkmeyer JD, Siewers AE, et al. Hospital volume and surgical mortality in US. NEJ medicine 2002:346:1128–37.
31. Wouters MW, Karim-Kos HE. Centralization of Esophageal Cancer Surgery: Does it Improve Clinical Outcome? Ann Surg Oncol 2009;16: 1789–98.

9

Hand Sewn Esophagogastric Anastomosis

Praful Desai, Ratna Parikh

Efficient and safe esophagogastric anastomosis after resection for esophageal cancer is the most vital step in preventing major surgical complications and long-term morbidities after this procedure (Figs 9.1 and 9.2). The most feared postoperative complication is a major anastomotic disruption, which can lead to significant morbidity and even on occasions mortality. Minor anastomotic disruptions, which heal with fibrosis is the cause of delayed dysphagia due to stenosis, which require repeated dilatation. Appropriately done anastomosis based on conventional surgical principles should lead to an optimal result with efficient deglutition until patient's survival, which is the main objective to be achieved in most cases of esophageal resections for cancer. Based on experience over a period of 50 years, the author is content to use the following technique to achieve a satisfactory result. The current disruption rate ranges around 5% and salvage from this complication is close to 100%, if diagnosed early.

The surgical principles for a good and safe anastomosis are:

1. Ensuring vascular ends of the esophagus and stomach (Fig. 9.3).
2. Tensionless, loose and easily movable anastomosis.
3. Use of absorbable 3–0 or 4–0 vicryl sutures.

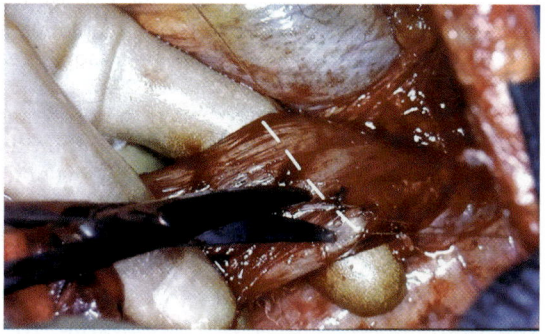

Fig. 9.1: Shows the hooked up esophagus with the surgeon's finger. The muscle layer of the esophagus is being cut with scissors, before actually sectioning the esophagus. Two stay sutures on either side of the esophageal margin are taken at the line of transection

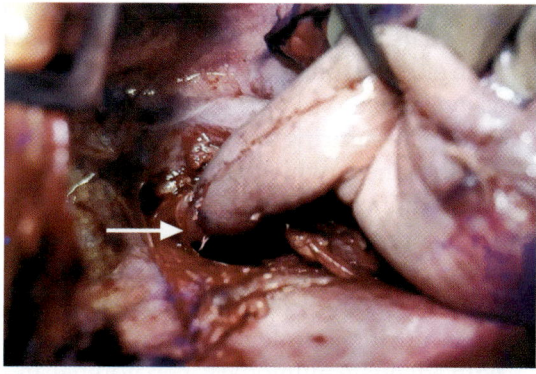

Fig. 9.2: Esophagogastric anastomosis after resection of an esophageal cancer. Arrow showing anastomotic suture line

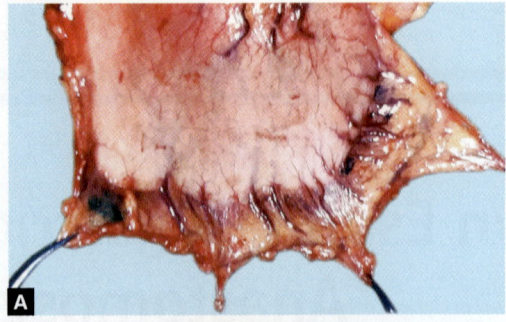

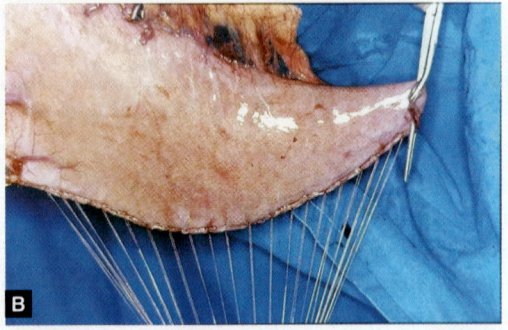

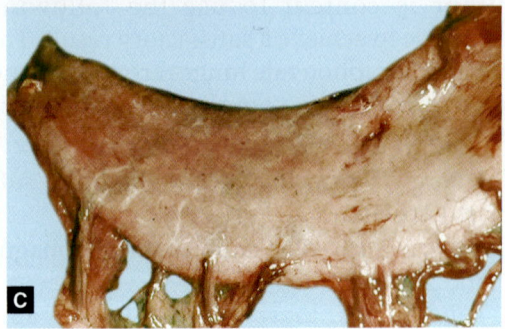

Fig. 9.3: (A) Importance of maintaining stomach vascularity by preserving the gastroepiploic arch. (B and C) Gastric tube ready for anastomosis

4. Adequate coverage of the anastomotic area with either an omental flap or pleural tissue as available.
5. Adequate suturing and covering of anastomotic corners, which is a common site for anastomotic leakage.
6. To ensure efficient gastric emptying with a pyloromyotomy or pyloroplasty is crucial.
7. An adequately prepared patient vis-à-vis good nutrition, proteins (albumin 3 gm %), with adequate pulmonary, hepatorenal and cardiac functions are mandatory.

Points in Surgical Technique

Unlike the stomach, the esophagus is devoid of any serosa, though partly this is compensated by a longitudinal muscle and a strong mucosal layer. Unlike the stomach, which has profuse blood supply, the esophagus has unnamed tiny vessels from the mediastinum, which nourishes the muscular layer of the esophagus. Hence, the esophagus should not be extensively mobilized off the mediastinum proximal to the anastomotic site. The author recommends and prefers one layer through and through inverting sutures taking care that only 1 or 2 mm bite of the esophageal mucosa is taken. Taking large bites of the mucosa is conducive to the formation of a diaphragm which can produce later stenosis. It can also jeopardize tiny transversely coursing vessels supplying the esophageal mucosal edge. The stitches taken on the esophageal wall should not be vertical but transverse as the muscle layer runs vertical. The sutures help only to keep the anastomotic ends together till nature unites the two segments (Fig. 9.4).

Prevention of Hematoma on Stomach or Esophageal Mucosal Ends

Careful submucosal gentle cauterization of tiny vessels in the stomach and esophageal end is important, as unattended, this oozing tends to diffuse in the serosa and can produce a hematoma which is inimical to a safe anastomosis. Occasionally submucosal ligation on either side may be necessary for a large vessel. After satisfactory completion of one layer anastomosis, either corners (most vulnerable to disruption) may be reinforced by a good figure of 8 suture taking a good bite of the esophageal muscle and gastric serosa. Further sutures are unnecessary; however, couple of similar sutures on the anterior and posterior surface will reinforce the main layer (Fig. 9.5). If available, the omentum (carrying the GE arch) can be wrapped around the anastomosis, though not necessary. If the opposite pleura is accidentally opened it is stitched after adequate

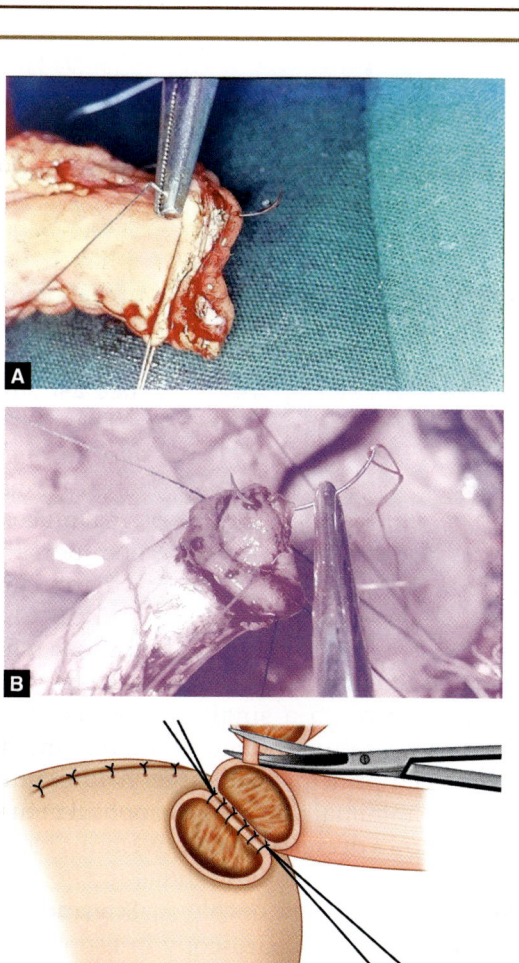

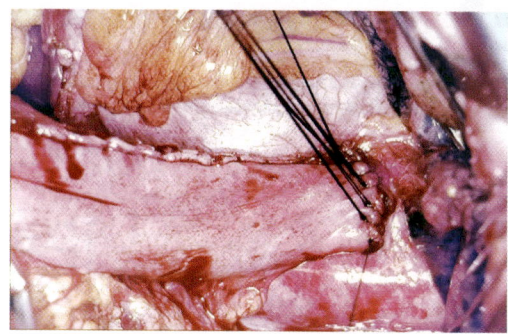

Fig. 9.5: Completed esophagogastric anastomosis with sutures still *in situ*

suction of the opposite thorax so that, in the event of a leak, the virgin chest is not insulted. An indwelling Ryle's tube is passed by the anesthetist beyond the anastomotic site into the stomach segment to keep it deflated during the first 72 hours. An efficient and appropriate anastomosis will allow a smooth passage of the tube into the stomach.

The anastomosed segment is replaced back in the mediastinum; a tiny anchoring stitch ensures that the stomach tube lies snugly in the mediastinum. No other special tricks or stitches are necessary. Lung expansion is ensured and the thorax is closed around an intrathoracic drainage. A feeding jejunostomy is performed only if one is concerned about the safety of the anastomosis. With adequate experience, routine jejunostomy can generally be avoided; nevertheless a jejunostomy is often routinely performed by most surgeons to ensure adequate fluid intake and maintain good nutrition. This helps in safer anastomotic healing.

Postoperative pyloric efficiency (emptying) is gauged by checking the stomach motility and its emptying time by performing a contrast with a thin barium between 5 and 7 days. This helps to confirm good anastomotic healing and restoration of normal swallowing. The indwelling tube can be removed within the next 48 hours after ensuring pyloric efficiency. The patient can start small frequent feeds and soft diet by 8th or 9th day and can return home by 11th or 12th postoperative day.

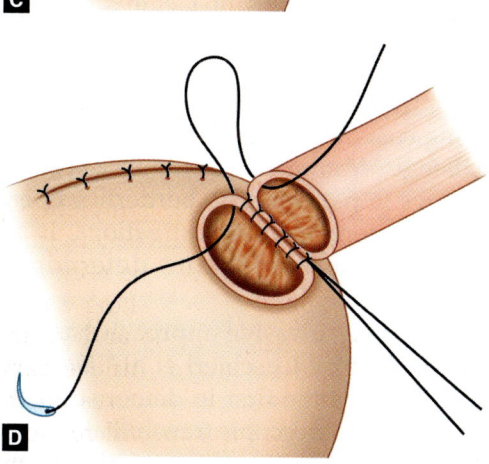

Fig. 9.4: (A) Beginning of the anastomosis; stomach serosa with a good mucosal margin ready for anastomosis with the esophageal lumen. (B) Anastomosis in progress. (C and D) Diagramatic representation of an esophagogastric anastomosis

10

Laparoscopic and Robotic Surgery for Esophageal Cancer

Shailesh Puntambekar, Advait Jathar, Manoj Manchekar, Mihir Chitale, Mangesh Panse,
Raveindra Sathe, Aishwarya Puntambekar

INTRODUCTION AND HISTORY

Esophageal cancer is the sixth leading cause of cancer death with a median survival of 11 months. Controversies about management are prevalent. Czerny first successfully resected cancer of the cervical esophagus in 1877. Surgical resection became the primary form of therapy for loco-regional disease because of its superior and more durable quality of swallowing as compared with non-operative modalities. Short-term outcome of surgical resection improved between 1970 and 1993 because of improvement in periopera-tive surgical management. Traditionally esophagectomy has been performed either by a thoracoabdominal, transhiatal or trans-thoracic approach. However, these methods have a high intraoperative and postoperative morbidity. Goldmine et al in 1993 conducted a prospective randomized trial of 67 patients undergoing esophagectomy by either a transhiatal approach or a right-sided thoraco-tomy. They concluded that long-term survival was unaffected by the type of surgery perfor-med. Minimizing complications and rapid return to routine are the main goals of surgery.

Minimal access surgery for esophageal cancer is indeed a paradigm change in the management of esophageal cancers since the 1980's. The common denominator in minimal access surgery is to perform the same surgery through a smaller incision. This reduces operative trauma without compro-mising the principles of surgery. Literature data on minimally invasive esophagectomy (MIE) shows decreased operative time, blood loss, postoperative complications and hospital stay with comparable oncological clearance.[1,2]

Application of laparoscopy in esophagec-tomy, however has been slow because of associated complexities, no tactile control and the risk of injuring adjacent vital structures. In a compromised space, inadequate lymph node retrieval is another challenge. A steep learning curve associated with MIE has been a challenge.[3] Minimal access approach has an advantage in patients with borderline opera-bility on preoperative investigations. It is a useful tool for staging and determining operability.

A minimally invasive approach has been described first by Cuschieri et al.[4] De Paula et al (1995) was the first to demonstrate the feasibility of laparoscopic transhiatal esopha-gectomy (THE) in a series of 12 patients.[5] Shmuel Avital et al in 2005 published a retrospective analysis of 22 patients under-going THE.[6] Simon Law et al (2005) retro-spectively analysed 29 patients and mentioned the advantages of magnified dissection in laparoscopic THE, especially of gastroesophageal junction.[7]

In 1998 Luketich and colleagues described the combined thoracoscopic and laparoscopic approach overcoming the disadvantage of laparoscopic transhiatal approach mainly the difficulty in mobilizing the middle third esophagus.[8] Martin et al (2005) promoted the prone position as the deflated lung lies in front of the operating field and does not require an extra port for a lung retractor. Smithers et al (2001) reported their experience with 162 patients who underwent laparoscopic transthoracic esophagectomy (TTE) in prone position. The median survival time was 29 months similar to the same group's experience with an open Ivor-Lewis technique.[9] Nguyen et al used thoracoscopy instead of thoracotomy and laparoscopy instead of laparotomy.[10] The advantages of thoracoscopy include improved visualization with better hemostasis, and the ability to evaluate proximal and middle third lesions for possible extension to other mediastinal structures.

The use of hand-assisted laparoscopic and thoracoscopic surgery in radical esophagectomy with a three-field lymphadenectomy for a thoracic lesion was described by Suzuki et al in 2005.[11] It fell into disrepute because of longer operative time.

Type of Procedure and Technique

The objectives of surgical management in carcinoma esophagus are:
• A complete resection of the esophagus
• Adequate lymph node clearance
• Replacement of the esophagus by a suitable conduit (Ideally the stomach)
• Minimum morbidity

The choice of operative approach depends on:
• Tumor location and histology of the disease (squamous cell carcinoma or adenocarcinoma)
• Stage of the disease
• Fitness of the patient.

Choice of anesthesia: For a transthoracic approach, single lumen tube ventilation is preferred in a prone position. Traditionally a double lumen tube was used for thoracoscopic approach; however, in prone position approach for thoracoscopy, single lumen tube is preferred. This leads to better ventilation of both lungs. The lungs are kept minimally inflated by increasing the respiratory rate and lowering the tidal volume, thereby maintaining minute volume. Both lungs are ventilated with this technique, decreasing ventilation-perfusion mismatch. Also this technique is easier than dual lumen ventilation which is difficult technically and a possible dislodgment of the tube endangering the procedure is avoided.

Indications of transhiatal approach:
• Tumors with TNM staging—T_1–T_3/N_0/M_0
• Lower one-third tumors
• Gastroesophageal junction tumors
• Barrett's esophagus
• Lower middle one-third tumors with low FEV1

Indications of transthoracic approach:
• Tumors with TNM staging T_1–T_3/N_0 and T_1–T_3/N_1
• Middle one-third tumors (infra-azygous)
• Lower one-third tumors (squamous cell cancer)
• Post chemoradiation patients.

For squamous cell carcinomas, the choice of surgery is usually a combined thoracoscopy-laparoscopy approach irrespective of site of lesion as these are more prone to have long segment lesions and double lesions. Poor pulmonary reserve patients are more suitable for transhiatal approach but the site of lesion still dictates the approach. Heavy nodal burden in the mediastinum is a contraindication for transhiatal approach. Patients are admitted 2 days prior to surgery for preoperative preparation, spirometric exercises to prognosticate and improve lung function. Central venous pressure line is inserted.

Transthoracic Approach

Patient Position

The patient is placed in prone position. Two bolsters are used, one to support the pelvis and the other beneath the chest to decrease concavity of the spine. The surgeon stands on the right side. Camera assistant stands to the left of the operating surgeon. The assistant surgeon stands on the left side of the patient.

Port Position

The primary port is inserted in the 6th or 7th intercostal space in the posterior axillary line remaining close to the upper border of the lower rib inferior to the angle of the scapula. This port entry is by open method. On entering the pleura, the anesthetist lowers the tidal volume leading to partial deflation of the lung. The pressure is maintained at 7 mmHg. The secondary ports are inserted under vision. The secondary ports are placed to achieve a triangulation. These are placed at 4 fingers distance from the camera port. The superior port is 1 cm medial to the medial border of scapula. The inferior port is in the same line of the superior port 4 fingers anterior to the camera port. A diagnostic thoracoscopy is first performed to inspect the pleural cavity and the lung for any suspicious lesions.

Procedure

Infra-Azygous Dissection

A. *Dissection anterior to the Esophagus:* The visceral pleura that covers the esophagus is grasped and the esophagus is pulled anteriorly. This exposes the anterior space between the esophagus and the pericardium. A Pleural cut is taken with the bipolar forceps or the Harmonic (Ethicon Endosurgery Inc. Cincinnati, OH) and the cut is extended cranially and caudally remaining parallel to the esophagus. The principle of dissecting "outside and lateral" to the vagus and not between the esophagus and vagus is applied. This achieves the removal of paraesophageal nodes.

B. *Dissection of the right hilar, subcarinal, and left hilar nodes:* The vagus is pushed anteriorly and its cardiac fibers which pass anteriorly and to the left are cut. The right main bronchus is identified passing downward. Further anterior retraction of the vagus and esophagus exposes the right hilar and subcarinal nodes. These nodes are dissected with the bipolar forceps. The nodes are supplied by small veins and these have to be coagulated carefully. The dissection between the esophagus and the pericardium is continued caudally. The paraesophageal nodes are dissected and removed along with the esophagus because they lie under the mesoesophagus. The pericardium is completely stripped of fibro-fatty tissue and the pericardial nodes. The left pleura is again seen in this region as a shining membrane and is prone to injury. By retracting the esophagus anteriorly, a clear plane between the pleura and esophagus can be seen. There are a few nodes at this level and these are included in the dissection. The esophagus is continuously pulled anteriorly with the left hand while the right hand performs the dissection. The caudal end point of dissection is the hiatus.

C. *Dissection posterior to the esophagus:* The procedure starts by taking a cut on the visceral pleura between the esophagus and the aorta in the infra-azygous part. The CO_2 insufflation helps in opening the plane between the esophagus and the aorta. The pleural cut is extended caudally up to the level of the diaphragm. The plane of dissection always lies outside the vagus and not between the vagus and the esophagus. This is the oncologically correct plane and results in complete mesoesophageal resection. This plane is relatively avascular and so bleeding is minimized. The vagus can be used for anterior traction, so that tethering of the esophageal muscle fibers is avoided. The vagus is held down with the left hand and the fibro-fatty tissue and the lymphoid tissue is swept towards the esophagus. Thus all the paraesophageal nodes are removed. Preferably a bipolar is used here, since it is better at coagulating the small blood vessels going to the aorta. They are clipped using vascular clips. These are usually two or three in number. The esophagus is separated anteriorly and cranially and the left inferior pulmonary vein is identified. It is more clearly seen medially when the anterior and posterior dissections are completed. The traction is always maintained by pulling on the pleura overlying the esophagus, or on the vagus to avoid tethering of the esophagus. This posterior dissection is continued further, cranially resecting all the fibro-fatty tissue till the aorta is bared. The direction of the aorta is followed cranially and the esophagus is lifted from the arch of the aorta. The arch lies at a level just below the azygous vein. The left main bronchus crosses anterior to the descending aorta. Utmost care is taken not to injure the posterior wall of the left bronchus while dissecting the esophagus from the arch of the aorta. The left hilar nodes are exposed at this level and can be dissected from the bronchus at this stage or at a later stage when the subcarinal nodes are removed.

Caudally, the dissection is continued toward the hiatus. At this stage, the opposite pleura is identified by careful blunt dissection using the suction cannula. The para-esophageal nodes and those at the hiatus are removed completely. The thoracic duct is identified as a white glistening structure over the descending aorta at the hiatus. This can be clipped or can be separated completely from the esophagus. This completes the posterior dissection. The sign of completed posterior dissection is absence of fibro-fatty tissue on the aorta, complete removal of paraesophageal nodes, clear visualization of the arch of aorta, the left main bronchus, and the inferior pulmonary vein.

D. *Medial and Circumferential dissection:* The esophagus at the level of the pericardium is retracted downwards with the left hand and a strip of gauze is pushed from the medial side of the esophagus to aid identification of the

plane of dissection. The dissection is continued bluntly using the suction cannula or the bipolar forceps. The tip of the grasper should rest on the vertebrae so that no vital structure is damaged. This helps in dissecting the esophagus on the medial side and freeing it further. The esophagus is manipulated by the left hand grasper and organ is separated along its length and all around.

Cranially, the anterior dissection ends at the level of azygous vein. The vagus is seen parallel to the esophagus. On completion of the anterior dissection, the carina is clearly seen with the left and right main bronchi. The infra-azygous dissection achieves complete removal of paraesophageal, subcarinal, hilar and hiatal nodes. The esophagus is also separated all around from the pericardium and the left pleura medially, arch of the aorta, and the descending aorta posteriorly, and the azygous vein laterally. At the end of dissection, all these structures should be identified. They should be free of any fibro-fatty and lymphoid tissue. Complete hemostasis is achieved before proceeding for the supra-azygous dissection. The thoracic duct area is inspected for any damage.

Supra-Azygous Dissection

The next step is the supra-azygous dissection. The pleura that covers the esophagus is lifted with the left-hand grasper and a cut is taken which is extended towards the root of the neck. The vagus nerve is identified. The vagal fibers going to the bronchus are preserved, and the rest of the vagus is cut at the level of the azygous vein. The dissection begins posterior to the esophagus; the right hand grasper pulls the esophagus downward and a plane is created between it and the vertebrae, This dissection is done either with the suction cannula or with the bipolar forceps. The use of bipolar is recommended, as small vessels can be easily coagulated. A few small vessels arising from the intercostal vessels and supplying the esophagus are coagulated and cut. The entire fibro-fatty tissue along with the nodes is pushed with the esophagus.

At this stage the infra-azygous esophagus is lifted, and dissection is performed in the posterior plane with a suction cannula. The left hand pulls the esophagus caudally and anteriorly; the supra-and infra-azygous planes are joined. Thus, the entire esophagus is freed posteriorly.

The pleura on the lateral wall of the azygous vein is held and cut. The lymphovascular tissues along the azygous vein are cleared at this stage. The azygous vein is freed along its entire length. The bronchial artery is posterior to the azygous vein and can be seen by retracting the vein downward. This allows complete separation of the vein. The vein is then retracted slightly and then the nodes along with the fibro-fatty tissue are removed. These nodes can be removed en block, or can be removed separately.

Once the azygous vein is freed or cut, the supra-azygous esophagus is pulled anteriorly, this exposes the plane between the posterior wall of the trachea and the esophagus. The dissection should be done with extreme caution; especially so, if the tumor involves the esophagus at this level. We recommend the use of a blunt dissector like a suction cannula, since the membranous trachea is to be protected against injury. The dissection should always be done parallel to the esophagus as well as to the trachea. A clear plane is identifiable, and this plane is further exposed by pulling the esophagus anteriorly. A strip of gauze can be used to complete the dissection. Once the infra-azygous esophagus has been freed completely, the dissection between the esophagus and the trachea is easier. A medial window, similar to that made earlier is made and the left-hand grasper pulls the esophagus further anteriorly. The entire esophagus is thus separated. There are few nodes in the paratracheal region which are dissected and removed. The esophagus is dissected around the circumference in the supra-azygous region and these planes are joined with those in the infra-azygous region, thus completely freeing the esophagus. This can be confirmed by pulling the esophagus craniocaudally ("the shoe-shine sign").

Once the esophagus is completely freed, it is pulled anteriorly to expose the left recurrent laryngeal nerve lying in the trachea-esophageal groove. Nodes along this nerve are removed. The use of bipolar or any other energy sources are not recommended near the nerve. The right recurrent laryngeal nerve is also identified at the thoracic inlet near the innominate artery.

The esophageal dissection is continued cranially to the root of the neck. The sign of complete dissection is the appearance of fat, as seen thoracoscopically or subcutaneous emphysema felt by the assistant in the left supraclavicular area. It is essential to dissect the esophagus completely from the posterior wall of the trachea and to the root of the neck, thus obviating the need of blind finger dissection in the neck. The esophagus is then moved craniocaudally and mediolaterally to confirm complete esophageal mobilization. The nodal areas are examined for the complete removal of the nodes. A thorough wash is given and the damage to the left pleura is checked under water. If damaged an intercostal drain needs to be placed on the left side too. Complete hemostasis is achieved by additional use of clips or bipolar energy.

On the right side, an intercostal drain is inserted through the working 10 mm port and is placed near the apex, with the help of the left-hand grasper. The 5 mm ports are removed under vision, as the intercostal vessels may have been damaged during the insertion of the ports and this is to be checked. The lung is inflated and the camera port is removed under vision. The intercostal drainage tube should be open and not clamped, to push out all the air during lung inflation. At the end of the thoracoscopic procedure, the drain is fixed and the incisions are closed. The patient is turned and positioned for the laparoscopic and neck dissection.

Stomach Mobilization and Nodal Dissection

The gastrocolic omentum is opened, taking care to remain outside the gastroepiploic arcade. The greater curve is mobilized from the pylorus to the spleen, the short gastric vessels are clamped close to the stomach wall, taking care not to injure the splenic hilum. These are taken with the harmonic. The left crus is again seen when the short gastric vessels are divided and the fundus is mobilized medially. The greater omentum is divided, but complete resection is not necessary. Congenital adhesions between the pancreas and stomach are released and the stomach is now completely lifted off the pancreas. Duodenal mobilization is performed only if the stomach is not of sufficient length. It is usually not necessary. The author does not routinely perform a drainage procedure. If deemed necessary, a pyloromyotomy can be performed laparosopically or extracorporeally during specimen removal.

The nodal dissection at the celiac axis is performed using the bipolar forceps of the harmonic. Nodes around the base of the left gastric vessels are dissected to delineate the left gastric artery and vein separately. The left gastric vein is clipped and cut. The common hepatic artery and the splenic artery are identified. The areolar tissue and nodes along the common hepatic artery are dissected and taken medially, along with the gastric nodes. There is sometimes some bleeding from the small vessels supplying the nodes. The bleeding usually stops once the node has been completely removed. This bleeding can be temporarily controlled by packing with a piece of gauze for some time alternatively, the bleeders can be coagulated or clipped. The nodes along the splenic artery are then taken. For this, the assistant on the left side has to gently depress the cranial part of the head of pancreas. This helps the camera to reach the celiac axis and show the splenic vessels well during the lymph node clearance. The para-aortic nodes in this region are cleared, again proceeding toward the hiatus. Complete nodal dissection bares the celiac axis entirely; this is seen as the "Mercedes Benz" sign. The magnification offered by the laparoscopic approach greatly aids the lymph node dissection and improves precision. The left

gastric artery is ligated or clipped and cut. The vessels along the lesser curve are clipped, for an adequate distance distally. This can also be done extracorporeally during specimen removal.

The stomach tube can be fashioned intracorporeally (using staplers) or extracorporeally. The author prefers the latter method, since the aim of the procedure is not to do everything laparoscopically, but to complete the operation with minimum morbidity.

Mobilization of the Esophagus in the Neck

The neck dissection is commenced by a second team, to mobilize the esophagus along the border of the left sternocleidomastoid muscle. The platysma and the omohyoid muscles are cut to expose the internal jugular vein. Dissection remains medial to the carotid sheath. The middle thyroid vein is divided and the thyroid gland is retracted medially. The esophagus is identified and dissection is continued posteriorly up to the prevertebral fascia. The posterior wall of the esophagus is separated from the prevertebral fascia. Anteriorly, the esophagus is gently separated from the trachea, remaining close to the esophageal wall, taking care not to injure the left recurrent laryngeal nerve. A cotton tape is passed around the esophagus. This sling helps to maintain traction on the esophagus for further mobilization in the mediastinum. A finger dissection, remaining close to the esophageal wall is used to mobilize the upper thoracic esophagus. Special care is taken anteriorly not to tear the membranous trachea. Deeper into the mediastinum, the pleura is separated from the esophagus as far as possible. The entire intrathoracic esophagus is thus freed and is accompanied by a give-away sensation perceived by the left hand pulling on the esophagus. The nasogastric (Levine) tube is removed and the esophagus is transected in the neck. On the proximal end, the mucosal and submucosal level of transection is kept 2–3 mm distal to the transection of the muscle layers. Two lateral stay sutures are placed on the proximal esophagus. The distal cut end of the esophagus is tied and a nasogastric tube is transfixed to it.

Specimen Delivery and Creation of the Stomach Tube

The pneumoperitoneum is re-established and the esophagus is pulled into the abdominal cavity. A small midline incision (usually 5 cm in thin patients) is used to deliver the specimen and the stomach outside the abdomen. The author prefers to fashion the stomach tube extracorporeally, using linear staplers. The lesser curve is excised in such a way that the stomach tube is of 5–6 cm width. The Levine tube attached to the esophagus and brought down through the thorax is now disconnected from the esophagus, and the specimen is removed. The staple-line is reinforced by continuous 3–0 running sutures (silk or PDS). A very wide stomach tube leads to gastric stasis, and is therefore avoided. The Levine

tube is transfixed to the upper end of the stomach tube. The conduit is thus pulled into the neck by rail-roading it to the Levine tube. We routinely perform a feeding jejunostomy in all patients. The abdomen is closed in layers.

Hand-Sewn Anastomosis in the Neck

The esophagus is anastomosed to the posterior wall near the apex of the gastric conduit to create an inverted ink-bottle effect. This prevents anastomotic leakages. The

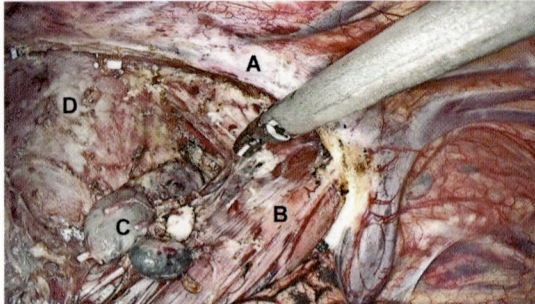

Fig. 10.3: (A) Azygous vein, (B) Esophagus, (C) Subcarinal lymph nodes, (D) Pericardium

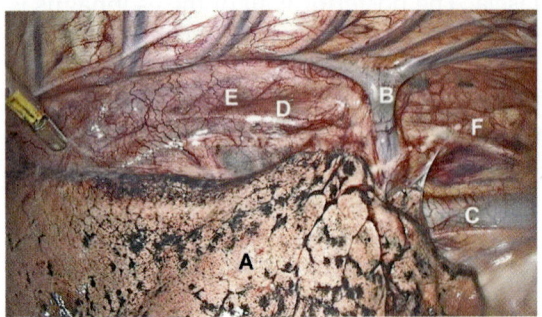

Fig. 10.1: (A) Right lung, (B) Azygous vein, (C) Superior vena cava, (D) Esophagus, (E) Aorta, (F) Trachea

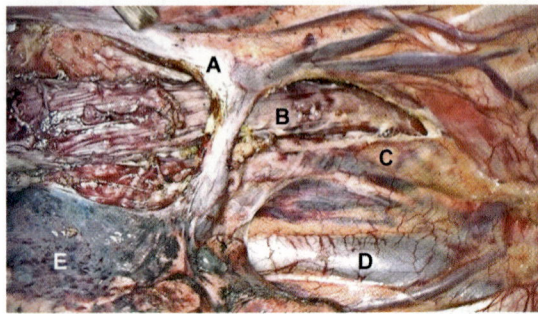

Fig. 10.4: (A) Azygous vein, (B) Esophagus, (C) Trachea, (D) Superior Vena Cava, (E) Right lung

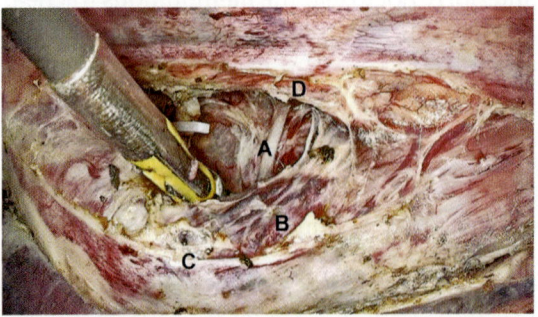

Fig. 10.2: (A) Direct branches from aorta, (B) Esophagus, (C) Vagus nerve, (D) Aorta

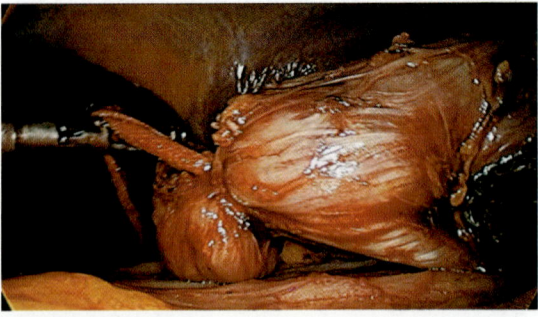

Fig. 10.5: Delivery of cervical esophagus into the abdomen

posterior seromuscular layer is taken using interrupted 3–0 silk sutures. An opening is made on the stomach wall with a diathermy. Continuous full-thickness sutures of 4–0 PDS/Vicryl are taken. This is the second layer and includes the full thickness of the posterior wall of the stomach and full-thickness of the posterior wall of the esophagus. A nasogastric tube is passed across the anastomosis and the second layer is continued anteriorly as the third layer. A fourth layer of interrupted 3–0 silk/PDS seromuscular sutures completes the anastomosis. A soft corrugated drain is placed adjacent to the anastomosis and the neck incision is closed (Figs 10.1 to 10.5).

Transhiatal Approach

Patient is given a combination of epidural and general anesthesia. Hypotensive anesthesia is important part of the procedure. Patient is given modified Llyod-Davies position with neck extension and 15° reverse trendelenburg position. The surgeon stands in between the legs, camera assistant on the right side of the patient and second assistant on the left side of the patient. The monitors are placed near the shoulders of the patient.

Steps

Veress needle introduced at palmers point and a pneumoperitoneum is created. The primary 10 mm camera port is inserted at the junction of upper two-thirds and lower third of the line joining the xiphisternum to the umbilicus. One 11 mm port on the left side and one 6 mm port on the right side are placed in the pararectal area in the midclavicular line with distance being approximately 4 finger-breadths from the camera port achieving triangulation at the hiatus. A 6 mm port is placed in the epigastrium for liver retraction and a 6 mm port is placed on the left side in the anterior axillary line at the level of the umbilicus.

The procedure starts by cutting the gastro-hepatic omentum in its avascular part and identifying the right crus of diaphragm. This can be visualized by retracting the left lobe of liver with an atraumatic grasper, inserted through the 5 mm port at the xiphisternum. This instrument is used like a stick, the tip supported against the diaphragm and the shaft lifting the liver. The esophageal mobilization is done prior to the stomach mobilization, so that the stomach acts as a natural retractor and steadies the esophagus during dissection. The assistant on the left pulls the stomach downward and to left, stretching the peritoneum over the right crus.

Defining the Hiatus

The peritoneum over the right crus is incised using a harmonic scalpel. The retroesophageal plane is entered by blunt dissection. The pneumoperitoneum helps to open this space further. The peritoneal cut over the right crus is extended upward, toward the apex of hiatus thus completely exposing the right crural fibers. The next step is to identify the posterior vagus. Once the vagus is identified, the dissection should continue posterior to the vagus and not between the vagus and esophagus. Dissection between the vagus and esophagus can lead to troublesome bleeding. The left hand grasper lifts up the esophagus along with the vagus and the dissection posterior to the vagus is continued till the left crural fibers are visualized. The posterior window is enlarged till the dome of the diaphragm is seen. The esophagus is continuously retracted anteriorly and caudally with the left-hand grasper during this dissection. This traction is further enhanced by the second assistant on the left, by pulling on the fundus of the stomach.

The dissection then proceeds to the right side of the esophagus. The right pleural reflection can be seen at this stage. The pleura is gently reflected off the esophagus. This dissection is better done with the left-hand grasper, or using the tip of a suction catheter, carefully pushing the pleura away as far as possible. CO_2 insufflation aids this dissection. Inadvertent pleural injury is managed by insertion of an ICD tube. However, a pleural injury at this stage can be extremely troublesome, since it leads to continuous loss of pneumoperitoneum. Once the right pleura and hiatus are defined, intrahiatal dissection is started.

Posterior Dissection

The esophagus is retracted anteriorly by the left-hand grasper along with the posterior vagus which is now clearly defined. Dissection is begun between the aorta and esophagus, again remaining behind the nerve. The paraesophageal nodes are removed with the esophagus. The entire fibro-fatty tissue over the aorta is also removed. The posterior dissection is done either with the harmonic shears or with the suction cannula. The direction of the dissection should be from the aorta towards the esophagus, sweeping all the tissues towards the esophagus. A few direct branches of the aorta supplying the esophagus are seen as vertical strands. It is better to use clips to seal these vessels before cutting them, since these are direct aortic branches, and are under high pressure. The use of bipolar or harmonic is not recommended for this purpose. Dissection is continued proximally behind the esophagus. This is again facilitated by the CO_2 gas which enters the planes of dissection.

Dissection on the Right Side

Once the esophagus is completely mobilized on the posterior aspect, the same plane of dissection is used to push the right wall of esophagus further away from the pleura. During this dissection, the esophagus is retracted to the left side with a grasper to further dissect the plane on the right side, proceeding cranially. The upper limit of dissection is the right main bronchus which is better palpated than visualized. The hemiazygous may be seen at this stage to the right of the esophagus. The azygous vein is not seen, as it lies above the right main bronchus. Dissection above the level of carina is not possible due to the

presence of the aortic arch, which limits the dissection. The posterior vagus is cut at the level of right main bronchus. The esophagus can be pulled further to the left and the dissection continued further cranially on the right side. The traction on the esophagus toward the left is accomplished with the left-hand grasper but can also be maintained by the assistant on the left by pulling the cardio-esophageal junction.

Anterior Dissection

The esophagus is pulled caudally and posteriorly with the left hand. The anterior dissection, between the heart and esophagus is the easiest part of dissection, as no major vascular structures are encountered here. The pericardium is a tough structure and is rarely involved by the disease. The dissection can often be achieved with blunt tipped instrument such as suction cannula. The anterior space can be opened further by placing the assistant's grasper at the apex of hiatus for retraction. The carina is the upper limit of this dissection.

Left Sided Dissection

Once the right-sided, posterior, and anterior dissections are completed, the esophagus becomes mobile and thereby manipulation becomes more difficult. The left-sided dissection is commenced. The first assistant's grasper holds the left crus and pushes it to the left, to widen this space. The fundus and the entire stomach are rolled to the right side by the second assistant on the left. This exposes the cardioesophageal junction on the left side and the peritoneum overlying it is cut. The left pleura is closely adherent here and care has to be taken to protect it from damage. Once the pleura is seen it is carefully reflected away from the esophagus by using the right-hand grasper, while the left hand pulls the esophagus.

The anterior vagus can be seen on the left side of the esophagus and is again an important landmark for dissection. The plane of dissection lies between the vagus and the left pleura and not between esophagus and vagus. By pulling on the vagus, sufficient traction can be applied facilitating dissection further cranially. Thus, the vagus should not be cut early in the dissection. At this stage all paraesophageal nodes are removed with the esophagus. The dissection is done either with harmonic shears or with a suction cannula. The cranial limit of dissection is the left main bronchus. The anterior vagus is cut at this level. The esophagus is pushed to the right side and the sign of completed dissection is the visualization of descending aorta from the left side of esophagus. The esophagus is then pulled caudally and rolled to check that it is free all around its circumference.

Nodal Dissection

The nodal dissection at the celiac axis is performed using the bipolar forceps or the harmonic Ace (Ethicon Endo-surgery Inc. Cincinnati, OH). Nodes around the base of the left gastric vessels are dissected to delineate the left gastric artery and vein separately. The left gastric vein is clipped and cut. The common hepatic artery and splenic artery are identified. The loose areolar tissue and nodes along the common hepatic artery are dissected and taken medially, along with the gastric nodes. The small vessels supplying the nodes may bleed, but the bleeding usually stops once the node has been completely removed. The nodes along the splenic artery are removed. For this, the assistant on the left side has to gently depress the cranial part of the head of pancreas. This helps the camera to reach the celiac axis and show the splenic vessels well during the lymph node clearance. The para-aortic nodes in this region are cleared, again proceeding towards the hiatus. Completed nodal dissection bares the celiac axis entirely; this is seen as the "Mercedes Benz" sign. The magnification offered by the laparoscopic approach greatly aids the lymph node dissection and improves precision.

The left gastric artery is ligated or clipped and cut. The vessels along the lesser curve are clipped at an adequate distance distally. This can also be done extracorporeally during specimen removal. Stomach mobilization, mobilization of the esophagus in the neck, specimen retrieval and creation of the stomach tube, esophagogastric anastomosis in the neck, and the postoperative management are the same as described for thoracoscopic esophagectomy.

Postoperatively, patients are shifted to ICU with endotracheal tube *in situ*. Jejunostomy feeding is started within 24 hours. Intercostal drainage tubes placement is confirmed on chest X-ray and removed sequentially on 2–4th postoperative day. Corrugated drain in the neck is removed on the postoperative 5th day, any leak would be picked up at this point. Patients are generally discharged with Ryle's tube *in situ* on 6–7th postoperative day and oral trial given on the 10–12th postoperative day on 1st follow-up visit. We do not do a gastro-grafin study on a routine basis (since the anastomosis is done in layers, is tension free and done on the posterior wall of the stomach) (Figs 10.6 to 10.9).

Discussion

The evolution of laparoscopic techniques for esophagectomy has drastically improved patient and oncological outcomes in recent years. The laparoscopic approach to esophageal malignancies was heralded by Cuschieri et al. The landmark study by Luketich et al combining thoracoscopic and laparoscopic approach with cervical anastomosis in 2003 paved the way for a change in paradigm for the minimal access approach to such diseases. Our experience in MIE is extensive, having published data of 68 geriatric MIE procedures, 112 patients of MIE via lateral position in thoracoscopic part and 83 robotic assisted transthoracic procedures.[12–14] Out of 68 geriatric MIE procedures we performed between 2009 and 2012, mean age of patients was 75. Fifty-seven were middle third and 17 were

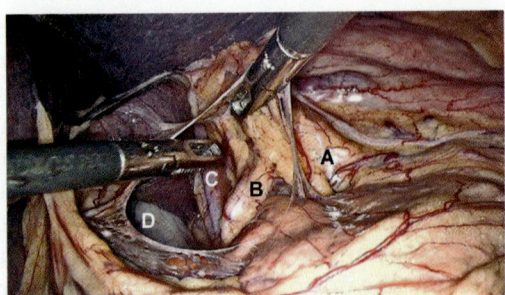

Fig. 10.6: (A) Esophagus, (B) Left gastric artery, (C) Right crus of diagram, (D) Inferior vena cava

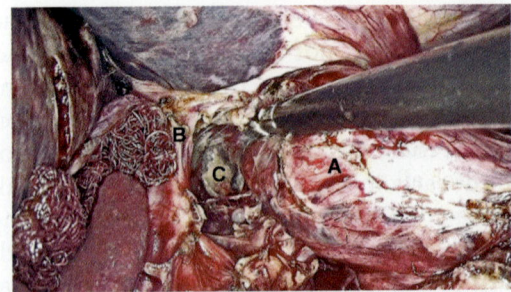

Fig. 10.8: (A) Esophagus, (B) Right crus of diaphragm, (C) Pleura

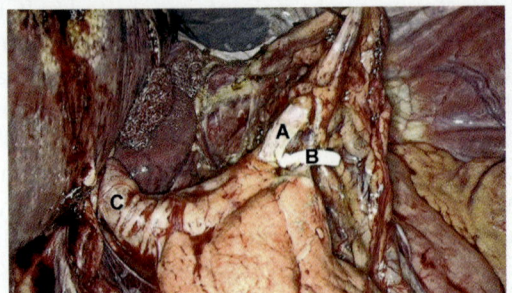

Fig. 10.7: (A) Left gastric artery, (B) Left gastric vein, (C) Common hepatic artery

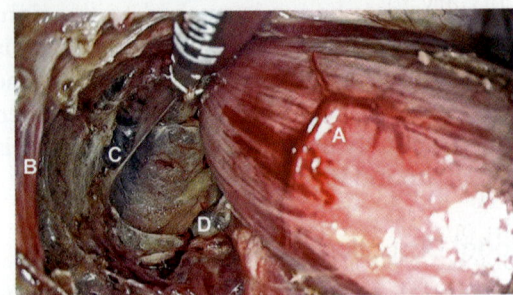

Fig. 10.9: (A) Esophagus, (B) Right crus of diaphragm, (C) Right pleura, (D) Preaortic tissue

lower third tumors. Twenty-one patients had stage I disease and 47 patients had stage II disease. Upfront surgery was offered to those patients according to the National Comprehensive Cancer Network (NCCN) guidelines. Fifty-seven patients had squamous cell carcinoma. The average total operating time was 179 minutes (90–240) and the thoracoscopic mobilization took about 67 minutes (45–110). The average lymph node yield was about 15 (9–23). Average blood loss was about 143 ml (32–450).[12] Our surgical outcomes are comparable to series published by Luketich, Berger, Smither and Dexter et al. (Table 10.1).

Table 10.1 Surgical outcomes of laparoscopic esophagectomy: A comparative study

	Our present series N = 68	Luketich et al. N = 481	Berger et al. N = 65	Smither's et al. N = 23	Dexter et al. N = 24	Puntambekar et al. (Lateral position N = 112
Mean age	75.76	65	61	61	62	54
Conversion%	0%	5%	9%	7%	4.2%	1.7%
Recurrent LN palsy	4.4%	8%	–	5%	36%	3.6%
Respiratory complications	10.3%	10%	15–20%	27%	59%	7.2%
Anastomotic leak	10.3%	5%	14%	4%	9%	2.7%
Chyle leak	0%	–	–	2.4%	9%	0%
Total LN harvested (Mean)	15.1	19	20	–	13	23
Mean blood loss	143 ml	–	182 ml	165 ml	–	200 ml
Mean operating time (total)	179	–	–	299	–	185
Mean thoracic operating time	67	–	–	104	183	85
Mortality (%)	4.4%	2.5%	7.7%	8%	14%	2.7%

Minor complications such as wound infections were seen in 6 patients. Anastomotic leaks occurred in 6 patients. They were contained to the neck. Hoarseness of voice due to recurrent laryngeal nerve damage was seen in 3 cases all of which had complete recovery after 6 weeks. The transthoracic approach helps in visualizing the recurrent laryngeal nerve (RLN) in the mediastinum during the supra-azygous dissection of the esophagus. Three patients died, two due to mediastinitis secondary to anastomotic leak and one due to myocardial infarction. Other complications of chylothorax, airway injuries and gastric tube necrosis did not occur in any of our patients. Pneumonia was seen in 10.3% of our patients. Table 10.2 enumerates the complications in the geriatric series.

In our study of 112 patients undergoing thoracoscopic esophagectomies in left lateral position, the average age of patients was 54. Of these patients, 80 patients had middle-third esophageal cancer. The pathology of 100 patients showed squamous cell carcinoma. The average thoracoscopic operating time was 85 minutes (40–120 min). The average blood loss was 200 ml, and the average number of harvested mediastinal nodes was 23 on par with open esophagectomies. Conversion to open was done in 1.7% of cases. The median follow-up period was 18 months. Postoperative morbidity occurred

for 16 patients, with 8 patients (7.27%) experiencing respiratory complications. Recurrent nerve palsy was seen in 3.6% of cases. Anastomotic leaks were seen in 2.7%. Postoperative mortality was seen in 2.7%. Table 10.1 compares our study with MIE study by Luketich et al and other open esophagectomy series.

In our robotic series of 83 patients, most commonly involved site (50 cases, 60.24%) was lower third of the esophagus. The predominant histology (67 cases, 80.72%) was squamous cell carcinoma. A total of 21.69% of patients presented with at least one comorbid condition, hypertension and diabetes was observed as most common comorbidities. The mean operative time was 204.94 minutes (180–300). The size of the tumor did not significantly affect operative times. The mean blood loss was 86.75 ml (50–200). The mean number of lymph node yield was 18.36 (13–24). Only two patients showed positive circumferential margin. None of the patient required conversion to thoracoscopic or open surgery. The mean ICU stay was 1 day (1–3) and the mean hospital stay was 10.37 days (10–13) Table 10.3.

Lymph node yield in our MIE procedures on average was 15–20 on par with series of 481 cases by Luketich et al (lymph node yield-19) in the mediastinum.[8,12,13] Such a high-yield was possible due to magnified view through endoscope, better electrosurgical devices ensuring bloodless fields. Our robotic series showed a lymph node yield of 18.36 comparable to other series.

MIE has reduced operative blood loss but increased operation time in comparison with open esophagectomy. Patients get less respiratory complications and are better overall in the MIE group than the open esophagectomy group. Hu W et al did not find any statistical difference between the two groups in terms of lymph node harvest, R_0 resection, and other major complications.[15] In a study of 1000 patients by Luketich J et al

Table 10.2 Geriatric series N = 68	
Major complications	
Tracheal tear	01
Pneumonia	06 (10.3%)
Anastomotic leak	06 (10.3%)
Hoarseness of voice	03 (4.4%)
Myocardial infarction	01
Chylous leak	00
Mediastinitis	02
Minor complications	
Wound infections	06 (10.3%)
Cardiac arrhythmia	11 (17%)
Mediastinitis secondary to anastomotic leak	02 (3.8%)
30 day perioperative mortality	03 (4.4%)

Table 10.3	Robotic series N = 83
Variable	Mean (range) or no. (%)
Total operative time (mins)	204.94 (180–300)
Docking time (mins)	9.06 (5–30)
Undocking time (mins)	5 (2–10)
Time for esophageal mobilization (mins)	104.08 (80–170)
Estimated blood loss (ml)	86.75 (50–200)
Lymph node yield	18.36 (13–24)
ICU stay (days)	1 (1–3)
Hospital stay (days)	10.37 (10–13)
Nil by mouth (days)	9.40 (8–12)
Conversion	Nil
Margin positivity	2 (2.41)
Adjuvant chemotherapy	15 (18.07)
Complications	
Dysphagia for solids	6 (7.23)
Pleural effusion	3 (3.61)
Aspiration pneumonia	1 (1.20)
Recurrent palsy	2 (2.41)
Anastomotic leak	3 (3.61)
Chyle leak	1 (1.20)
Port site metastasis	1 (1.20)
Surgical site infection	1 (1.20)
Sepsis	1 (1.20)

MIE was proven safe, with low mortality, acceptable morbidity, and a short length of stay.[8]

In a landmark study by Miguel E Cuesta et al the TIME trial compares the traditional transthoracic esophageal resection (right thoracotomy and laparotomy) with MIE (right thoracoscopy in prone and laparoscopy) followed by intrathoracic or cervical anastomosis between June 2009 and March 2011. It showed a lower incidence of pulmonary infections, a shorter hospital stay, and a better short-term quality of life without compromise of the quality of the resected specimen.[16]

In a single centre study of 142 patients by Baofu chen et al the average number of harvested mediastinal lymph nodes was 13.5 (3–30). Average total procedure time was 270.5 ± 28.1 minutes (196–320 min). The median operation time for thoracoscopy was 81.5 ± 14.6 minutes (60–130 min) and for laparoscopy it was 63.8 ± 9.1 minutes (40–90 min). The mean blood loss associated with thoracoscopy was 123.8 ± 39.2 ml (60–310 ml), and that of the laparoscopic procedures was 49.9 ± 14.3 ml (30–100 ml). Median postoperative duration of hospital stay was 12.2 days (9–45 days). The 30–day mortality rate was 0.7% (n = 1).[17]

Table 10.4 compares our series of thoracoscopic esophagectomies in geriatric age group and lateral position with other reputed MIE trials.

The postoperative morbidity has significantly reduced as seen by shorter ICU and hospital stay and decreased complication rates. A randomized controlled trial consisting of 56 patients randomly assigned to open vs MIE technique by Biere et al showed short-term benefits of MIE such as faster recovery and quality of life over open technique.[18] In a study by Kubo et al involving 209 patients, the incidence of pulmonary complications was significantly reduced (p = 0.015) in the total-MIE group (8/93 : 8.5%) compared with the total-open group (16/74 : 21.6%).[19] A study by Avital S et al involving 22 patients who underwent laparoscopic transhiatal esophagectomy showed decreased intraoperative blood loss, a smaller incision, and a potentially faster postoperative recovery were seen. Immediate oncologic goals of adequate margins and lymph node dissection can be achieved, and long-term outcome appears to be similar to that found with open approaches.[20]

A meta-analysis of 13 prospective and retrospective studies of open versus laparoscopic esophagectomies by Wang B et al showed blood loss in the thoracolaparoscopic esophagectomy group had a clear advantage compared with open esophagectomy group, however, anastomotic leakage and the number of lymph nodes harvested did not show any difference.[21] In a review of 8 studies by G Sgourakis et al there were significantly fewer total complications in the minimally

Table 10.4 Comparison of the author's series of thoracoscopic esophagectomies in geriatric age group and lateral position with other reputed MIE trials

	Luketich et al 2013	Puntambekar et al 2013 (Geriatric)	Puntambekar et al 2013 (Lat. transthoracic)	Puntambekar et al (Robotic)	Miguel Cuesta et al (TIME trial MIE group)	Baofu Chen et al
Surgical outcome	N = 222	N = 68	N = 112	N = 83	N = 59	N = 142
Lymph node harvest	19	15.1	23	18.36		13.5
Mean operative time	NR	179 min	185 min	178.84 min		270 min
Blood loss		143 ml	200 ml	86.75 ml		173 ml
ICU stay	NR	3.84	1	1		1
Vocal cord palsy	3.60%	4.40%	3.60%	2.41%	2%	5.60%
Anastomotic leak	11.70%	10.30%	2.70%	3.61%	12%	6.30%
Pneumonia	7.70%	10.30%	7.20%	1.20%	12%	11.30%
Mortality	1.40%	4.40%	2.70%	0%	3.40%	0.70%

NR: Not recorded

invasive esophagectomy group and fewer anastomotic strictures in the open thoracotomy arm. The two procedures had comparable outcomes for other measures (removed lymph nodes, 30-day mortality, three-year survival).[22]

Robotic Transthoracic Esophagectomy

Robotic assisted transthoracic esophagectomy has accelerated the learning curve of MIE with the help of magnified three dimensional view, improved articulation of instruments with seven degrees of freedom, improved dexterity and enhanced ergonomics.[23,24] The patient placement is similar to its conventional thoracoscopic counterpart. Additional 10 mm port is placed anteriorly to the camera port for the assistant for suctioning and application of clips (Fig. 10.10).

The procedural steps in the robot assisted thoracoscopic part are similar to the thoracoscopy explained in detail earlier. The abdominal part is conducted laparoscopically and proceeds similar to routine combined thoracoscopic–laparoscopic technique. The

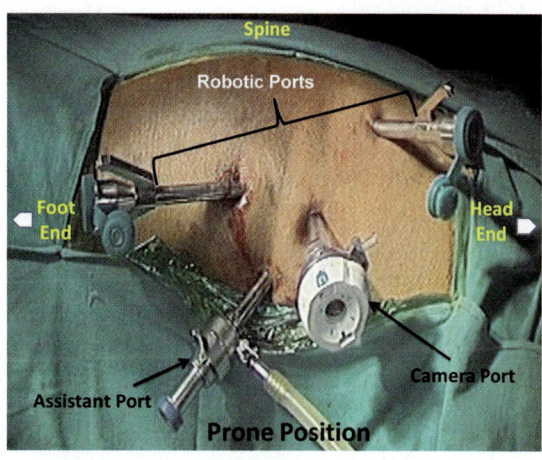

Fig. 10.10: Robotic transthoracic esophagectomy

robot assisted transthoracic approach has enabled us to be versatile in the confined cage of the thorax. The dexterity and articulated instruments enable 7 degrees of movement–in/out, rotation, pitch at wrist, yaw at wrist, pitch at fulcrum, yaw at fulcrum and grip strength. The improved tremor free hand movements facilitate a precise dissection and suturing in confined spaces. A study from van Hillegersberg R et al harvested a median of 20 lymph nodes (9–30) through robot-assisted thoracoscopic esophagectomy.[23] Cerfolio et al reported median number of 20 lymph nodes through the same approach.[25] Galvani et al achieved mean lymph nodes yield of 12 (7–27) using robot-assisted transhiatal esophagectomy.[26] The same approach was utilized by Dunn et al who harvested a median of 20 lymph nodes (3–38).[27] Sarkaria et al reported median number of 20 lymph nodes (10–49) using combined thoracoscopic and laparoscopic robotic-assisted approach.[28] Better quality lymphadenectomy could be achieved in robotic esophagectomy although survival benefit was not clear.[29]

The first performed robotic-assisted esophagectomy in 2003 reported total operative time of 246 minutes. Subsequent case series by van Hillegers et al reported total operative time of 450 minutes (370–550) and thoracoscopic time of 180 minutes (120–240) from experience in 21 patients.[23] Boone et al reported median operative time of 450 minutes in a series of 47 patients.[23] In the report from Sarkaria et al the median total operative time was 556 minutes (395–807).[28]

Our experience of 83 cases of robotic transthoracic esophagectomy showed that, with the use of robotic arms, we were able to achieve the mean lymph node yield of 18.36 (13–24). The total operating time of the procedure in our series was 204.94 minutes. The relatively low total operative time in our series was a result of increased experience in robotic surgery, a well-focused operating team, as well as nursing staff's familiarity with the procedures and equipment. The advantages of robotic system helped us to minimize operative time, blood loss and complications in our center.

CONCLUSION

The acceptance of MIS in esophageal cancer is increasing as more and more surgeons are gaining experience. The biggest advantage is avoiding thoracotomy. The quality of thoracoscopic esophagectomy is comparable to that of open esophagectomy. The morbidity in terms of lung complication is definitely low. TIME trial has conclusively shown an advantage of MIS over open surgery. A large multicentric trial is needed to prove a clear advantage of MIE over open esophagectomy.

REFERENCES

1. Nafteux P, Moons J, Coosemans W, Decaluwé H, Decker G, De Leyn P, et al. Minimally invasive oesophagectomy: a valuable alternative to open oesophagectomy for the treatment of early oesophageal and gastro-oesophageal junction carcinoma. Eur J Cardio-Thoracic Surg [Internet]. 2011 Apr [cited 2018 Jun 22];40(6):1455–63; discussion 1463–4. Available from: http://www.ncbi.nlm.nih.gov/pubmed/21514837

2. Verhage RJJ, Hazebroek EJ, Boone J, Van Hillegersberg R. Minimally invasive surgery compared to open procedures in esophagectomy for cancer: a systematic review of the literature. Minerva Chir [Internet]. 2009 Apr [cited 2018 Jun 22];64(2):135–46. Available from: http://www.ncbi.nlm.nih.gov/pubmed/19365314

3. Law S. Minimally invasive techniques for oesophageal cancer surgery. Best Pract Res Clin Gastroenterol [Internet]. 2006 Jan [cited 2018 Jun 22];20(5):925–40. Available from: http://www.ncbi.nlm.nih.gov/pubmed/16997170

4. Cuschieri A. Thoracoscopic subtotal oesophagectomy. Endosc Surg Allied Technol [Internet]. 1994 Feb [cited 2018 Jun 22];2(1):21–5. Available from: http://www.ncbi.nlm.nih.gov/pubmed/8081911

5. DePaula AL, Hashiba K, Ferreira EA, de Paula RA, Grecco E. Laparoscopic transhiatal esophagectomy with esophagogastroplasty. Surg Laparosc Endosc [Internet]. 1995 Feb [cited 2018 Jun 28];5(1):1–5. Available from: http://www.ncbi.nlm.nih.gov/pubmed/7735533

6. Avital S, Zundel N, Szomstein S, Rosenthal R. Laparoscopic transhiatal esophagectomy for esophageal cancer. Am J Surg [Internet]. 2005 Jul [cited 2018 Jun 28];190(1):69–74. Available from: http://www.ncbi.nlm.nih.gov/pubmed/15972176

7. Law S. Optimal Surgical Approach for Esophagectomy: The Debate Still Goes on? Transthoracic versus Transhiatal Resection. Ann Thorac Cardiovasc Surg [Internet]. 2009 [cited 2018 Jun 28];15(5). Available from: https://pdfs.semanticscholar.org/4421/dcda111a32dd0f808bca81ce916fd807fb7a.pdf

8. Luketich JD, Pennathur A, Awais O, Levy RM, Keeley S, Shende M, et al. Outcomes after minimally invasive esophagectomy: review of over 1000 patients. Ann Surg [Internet]. 2012 Jul [cited 2018 Jun 22];256(1):95–103. Available from: http://www.ncbi.nlm.nih.gov/pubmed/22668811

9. Smithers BM, Gotley DC, Martin I, Thomas JM. Comparison of the Outcomes Between Open and Minimally Invasive Esophagectomy. Ann Surg [Internet]. 2007 Feb [cited 2018 Jun 28];245(2):232–40. Available from: http://www.ncbi.nlm.nih.gov/pubmed/17245176

10. Nguyen NT, Roberts P, Follette DM, Rivers R, Wolfe BM. Thoracoscopic and laparoscopic esophagectomy for benign and malignant disease: lessons learned from 46 consecutive procedures. J Am Coll Surg [Internet]. 2003 Dec [cited 2018 Jun 28];197(6):902–13. Available from: http://www.ncbi.nlm.nih.gov/pubmed/14644277

11. Suzuki Y, Urashima M, Ishibashi Y, Abo M, Omura N, Nakada K, et al. Hand-assisted laparoscopic and thoracoscopic surgery (HALTS) in radical esophagectomy with three-field lymphadenectomy for thoracic esophageal cancer. Eur J Surg Oncol [Internet]. 2005 Dec [cited 2018 Jun 28];31(10):1166–74. Available from: http://www.ncbi.nlm.nih.gov/pubmed/16055298

12. Puntambekar S, Kenawadekar R, Pandit A, Nadkarni A, Joshi S, Agarwal G, et al. Minimally Invasive Esophagectomy in the Elderly. Indian J Surg Oncol 2013.

13. Puntambekar SP, Agarwal GA, Joshi SN, Rayate NV, Sathe RM, Patil AM. Thoraco-laparoscopy in the lateral position for esophageal cancer: the experience of a single institution with 112 consecutive patients. Surg Endosc [Internet]. 2010 Oct 5 [cited 2018 Jun 23];24(10):2407–14. Available from: http://www.ncbi.nlm.nih.gov/pubmed/20204415

14. Puntambekar SP, Rayate N, Joshi S, Agarwal G. Robotic transthoracic esophagectomy in the prone position: Experience with 32 patients with esophageal cancer. J Thorac Cardiovasc Surg 2011.

15. Lv L, Hu W, Ren Y, Wei X. Minimally invasive esophagectomy versus open esophagectomy for esophageal cancer: a meta-analysis. Onco Targets Ther [Internet]. 2016 Oct [cited 2018 Jun 22];Volume 9:6751–62. Available from: http://www.ncbi.nlm.nih.gov/pubmed/27826201

16. Cuesta MA, Biere SSAY, van Berge Henegouwen MI, van der Peet DL. Randomised trial, Minimally Invasive Oesophagectomy versus open oesophagectomy for patients with resectable oesophageal cancer. Journal of Thoracic Disease 2012.

17. Chen B, Zhang B, Zhu C, Ye Z, Wang C, Ma D, et al. Modified McKeown minimally invasive esophagectomy for esophageal cancer: a 5-year retrospective study of 142 patients in a single institution. PLoS One [Internet]. 2013 [cited 2018 Jun 23];8(12):e82428. Available from: http://www.ncbi.nlm.nih.gov/pubmed/24376537

18. Biere SS, van Berge Henegouwen MI, Maas KW, Bonavina L, Rosman C, Garcia JR, et al. Minimally invasive versus open oesophagectomy for patients with oesophageal cancer: a multicentre, open-label, randomised controlled trial. Lancet [Internet]. 2012 May 19 [cited 2018 Aug 4];379(9829):1887–92. Available from: http://www.ncbi.nlm.nih.gov/pubmed/22552194

19. Kubo N, Ohira M, Yamashita Y, Sakurai K, Toyokawa T, Tanaka H, et al. The impact of combined thoracoscopic and laparoscopic surgery on pulmonary complications after radical esophagectomy in patients with resectable esophageal cancer. Anticancer Res [Internet]. 2014 May [cited 2018 Aug 4];34(5):2399–404. Available from: http://www.ncbi.nlm.nih.gov/pubmed/24778050

20. Avital S, Zundel N, Szomstein S, Rosenthal R. Laparoscopic transhiatal esophagectomy for esophageal cancer. Am J Surg [Internet]. 2005 Jul [cited 2018 Aug 4];190(1):69–74. Available from: http://www.ncbi.nlm.nih.gov/pubmed/15972176

21. Wang B, Z Z, Qiu CH, Du B, Gao Y, Gao Y. The comparison of thoracoscopic‑laparoscopic esophagectomy and open esophagectomy: A meta‑analysis. Indian J Cancer 2017;115.

22. Sgourakis G, Gockel I, Radtke A, Musholt TJ, Timm S, Rink A, et al. Minimally Invasive Versus Open Esophagectomy: Meta-Analysis of Outcomes. Dig Dis Sci [Internet]. 2010 Nov 26 [cited 2018 Jun 22];55(11):3031–40. Available from: http://www.ncbi.nlm.nih.gov/pubmed/20186484

23. van Hillegersberg R, Boone J, Draaisma WA, Broeders IAMJ, Giezeman MJMM, Rinkes IHMB. First experience with robot-assisted thoracoscopic esophagolymphadenectomy for esophageal cancer. Surg Endosc Other Interv Tech [Internet]. 2006 Sep 15 [cited 2018 Jun 22];20(9):1435–9. Available from: http://www.ncbi.nlm.nih.gov/pubmed/16703427

24. Kernstine KH. The first series of completely robotic esophagectomies with three-field lymphadenectomy: initial experience. Surg Endosc [Internet]. 2008 Sep 18 [cited 2018 Jun 22];22(9):2102. Available from: http://link.springer.com/10.1007/s00464-008-9959-z

25. Cerfolio RJ, Bryant AS, Hawn MT. Technical aspects and early results of robotic esophagectomy with chest anastomosis. J Thorac Cardiovasc Surg [Internet]. 2013 Jan [cited 2018 Jun 22];145(1):90–6. Available from: http://www.ncbi.nlm.nih.gov/pubmed/22910197

26. Galvani C, Gorodner M, Moser F et al. Robotically assisted laparoscopic transhiatal esophagectomy. Surgical endoscopy 2008;22(1):188–95.

27. Dunn DH, Johnson EM, Morphew JA, Dilworth HP, Krueger JL, Banerji N. Robot-assisted transhiatal esophagectomy: a 3-year single-center experience. Dis Esophagus [Internet]. 2013 Feb [cited 2018 Jun 22];26(2):159–66. Available from: http://www.ncbi.nlm.nih.gov/pubmed/22394116

28. Sarkaria IS, Rizk NP, Finley DJ, Bains MS, Adusumilli PS, Huang J, et al. Combined thoracoscopic and laparoscopic robotic-assisted minimally invasive esophagectomy using a four-arm platform: experience, technique and cautions during early procedure development†. Eur J Cardio-Thoracic Surg [Internet]. 2013 May [cited 2018 Jun 22];43(5):e107–15. Available from: http://www.ncbi.nlm.nih.gov/pubmed/23371971

29. Park S, Hwang Y, Lee HJ, Park IK, Kim YT, Kang CH. Comparison of robot-assisted esophagectomy and thoracoscopic esophagectomy in esophageal squamous cell carcinoma. J Thorac Dis. 2016.

11

Postoperatiave Care, Complications and Management

RK Deshpande, Tanveer Abdul Majeed, Prriya Espuniyani

INTRODUCTION

Esophagectomy irrespective of approaches used is an operation associated with physiological violation of two body cavities (thorax and abdomen) and occasionally the neck, disrupting various internal systems, i.e. pulmonary, cardiovascular, fluid and electrolyte compartments and also body's protective mechanisms (cough reflex, albumin synthesis and bone marrow response). This can result in severe side effects and complications further aggravated by existing comorbidities. It encompasses wide field radical mediastinal dissection causing excessive shift of fluids between intracellular and extracellular compartments, worsened if thoracic duct is ligated. Morbidities up to 70% and mortality from 0 to 22% have been reported, while studies by Metzer and Rodgers have clearly shown the successful effect of well-oiled machineries of structured execution of this exercise resulting into reduced mortality by experienced esophageal surgery centers from 18% (<5 cases per year) to <5% (>20 cases per year). A careful pretherapy evaluation, optimization (cessation of smoking and incentive spirometry), selection of patients, appropriate approach and surgery diligently performed (minimizing blood loss, preventing recurrent nerve injury, fracture of ribs) enables the post-operative course to be smoother with superior outcomes. Recent advent of minimally invasive surgery has decreased the incidence of pulmonary complications (by 20%), intensive care stay, ventilatory time[1] and has shown a trend towards better survival as compared to open esophagectomy. Despite all precautions and experiences that one brings to bear in esophageal surgery, the medical team has to contend and deal with the problems ranging from anastomotic breakdowns, pneumonias to arrhythmias the worst being complication of esophageal leaks. The incidence of esophageal leaks as reported ranges from 10 to 44%[2,3] or as low as 2% or even 0%[4,5] in experienced hands. Currently in most centers of excellence, dehiscence rate of around 5% is well acceptable, early diagnosis and effective management is the key as most of these patients are salvageable.

Perioperative Care

Perioperative care of patients undergoing esophagectomy should be individualized as intraoperative course influences morbidity, mortality and outcomes. Postoperative monitoring for the first 1–2 days in surgical ICU of vital signs, with a possible ventilator support for first 12 hours in deserving patients, intake output chart, raised position while nursing for better respiratory care, initial nutrition maintenance through the intravenous route and the use of nasogastric tube/jejunostomy feeds are followed in some centers. A radiologic study from 5th to 9th day confirming a good anastomotic healing and gastric emptying when oral feeds are started in a gradual manner, graduating to full diet within 2 weeks of surgery is the usual protocol in most centers. All the while respiratory toilet and careful monitoring to rule out complications–respiratory, cardiac/vascular or anastomotic is essential. The relationship of intraoperative anesthetic management and postoperative outcomes is clearly established,[6,7] hence preoperative optimization is the key to successful outcome.

Cardiovascular Considerations in Esophageal Surgery

Arrhythmias: Intraoperative and early postoperative arrhythmias are commonly seen during esophageal resections possibly due to manipulation in the pericardiac area and due to vagal resection. The supraventricular and ventricular ectopics are seen in 30 to 65% patients undergoing transhiatal esophagectomy.[8] These are usually transient requiring no treatment; however, persistent atrial fibrillation is the most common form of arrhythmia (30%) seen in the postoperative period.[9] This is often associated with severe morbidity and poor survival.[10] Atrial fibrillation usually responds to antiarrhythmic medications and electrolyte correction.

Hypotension: About 20% decrease in systolic blood pressure from baseline just prior to start of mediastinal dissection of esophagectomy[8] is commonly seen (75%) and is usually transient. The combination of hypotension and arrhythmias adversely affects outcomes and is to be recognized and treated early, however transient arrhythmias and hypotension revert to normal once the offending agent (surgeons hand in the mediastinum) is removed. Patients on long-term beta-blockers need special protection from prolonged hypotension to avoid neurological complications.

Pulmonary Considerations During Esophageal Surgery

Preoperative pulmonary function has a very significant bearing in deciding treatment approaches for esophageal resections. A poor pulmonary function test reflected by low FVC and FEV1 with anatomical alterations in spine, rib cage and chest wall is an absolute contraindication to transthoracic approach. Carbon monoxide diffusion testing is imperative in high-risk patients. Cessation of smoking and incentive spirometry play an important role in decreasing morbidities associated by facilitating early extubation, decreased ventilatory requirement, bronchoscopic lavage, hospital stay and reintubation. Although single lung ventilation is favored by most thoracic surgeons its use is associated with high fractional FiO_2 which aggravates atelectasis, decreased mucociliary clearance and diffuse alveolar damage,[11] a suitable alternative being both lung ventilation with decreased tidal volume and increase in respiratory rate thus maintaining constant respiratory minute volume and simultaneous use of low pressure CO_2 intrathoracic (8 mmHg) insufflation, all the while maintaining circulatory volume to avoid hypotension. Minimally invasive thoracic esophageal mobilization in prone position avoids lung deflation and improves pulmonary parameters.[12]

Early weaning off the ventilator is the key to reduce complications and early recovery, decreased intensive care stay, prevention of systemic inflammatory reaction and pneumonia. Intraoperative fluid restriction prevents excessive third spacing, thereby preventing pulmonary edema and promoting early extubation. Although early extubation is the key to successful outcomes postesophagectomy in certain situations elective ventilation is advocated especially after prolonged surgery, excessive blood–fluid loss with volume replacement , inability to restrict fluid intake intraoperatively (thoracic duct ligation and excessive mediastinal dissection) and poor respiratory efforts.

Fluid Management

Hyper-hydration increases pulmonary and cardiac complications during esophageal resections, hence fluid restriction plays an important role in intraoperative and post-operative management of patients under-going esophagectomy. Fluid overload can compound effects of excessive mediastinal dissection, impaired cough reflex, pain of thoracotomy, pulmonary edema, decreased cardiac index and left ventricular stroke work index and increased pulmonary vascular resistance leading to unstable cardiorespi-ratory period. Excess fluid intake leads to aggravating of unstable cardiac period and its sequelae, hence fluid restriction is of utmost importance. It is very difficult to formulate guidelines of adequate fluid therapy, but hemodynamic stability and urinary output of 1 ml/kg/hour, appears to be a reasonable surrogate marker[13] in monitoring these patients. A larger fluid and cumulative fluid balance in the early postoperative period is significantly associated with adverse surgical outcomes,[14] needing tracheostomy, broncho-scopic suctioning and extubation failure.

The use of pulmonary arterial catheter (Swan Ganz), formerly the gold standard for monitoring preload, afterload, contractility and tissue oxygenation, is now out dated due to its invasive nature and associated complications. It is now a common practice to rely on a central line for central venous pressure monitoring and an arterial line for monitoring blood pressure while watching adequate urine output.

Intraoperative bleeding is a rare phenomenon in experienced hands, occasionally seen during resection of locally advanced eso-phageal cancers (postneoadjuvant therapy) and may include azygous vein injury (0.6% incidence and 0.2% mortality)[15] and aortic injury. Aortic injuries are usually small at the site of esophageal perforators originating in the aorta and usually require suture ligation, however azygous vein injuries may necessi-tate suture ligation of azygous vein and corresponding feeding intercostal veins. Pulmonary artery and vein injuries are generally rare due to protection offered by the pericardium.

Miscellaneous Complication

Pain: Thoracic epidural analgesia has been shown to provide adequate postoperative analgesia and decreased respiratory compli-cations postesophagectomy.[16,17] Epidural analgesia is associated with decreased inci-dence of esophageal leaks by improving graft microcirculation and preventing anastomotic insufficiency.[18]

Recurrent Laryngeal Nerve Injury is a dreaded complication following esophagectomy and ranges from neuropraxia to neurotmesis with an incidence of 20% in inexperienced surgeons,[19] Unilateral injury presents with hoarseness and inability to cough out pulmonary secre-tions, it is an important factor linked with aspiration and pulmonary complication. Bilateral recurrent laryngeal nerve (RCLN) injury causes airway obstruction and may necessitate tracheostomy.[20]

Tracheal Injury is quite uncommon, with a similar incidence in both transthoracic and transhiatal esophagectomy.[21,22] It is usually detected intraoperatively, associated with a drop in airway circuit pressure.[22] If detected intraoperatively the endotracheal tube must be advanced beyond the injury site for ventilation under bronchoscopic or surgeons guidance followed by repair of the rent. A very important intraoperative measure is to place the vascularized gastric conduit in the posterior mediastinum to buttress the injury site. A tracheostomy is performed and these patients are extubated post-surgery. Positive pressure ventilation is a contraindication in these patients.

Intensive care stay: It is not unusual for an esophagectomy patient to have a prolonged intensive care unit stay. High-risk patients who need prolonged ventilatory support include—unstable patients, those with multiple comorbidities, third space leaks, RCLN injury and those requiring massive blood transfusions. Elective ventilation is restricted to indications mentioned previously however most patients are extubated within 24 hours after prior assessment, T piece trial and arterial blood gas monitoring. A low PaO_2 <65 mmHg and PCO_2 >45 and a low pH <7.33 is a frequent reason for elective or prolonged ventilation. Various factors ranging from low tissue perfusion, hypotension, ischemic tube, lactic acidosis, pulmonary edema, poor respiratory efforts due to sedative or severe pain and poor cardiac function are well-established factors responsible for elective ventilation.

Early Postoperative Care

Postextubation after ensuring adequate analgesia patient is encouraged to perform incentive spirometry and optimal chest physiotherapy. Tenacious and excessive sputum production is taken care of by N-acetyl cysteine nebulization. The role of early enteral feeding is well-established and our protocol includes inserting no 12 French tube in proximal jejunum (Witzel submucosal valvular) to be used in the early postoperative period till esophagogastric anastomoses is well-healed. The submucosal approach is used to prevent leakage and narrowing at the site of jejunostomy. It is our practice to start test jejunostomy feeds using 20 ml ringer lactate/ hour, which is followed by increasing feeds at regular intervals as per patient's tolerance. Important precaution is slow feeding by siphoning method thereby decreasing the osmotic load and preventing diarrhea. It is also important to prevent colonization of feeding bag to prevent infective diarrhea. Prophylaxis for deep venous thrombosis is equally important in

esophagectomy patients and usually ranges from use of pneumatic compression device to use of low molecular weight heparin. All post-esophagectomy patients are advised early mobilization usually from the second postoperative day. The anastomotic integrity is tested usually on the 7th postoperative day using Gastrografin CT scan. Conray 240 is not used due to risk of aspiration pneumonitis more so in patient with RCLN injury. If Gastrografin CT confirms good anastomotic integrity with no out-pouching and leak (Figs 11.1 and 11.2), no hold-up of dye in mediastinum (gastroparesis), adequate filling of small bowel and decreased ryles tube aspirate following the day after Gastrografin, ryles tube is removed and patient encouraged gradual oral feeds. In unusual circumstances, if the ryles tube accidently slips out in the early

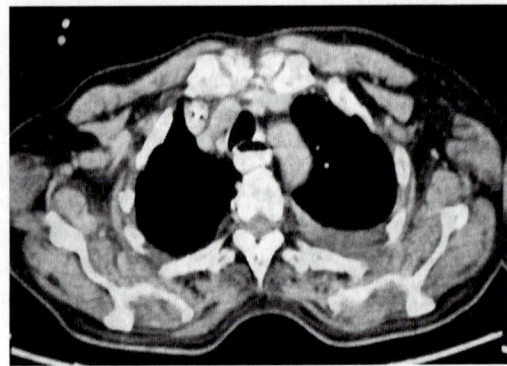

Fig. 11.1: Normal postesophagectomy CT Gastrografin study

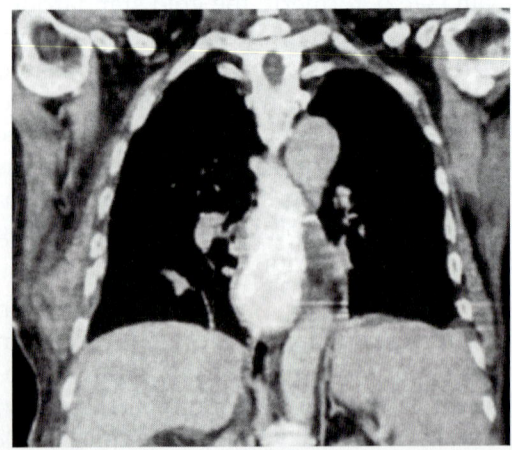

Fig. 11.2: Normal postesophagectomy CT Gastrografin study

postoperative period and if the mediastinum shows air fluid levels there is a high-risk of aspiration and in these circumstances ryles tube is reinserted under endoscopic guidance taking care not to insufflate air and aggravate anastomotic dehiscence.

Oral feeds are started once anastomotic integrity is well-established, small oral feeds (30 ml) is started every 2 hourly as pylorus takes time to regain function (in about 20%) and rapid feeding is associated with delayed emptying and a dilated stomach tube in the mediastinum, which is an important causal factor for aspiration pneumonia. Once pyloric emptying is normal a gradual increase in the quantum of fluid and initiation of small soft pureed diet is started by giving small frequent feeds every 3 hourly to maintain nutrition.

Complications of Esophageal Surgery

Esophagectomy is an operation associated with wide range of complications ranging from self-limiting atelectasis to florid pneumonia and major esophageal leaks necessitating major interventions. They are classified as Flowchart 11.1:

Irrespective of advancements of surgical technique, esophagectomy carries risk of severe complications and is associated with highest mortality rate, ranging from 3–22%,[2,3] among all elective gastrointestinal procedures. Important factors contributing to esophageal leaks include segmental esophageal blood supply, prone for ischemic necrosis, negative intrathoracic pressure which sucks the gastric fluid across the anastomoses preventing healing of the anastomoses, variations in intramural arterial vasculature of stomach tube distal to the last branch of right gastroepiploic artery,[23] anastomotic site edema due to associated inflammatory response, absence of circular muscle-serosa leading to insufficient strength and poor healing. The key to successful outcomes are early recognition of complications followed by prompt interventions. Cardiopulmonary complications are rare; most pulmonary complications, both minor and major, are secondary to a small, self-healing anastomotic disruption, recurrent laryngeal nerve injury and aspiration pneumonia. A major bronchopneumonia, collapse and hydropneumothorax are all secondary to major anastomotic dehiscence and this must be proven by contrast imaging and endoscopic evaluation of gastric conduits.

Flowchart 11.1: Complications of esophagectomy

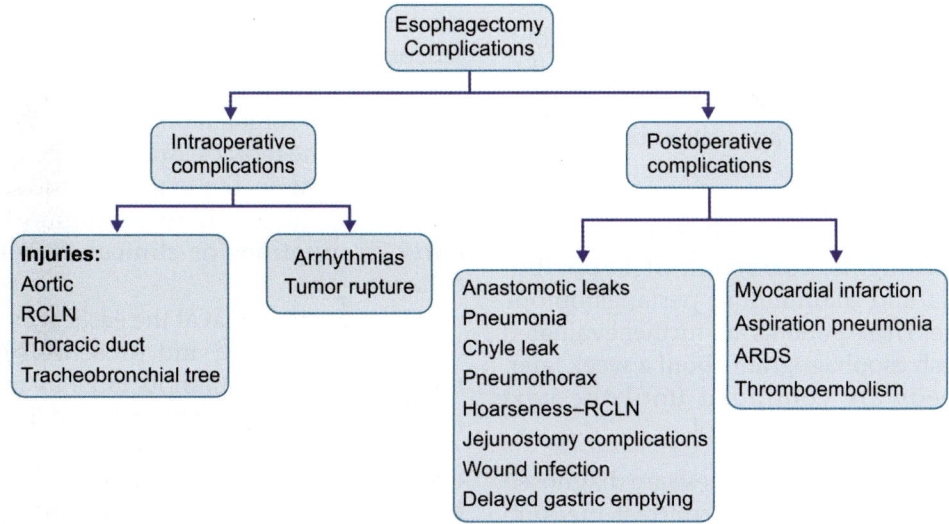

Anastomotic leaks which occur in post-esophagectomy patients are associated with very high mortality (40%),[2,3] if early interventions are not taken. Hence, a high degree of suspicion is necessary for diagnosing post-esophagectomy leaks. The incidence of cervical leaks and thoracic leaks are (10–25% cervical) and (3–25% thoracic) respectively with an associated mortality ranging from 10–60%.[24–27] Esophageal leak management is bereft of uniformity in management, ranging from aggressive surgical approach to conservative management comprising of perianastomotic drainage, nasogastric decompression, maintaining adequate nutrition and prolonged antibiotic therapy, however the use of self-expandable metal stents (SEMS) and metal clips is emerging in the recent times.[28]

Classification of Anastomotic Leaks and Management (Lerut)[29]

Grading	Definition
I Radiological	Subclinical leakage
II Minor clinical	Wound inflammation or leakage of contrast agent, fever, leukocytosis
III Major clinical	Sepsis
IV Conduit necrosis	Necrosis of bowel—(endoscopically confirmed)

Type I: It is usually diagnosed on routine postoperative esophagogram which confirms outpouching in an otherwise clinically stable patient. The "Radiologic outpouching" is due to slight asymmetric apposition between the esophagus and the substituted segment (stomach or colon). The management consists of delaying the onset of oral feeds, antibiotics and antifungals, correction of hypoalbuminemia and maintaining perianastomotic drainage. These patients are further evaluated with fresh esophagogram about a week later. Oral feeds are continued until the next negative radiological control.

Type II (Minor Clinical): These are diagnosed incidentally, when a thin contrast medium (Conray) is given before starting oral feeds. A thin streak of outpouching or a linear streak in the mediastinum is the commonest finding; often this streak empties out into the anastomotic area and into the stomach. Patients are generally asymptomatic, however mild bronchospasm, fever with leukocytosis are not uncommon. The management guidelines include that of Type I, in addition opening of surgical wound and drainage. It is mandatory to classify the leak by performing a contrast enhanced (intravenous and oral) CT scan thorax with Gastrografin/thin dilute barium and ruling out Type III and IV leaks as the outcome for these are invariably associated with delay in the onset of treatment.

Type III (Major Clinical): It is a common type of dehiscence and occurs during the same postoperative period (between 4 and 8 days). Stomach necrosis is the commoner site; occasionally, the sutured lesser curvature of the stomach gives way. Rarely, there can be a complete failure to heal at the anastomotic site.

The symptoms which should arouse suspicion to achieve an early diagnosis of this complication are a moderate spike in temperature, bronchospasm in not a known asthmatic, mild dyspnea for no apparent reason and persistent tachycardia. Generally, the cardiovascular profile is stable, though the leucocyte count shows an upward trend with high procalcitonin and chest X-ray showing patchy pneumonitis along with hydropneumothorax. The thoracic drain may or may not show increase in the exudates and auscultation of the lungs will reveal diminished air entry, crepitations or clinical evidence of collapse.

It is imperative that at the earliest evidence of clinical suspicion and presence of signs mentioned above, attempts must be made to prove or disprove a suture line dehiscence. As mentioned earlier CT esophagogram using Gastrografin/thin barium along with contrast CT scan chest are of utmost importance

(Figs 11.3 and 11.4), especially more in an unstable patient. Larger leaks with major clinical manifestations (grade 3) and conduit necrosis (grade 4) require immediate surgical intervention.[30,31] CT-guided drainage of an intrathoracic leak or an abscess may be used temporarily to allow decompression of the abscess cavity and clinical stabilization before surgical repair,[32] and can also be used for management of mediastinal collections and pneumothorax.[33] Generally, if a good lung expansion is ensured, the stomach segment is well-decompressed, nutrition can be effectively maintained by a jejunostomy or parenteral hyperalimentation and if the patient does not show any significant

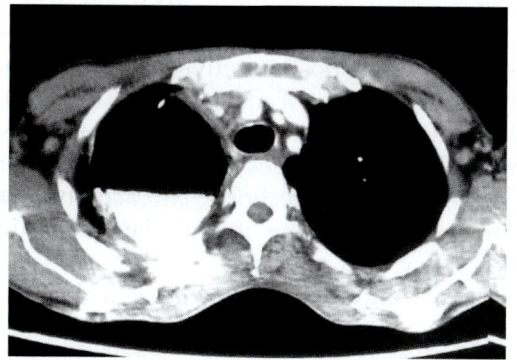

Fig. 11.3: Postesophagectomy CT Gastrografin showing esophageal leak with spillage in the right pleural cavity (Type III) leak

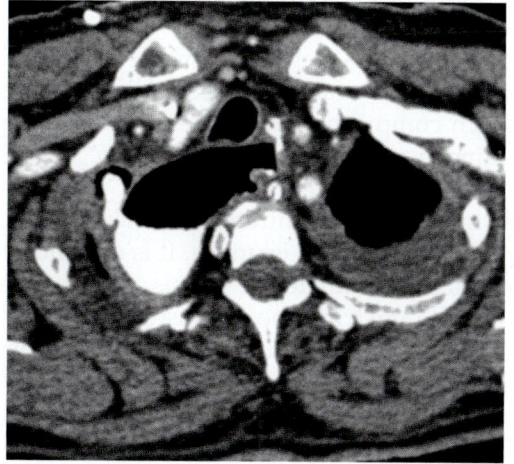

Fig. 11.4: Postesophagectomy CT Gastrografin showing site of esophageal leak (Type III) leak

evidence of septicemia, nearly all patients can be salvaged by conservative approach. The breakdown will heal in about 10 to 14 days during which the patient needs to be supported with appropriate and adequate antibiotics, physiotherapy, etc. Generally ventilatory supports are not indicated in this group of patients unless the PaO_2, pCO_2 levels continues to be abnormal. The chest picture will rapidly improve, pyrexia will settle and the overall clinical condition will steadily get better. A repeat Conray study can be done after two weeks and once the anastomosis has healed, oral intake can be gradually started. About 1/3rd patients will deteriorate within 24 to 48 hours after diagnosis. Thoracotomy aims to efficiently drain infected or loculated pockets and ensure complete lung expansion with adequate pleural drainage. Nutritional support is of utmost importance in management and may range from parenteral hyperalimentation to jejunostomy feeding.

Type IV (Conduit Necrosis): Usually occurs between the 4th and 8th postoperative day. The patient rapidly deteriorates with a breakdown of cardiopulmonary function with signs and symptoms of bronchospasm, shock, collapse and dyspnea, X-ray studies may reveal pneumothorax or collapse of the lung with pleural fluid; thoracic drain may or may not show sudden increase in drainage.

Immediate management will require urgent resuscitative measures, a thoracotomy for rapid evacuation of infected material from the chest with appropriate drains, ensure expansion of the lung, adequate antibiotic therapy, restoration of normovolemic state and ventilatory support as indicated. It is futile to re-anastomose disrupted necrotic ends and the stomach tube needs to be disconnected and brought out as a gastrostomy for feeding and fashion a cervical esophagostomy till a retrosternal substitution is carried out 3 or 4 weeks later when the patient settles. In 8 major disruptions, 6 (75%) were salvaged by adopting such quick, intensive surgical measures. A fatality is always at hand if such aggressive management is not instituted as an emergency measure.

Prevention of Anastomotic leaks[34]

1. Avoid excessive mobilization of proximal esophagus as excessive mobilized esophagus is prone for ischemia due to segmental blood supply of esophagus.
2. Removal of the distal inadequately perfused fundus of stomach.
3. Removal of excessive fundic area of stomach, responsible for acid secretion.
4. Avoid excessive handling and kneading of stomach tube to prevent hematoma formation.
5. Ensure adequate nutrition for prompt healing.
6. Check for adequacy of thoracic inlet and diaphragmatic hiatus.

Pulmonary complications, which are usually secondary to esophageal leaks, account for two-thirds of postoperative deaths.[3] As mentioned earlier any significant pulmonary complication (bronchospasm, collapse, pleural effusion, pneumothorax or bronchopneumonic patches) are all secondary to anastomotic breakdowns of Type I or Type II. Literature review,[35] of patient losses, reported due to pulmonary complications are mostly cases of undiagnosed anastomotic dehiscence. Based on our experiences, these are all salvageable. Very rarely a primary lung complication like collapse due to sputum retention or emphysema may occur because of a compromised lung function due to chronic tobacco usage. One important consideration is injury to the recurrent laryngeal nerve, which leads to inadequate tracheobronchial drainage due to inability to expel the sputum and leading to pulmonary complications. Elective tracheobronchial toileting and vigorous physiotherapy is the key to prevention, in these patients.

Cardiac: Less than 5% of patients suffer from major postoperative cardiac problems.

Surgery for esophageal cancer severely tests the patient's cardiopulmonary status. Pre surgical work-up and management should prevent this complication. Once diagnosed, effective measures should be instituted after a cardiac consultation. Hypervolemia or hypovolemia during the first 48 hours can become a problem, if adequate care is not taken in monitoring fluid therapy. Routine measurement of central venous pressure and diligently maintained cumulative fluid balance are specific preventive measures.

Chylothorax is a rare complication of esophagectomy and results due to thoracic duct injury more so in locally advanced middle third lesions and has an incidence of 1 to 5%.[36] If recognized intraoperatively thoracic duct can be ligated and clipped, however in the postoperative period thoracic duct injury can be a major cause of concern due to its associated decrease of lymphocytes, nutritional deficiencies and may eventually lead to systemic infections. Thoracoscopic or transthoracic clipping of injured duct may be necessary in patients associated with refractory and high volume chyle leak.

Herniation of the transverse colon and small bowel through the esophageal hiatus is a known complication very rarely seen, such patients present with acute intestinal obstruction and are usually diagnosed on contrast enhanced CT scan and need emergency intervention. A very tight hiatus opening is an important factor for esophageal leaks, which compromises the arterial and venous drainage of the right gastroepiploic vessels. A very lax hiatus is a cause of intestinal obstruction due to intrathoracic herniation of transverse colon or jejunum. It is our routine practice to evaluate the hiatus after railroading the gastric tube in posterior mediastinum. Rarely jejunostomy intussusception and volvulus is seen which needs operative intervention after appropriate imaging for diagnosis-usually a contrast enhanced CT scan of the abdomen.

Gastroparesis with delayed gastric emptying is seen in about 10% patients undergoing esophagectomy.[36] Vagotomy causes gastric paresis and inability of the pylorus to relax due to incoordinated and impaired gastric peristalsis. It is our routine practice to perform pyloromyotomy for all esophagectomy. These patients usually present with dilated gastric tube in the mediastinum with increased nasogastric aspirate, X-ray Gastrografin usually clinches the diagnosis (Fig. 11.5), and conservative measures such as use of prokinetics, prolonged nasogastric drainage and delayed oral feeding are usually sufficient. Occasionally these patients may require endoscopic balloon dilatation.

Anastomotic strictures have been reported ranging from 9 to 48%,[37] and are most common sequelae of healed anastomotic leaks. Diagnosis is based on imaging and endoscopic evaluation. Rarely, they can be associated with recurrent disease where biopsy may become mandatory. They are usually treated by endoscopic dilatation. Placement of the gastric conduit in retrosternal or subcutaneous planes can make dilatation difficult due to their tortuous planes.

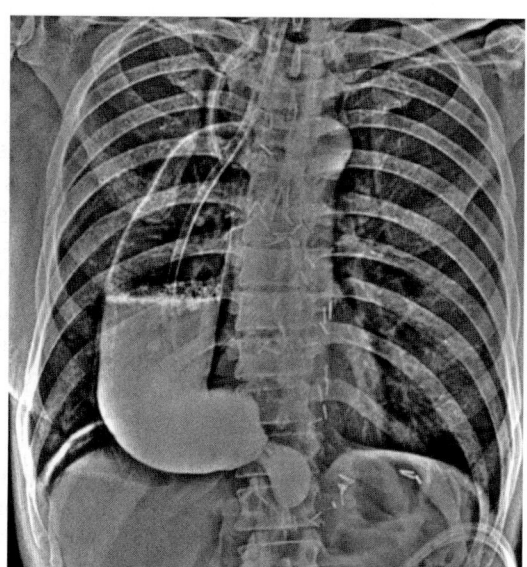

Fig. 11.5: Postesophagectomy gastroparesis

Antibiotic Therapy

In a study carried out at Tata Memorial Centre in 1993[38] antibiotics beyond 48 hours after a clean contaminated thoracic procedure is unwarranted. Patients with a large ulcerated fungating growth are prone to septicemia (Primary esophageal Sepsis—due to colonization of esophageal growth by various endogenous bacteria and yeast). The postoperative course of patients with Primary esophageal sepsis is stormy and associated with very poor outcomes. They usually respond to third generation cephalosporins, ureidopenicillins and carbapenems along with metronidazole in the immediate pre and postoperative periods.

Long-Term Sequelae of Esophagectomy

1. Esophagogastric resection results in loss of at least 40% of stomach capacity, loss of lower esophageal sphincter mechanism as gastroesophageal junction is resected and stomach is in the mediastinum instead of the abdominal cavity hence these patients are prone for aspiration pneumonia. They are advised to sleep with head end of bed elevated-45 degrees, small frequent feeds after every 4–6 hours and not to lie down at least 2 hours after eating feeds as a preventive measure for aspiration pneumonia.
2. Loss of intrinsic factor due to loss of fundic part of stomach, hence more prone for vitamin B_{12} deficiency, hence they are advised vitamin B_{12} supplementation every monthly.

Surgery for Palliation

The treatment of choice for majority of patients of squamous cell cancer of the esophagus which are resectable ($T_{1-3}N_1$) is surgery. Those beyond this stage are best treated by alternative methods (chemotherapy, radiotherapy, laserization, esophageal stenting, etc). Despite these alternative methods there will remain a core of cases where salvage surgery to restore deglutition will be indicated. The common examples are severe radiation fibrosis not amenable to dilatation and problems with prosthetic intubation at a higher level. In such a clinical setting if the patient's general condition is still good and no distant disease is documented, palliative surgical resection of the primary lesion may be considered. If the local tumor status precludes any excision, the lesion could be bypassed retrosternally.

REFERENCES

1. Miguel A Cuesta, Surya SAY Biere, et. al. Randomised trial, Minimally Invasive Esophagectomy versus open esophagectomy for patients with resectable oesophageal cancer. J Thorac Dis 2012;4(5):462–4.

2. Schieman C, Wigle DA, Deschamps C, et al. Patterns of operative mortality following esophagectomy. Dis Esophagus 2012;25(7):645–51.

3. Raymond D. Complications of esophagectomy. Surg Clin North Am 2012;92(5):1299–313.

4. Mathison DB, et al. "Transthoracic Esophagectomy—A safe approach to cancer of the Esophagus." Ann Th Surg 1988;45:137.

5. Ellis FH, Gibbs SP, et al."Esophago-Gastrectomy—A safe widely applicable and expeditious form of palliation for patients with cancer of the Esophagus & cardia." Ann Surg 1983;198:534–40.

6. Ng JM. Perioperative anaesthetic management for esophagectomy. Anesthesiol Clin 2008;26(2):293–304.

7. Orringer MB, Marshall B, Iannettoni MD. Transhiatal Esophagectomy for treatment of benign and malignant Esophageal disease. World J Surg 2001;25(2):196–203.

8. Williams VA, Watson TJ, et al. Esophagectomy for high grade dysplasia is safe, curative and results in good alimentary outcome. J Gastrointestinal Surg 2007;11(12):1589–97.

9. Hahm TS, Lee JJ, Yang MK, Kim JA. Risk factors for an intraoperative arrhythmias during esophagectomy. Yonsei Med J 2007;48(3):474–9.

10. Ma JY, Wang Y, Zhao YF, Wu Z, et al. Atrial fibrillation after surgery for Esophageal carcinoma: Clinical and prognostic significance. World J Gastroenterology 2007;12(13):449–52.

11. Tisdale JE, Wroblewski HA, Wall DS, et al. A randomized , controlled study of amiodarone for prevention of atrial fibrillation after transthoracic esophagectomy. J Thoracic Cardiovascular Surgery 2010;140(1):45–51.

12. Kita T, Mammoto T, Kishi Y. Fluid management and post-operative respiratory disturbances in patients with transthoracic esophagectomy for Carcinoma. J Clin Anesthe 2002;14(4):252–6.

13. Yap FH, Lau JY, Jyont GM, et al. Early extubation after transthoracic esophagectomy Hong Kong Med J 2003;9(2):98–102.

14. Holte K, Kehlet H. Fluid therapy and surgical outcomes in elective surgery: Need for reassessment in fast track surgery. J Am Coll Surg 2006; 202(6):971–89.

15. Michelet P, Roch A, D Journo XB, et al. Effect of thoracic epidural analgesia on gastric blood flow after esophagectomy . Acta Anesthesiol Scand 2007;51(5):587–94.

16. Lanuti M, Delva PE, Maher A, et al. Feasibility and outcomes of an early extubation policy after esophagectomy. Ann Thorac Surg 2006;82(6); 2037–41.

17. Safranek PM, Cubitt J, Booth MI. Review of open and minimally access approaches to esophagectomy for cancer. Br J Surg 2010;97(12):1845–53.

18. Lazar G, Kaszaki J, Abraham S, Horvath G, et al. Thoracic epidural anaesthesia improves gastric microcirculation during experimental gastric tube formation. Surgery 2003;134(5):799–805.

19. Gupta V, Gupta R, Thingam SK, et al. Major airway injury during esophagectomy: Experience at a tertiary care center. J Gastrointestinal Surg 2009;13(3):438–41.

20. Wright CD, Zeitels SM. Recurrent laryngeal nerve injuries after esophagectomy. Thorac Surg Clin 2006;16(1):23–33.

21. Brown MJ, Kor DJ, Allen MS, et al. Dual epidural catheter technique and perioperative outcomes after Ivor Lewis esophagectomy. Reg Anesth Pain Med 2013;38(1):3–8.

22. Hulscher JB, Tjissen JG, Obertop H. Transthoracic versus transhiatal resection for carcinoma of the Esophagus: a metanalyses. Ann Thorac Surg 2001;72(1):306–13.

23. J̈org Zehetner, Steven R DeMeester, Evan T Alicuben, et al. Intraoperative Assessment of Perfusion of the Gastric Graft and Correlation With Anastomotic Leaks After Esophagectomy. Annals of Surgery, 2015;262(1):74–8.

24. Orringer MB, Marshall B, et al. Transhiatal eso-phagectomy Clinical experience and refinement. Ann Surg 1999;230:392–400.

25. Urshel JD. Esophagogastrostomy anastomotic leaks complicating esophagectomy: A review. Am J Surg 1995;169(6):634–40.

26. Whooley BP, Law S, et al. Critical appraisal of the significance of intrathoracic anastomotic leakage after esophagectomy for cancer. Am J Surg 2001;181(3):198–203.

27. Sauvanet A, Baltar J, et al. Diagnosis and conser-vative management of intrathoracic leakage after esophagectomy. Br J Surgery 1998; 85:1446–9.

28. Mohammed A Qadeer, John A, et al. Endoscopic clips for closing Esophageal perforation. Gastro-intestinal Endoscopy 2007;66(3):605–10.

29. Lerut T, Coosemans W, Decker G, De Leyn P, Nafteux P, van Raemdonck D. Anastomotic complications after esophagectomy. Dig Surg 2002;19(2):92–8.

30. Cassivi SD. Leaks, strictures, and necrosis: A review of anastomotic complications following esophagectomy. Semin Thorac Cardiovasc Surg 2004;16(2):124–32.

31. Stefano Cafarotti, Alfred Cesario, Venanzio-Porziella, et al. Post esophagectomy anastomotic leaks. Ann Ital Chir 2013;84:137–41.

32. Maher MM, Lucey BC, Boland G, Gervais DA, Mueller PR. The role of interventional radiology in the treatment of mediastinal collections caused by Esophageal anastomotic leaks. AJR Am J Roentgenol 2002;178(3):649–53.

33. LeBedis CA, Penn DR, Uyeda JW, Murakami AM, Soto JA, Gupta A. The diagnostic and therapeutic role of imaging in postoperative complications of Esophageal surgery. Semin Ultrasound CT MR 2013;34(4):288–98.

34. Ke - Neng Chen. Managing Complications: leaks, strictures, emptying, reflux, chylothorax. J Thorac Dis 2014;6(S3):S355–63.

35. Patrick Lozach, Phillipe Topart. "Ivor-Lewis procedure for epidermoid cancer of the eso-phagus. A series of 264 patients"—Seminar Surg Oncology 1997;13:238–44.

36. Paul S, Bueno R. Complications following esophagectomy: Early detection, treatment, and prevention. Semin Thorac Cardiovasc Surg 2003;15(2):210–5.

37. Park JY, Song HY, Kim JH, et al. Benign anasto-motic strictures after esophagectomy: Long-term effectiveness of balloon dilation and factors affecting recurrence in 155 patients. Am J Roentgenol 2012;198(5):1208–13.

38. Bhansali M, Badwe R, et al. Randomised trial for duration of antibiotic prophylaxis in clean thoracic surgery. An interim report. Indian J Surgery 1993;55:589–94.

12

Chemotherapy for Esophageal Cancer

Suresh Advani

Esophageal cancer (EC) is the eighth most common cancer responsible for 450000 deaths per year worldwide.[1] Despite recent advances in surgical, medical and radiation treatment, the outcome of Esophageal cancer (EC) remains dismal with 5 years survival ranging from 15–25%.[2,3] Esophageal cancer manifest as adenocarcinoma in Caucasians associated with obesity, gastroesophageal reflux disease (GERD) and Barrett's esophagus. Squamous cell carcinoma of esophagus is dominant in Asians mainly related to smoking and alcohol consumption. Both histology exhibit equally poor outcome.[4]

Surgery alone may be enough for an early stage EC; however, survival has not improved as most patients die due to either local recurrence or distant metastasis after surgery. Data confirms occurrence of early micro-metastasis even before the clinical diagnosis is made.[5] Also, 50% of patients with esophageal cancer have overt metastatic disease at diagnosis and need systemic treatment with chemotherapy. It is evident that chemotherapy has to be integrated in early stage as well as locally advanced disease and metastatic esophageal cancer. Today, trimodality therapy has become standard treatment in controlling both metastatic and local disease.[6] Chemotherapy, therefore, has

to be used at different stages during the treatment for EC as indicated below.

- **Adjuvant chemotherapy:** After surgery in order to control and hopefully eradicate micrometastasis which is generally present in most cases beyond stage I disease. It has not significantly improved survival in EC.
- **Neoadjuvant chemotherapy/chemoradio-therapy:** Chemotherapy is given alone or with radiation before surgery to control micrometastasis and to shrink the primary cancer.
- **Chemotherapy for advanced esophageal cancer:** Chemotherapy is used in patients with disseminated disease to help shrink the tumor and relieve symptoms (Fig. 12.1).

Trimodality therapy in locally advanced disease with preoperative chemotherapy or chemoradiotherapy followed by surgery has resulted in improvement of disease control. Over last 2–3 decades, systemic chemotherapy has transformed from single agent chemo-therapy to combination chemotherapy to neo-adjuvant chemotherapy and concurrent chemoradiotherapy followed by surgery.

Single Agent Chemotherapy

Essentially, single agents effective in EC include older and newer agents. Broad range

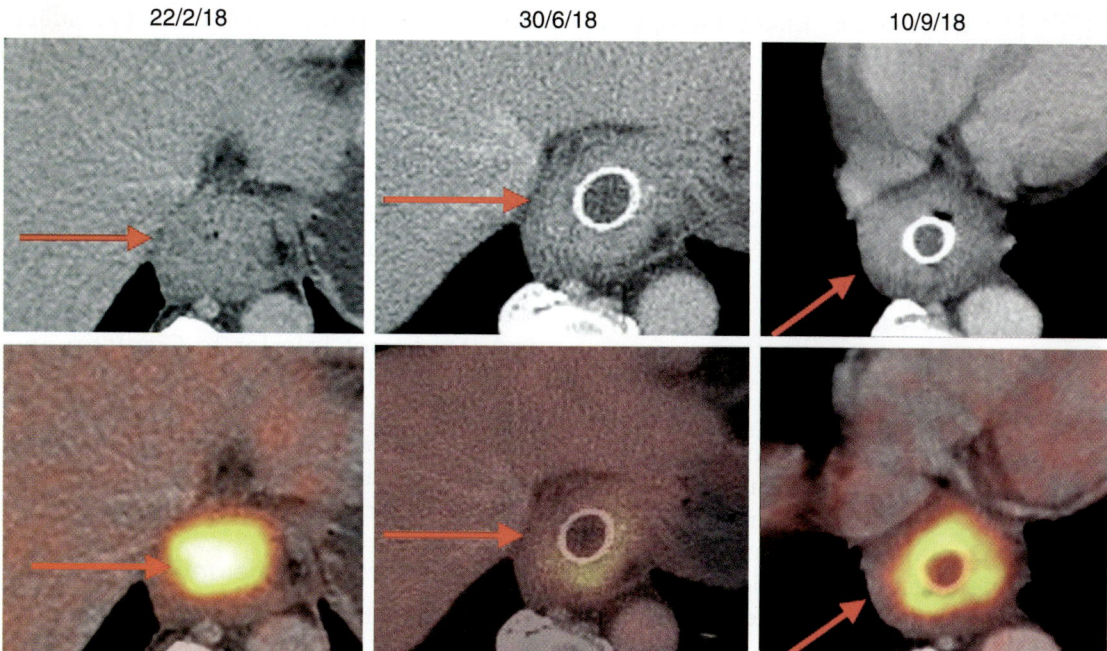

Fig. 12.1: 66-year-old male with mass lesion in the distal esophagus and FDG uptake in the PET-CT. PET-CT done at the time of diagnosis on 22/2/18, after 4 months of chemotherapy on 30/6/18 and finally after another 3 months on 10/9/18. The initial PET-CT shows a distal esophageal mass. Second PET-CT demonstrates a stent *in situ* with regression in the size of mass and FDG uptake. The third PET-CT demonstrates increase in the mass size and uptake indicating an initial response and subsequently a recurrence. (*Courtesy* Dr. Anirudh Kohli)

of single agent chemotherapy used in EC has produced mild antitumor response of short duration (Table 12.1). Among newer agents, Paclitaxel as single agent revealed response rate from 15–30%.[7] Similarly, Docetaxel has

Table 12.1	Single agent chemotherapy in esophageal cancer
Drug name	**Response rate**
5 Fluorouracil Bolus	5%
5 Fluorouracil Continuous Infusion	10%
Cisplatin	18%
Carboplatin	10%
Mitomycin	10%
Capecitabine	26%
Vinorelbine	15%
Vindesin	20%
Paclitaxel	15–30%
Docetaxel	20–25%
Etoposide	0–19%
Irinotecan	15%
Intermediate dose Methotrexate	50%

been evaluated at doses of 70 to 100 mg/m^2 with response rate of 20–25%.[8] Of course, hematologic toxicity was high with Grade 3 and 4 neutropenia. Oral Capecitabine mimicking continuous infusion of 5FU has shown response rate of 26% as seen in Japanese trials. The Topoisomerase I inhibitor (Etoposide) and Topoisomerase II inhibitor (Irinotecan) have also been evaluated with response rate of 19% and 15% respectively.[9]

Combination Chemotherapy

Combination chemotherapy was designed to improve the efficacy and reduce the chances of resistant disease (Table 12.2). Combination chemotherapy with Cisplatin along with infusional 5FU has consistently shown 40–50% response rate although associated with substantial but tolerable mucositis and myelosuppression.[10] In one study, Cisplatin, 5FU and Mitomycin combination produced 60% response rate. Epirubicin, Cisplatin and

Table 12.2	Combination chemotherapy in esophageal cancer	
Drugs		**Response rate**
Cisplatin and 5FU		42%
Carboplatin and Paclitaxel		44%
Epirubicin, Cisplatin and 5FU (ECF)		45%
Docetaxel, Cisplatin and 5FU (DCF)		54%
Methotrexate and Cisplatin		80%
Oxaliplatin and Capecitabine		40%
Irinotecan, 5FU and Cisplatin		26%
Irinotecan and Cisplatin		57%

5FU (ECF) having 3 drug combination by Royal Marsden Hospital resulted in better response rate of 45% as compared to Cisplatin and 5FU combination. Taxanes with substantial single agent activity did show further improvement with combination of Cisplatin and 5FU resulting in 46–50% response rate. Paclitaxel/Cisplatin with 5FU infusion achieved 50% response rate. Two drug combination of Paclitaxel and Cisplatin with G-CSF (Granulocyte-colony stimulating factor) support showed 44% response rate. Also Irinotecan and 5FU infusion showed 25 to 30% response rate. Similarly, Oxaliplatin and 5FU showed 40% response rate.

Paclitaxel in combination with Carboplatin also showed 54% response rate. Docetaxel along with Cisplatin and 5FU (DCF) resulted in higher, 36% response rate and longer time to progression. DCF regimen appears to be superior as compared to ECF. However, median survival improvement was marginal.[11] Combination of Irinotecan and infusional 5FU may represent active but better tolerated regimen as compared to 5FU and Cisplatin. Response rate of 40% was also observed with Oxaliplatin and Capecitabine and it was not inferior to Cisplatin and infusional 5FU. Combination of Irinotecan and Cisplatin resulted in 57% response in patients with adenocarcinoma and squamous cell carcinoma of esophagus. Irinotecan and 5FU has superior toxicity profile.

Neoadjuvant Chemotherapy

Majority of patients with operable EC present with locally bulky disease. The neoadjuvant chemotherapy consisting of either chemotherapy, radiation therapy or combination of these two have shown promising results (Table 12.3). Surgery, radiation and chemotherapy individually do not impact the survival in EC. The pattern of local and systemic failure highlights the need for complimentary modalities of treatments to prevent local recurrence and metastasis. Over the past 3 decades integration of surgical,

Table 12.3	Randomized clinical trials. (Surgery for esophageal cancers with and without neoadjuvant chemotherapy)			
			Overall survival rate	
Authors	**Trial**	**Drugs**	**Chemotherapy + Surgery**	**Surgery**
Boonstra[12]		Cisplatin, Etoposide	26%	17%
Allum WH, et al. (2009)[13]	European (OEO$_2$)	Cisplatin, 5FU	23%	17%
Kelsen DP, et al. (2007)[14]	North American (USA Intergroup 113)	Cisplatin, 5FU	20%	20%
Medical Research council esophageal group[15]		Cisplatin, 5FU	43%	24%
Cunningham D, et al. (2006)[16]	MAGIC	Cisplatin, 5FU	36%	23%
Ychou M, et al. (2011)[17]	FNCLCC/FFCD Multicenter phase III	Cisplatin, 5FU	38%	24%

radiation and systemic treatment has greatly improved the disease outcome. The effect of preoperative chemotherapy is confirmed by enhancing loco-regional disease control and eliminating micrometastasis. Preoperative Cisplatin based chemotherapy has been the choice of therapy for locally advanced esophageal cancer. Many trials have shown survival benefit of neoadjuvant chemotherapy in patients with operable EC without increasing postoperative complications.

Neoadjuvant chemotherapy alone appears to offer a limited benefit at best. A North American randomized trial[14] found that preoperative combination chemotherapy of Cisplatin and Fluorouracil did not improve overall survival among patients with squamous cell carcinoma or adenocarcinoma of the esophagus. In a larger trial, British investigators[13] found that preoperative chemotherapy with those two agents resulted in a 5 year survival rate of 23.0%, compared with 17.1% for surgery alone. Cunningham et al[16] in MAGIC trial showed 5 years survival 36.3% in preoperative chemotherapy as compared to 23% in surgery alone. FNCLCC[17] also reported 5 year overall survival of 38% in chemotherapy and surgery group compared to 24% in surgery alone. A meta-analysis on preoperative chemotherapy trials in esophageal cancers, including nine randomized comparisons of neoadjuvant chemotherapy versus surgery alone confirmed the advantage of better survival with neoadjuvant chemotherapy as compared to surgery alone. Also Cochrane review demonstrated longer overall survival with neoadjuvant chemotherapy. Few authors have shown that preoperative chemotherapy can downstage the disease and improve the survival and local recurrence rate. Advani et al[18] and Desai et al[19] have emphasized the role of neoadjuvant chemotherapy with high response rate using Cisplatin and Methotrexate combination in patients with proliferative growth in EC. Proliferative, non-infiltrating (even bulky size) types of lesions respond much better to chemoradiotherapy (including complete pathologic response) than the obstructive, infiltrative and stenosing (stricture) types of EC's. Surgery in this group should therefore be considered per primum, if feasible (Figs 12.2 to 12.4 and Table 12.4).

A review has also shown higher rate of R_0 resection following preoperative chemo-

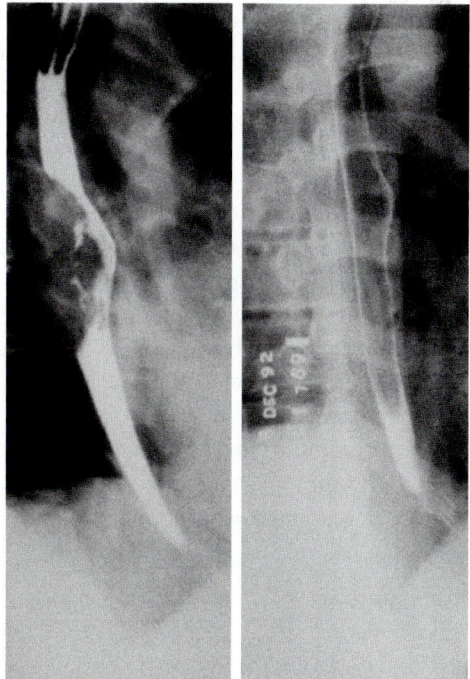

Fig. 12.2: Barium swallow of a patient with locally advanced proliferative lesion in the mid-esophagus showing very satisfactory response with chemoradiotherapy. Prolonged palliation extending to 4 years. Proliferative lesions respond well to chemo-radiotherapy. (*Courtesy* Dr. Praful Desai)

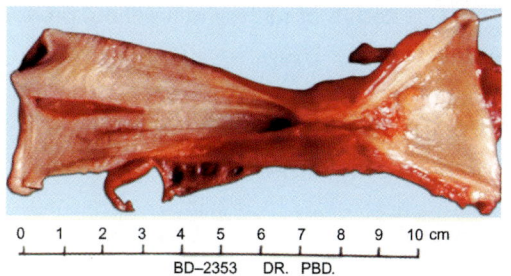

Fig. 12.3: Surgical specimen of a strictured lesion. These lesions respond poorly to chemoradiotherapy, hence these patients should be considered for surgery per primum, if feasible. (*Courtesy* Dr. Praful Desai)

Table 12.4 Chemotherapy/radiotherapy response in cancer esophagus

Type of lesion	N = 200	Responses			(%)
		CR	PR	NR	
Ulcerative: Stenotic, infiltrative	65	0	10	55	15
Proliferative	101	20	54	27	73* (CR/PR)
Ulceroproliferative	34	0	15	19	44

*p ≤0.02

CR: Complete response; PR: Partial response; NR: No response (*Desai et al. Personal series*)

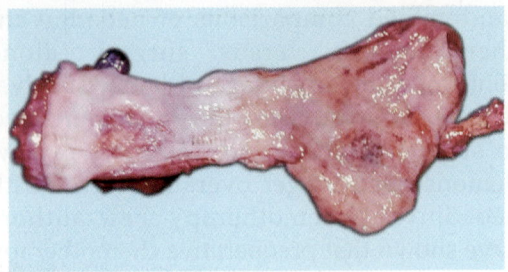

Fig. 12.4: Resected specimen of an esophageal carcinoma post chemoradiotherapy. Persistent residual disease which mandated surgery. (*Courtesy* Dr. Praful Desai)

therapy. A meta-analysis has also shown that preoperative chemotherapy for EC did not increase risk of perioperative mortality and postoperative morbidity. Overall, evidences favor preoperative chemotherapy over surgery alone.

Preoperative Chemoradiotherapy

Local and systemic relapse constitute most frequent reasons for failure of therapy. The use of preoperative radiotherapy followed by surgery or surgery alone showed no benefit of radiotherapy. Logically, neoadjuvant radiotherapy along with neoadjuvant chemotherapy is expected to increase local control of disease thus taking care of local relapses and metastatic disease by radiotherapy and chemotherapy respectively (Table 12.5). Use of concurrent chemoradiotherapy also reduces the bulk of primary tumor before surgery to facilitate higher curative resection. Preoperative chemoradiotherapy consists of radiotherapy (45 Gy) and chemotherapy with Cisplatin and 5FU. Radiotherapy acts on the local tumor, while the chemotherapy affects the tumor cells locally as well as the micrometastasis. This combination is usually given in 45 days and surgery is performed within 4–6 weeks.

In CROSS study,[23] reported that chemoradiotherapy followed by surgery increased the 5 years survival from 34 to 47%. The R_0 resection rate was high (92%) in chemotherapy, radiotherapy and surgery (CRS) group versus 69% with surgery alone. CRS has increased 5 year survival from 33 to 47%.

Table 12.5 Results of surgery with/without preoperative chemoradiotherapy in esophageal cancer

Authors	Drugs	Surgery	Chemotherapy + Radiotherapy + Surgery
Bosset[20]	Cisplatin, Radiotherapy	69% Resection rate	81%
Burmeister[21]	Cisplatin, 5FU, Radiotherapy	59% Resection rate survival equal	80%
Walsh et al[22]	Cisplatin + 5FU, Radiotherapy	6%	32%
CROSS[23]	Paclitaxel, Carboplatin	34%	47%
Meta-analysis[24]	Radiotherapy + Chemotherapy		13% benefit
Meta-analysis[24]	Chemotherapy		7% benefit

Overall recurrence rates was 35% with preoperative chemoradiotherapy and surgery, while 58% relapsed in surgery alone arm. In a comparative trial 3 years survival was 43.4% for preoperative chemoradiotherapy compared to 27% for preoperative chemotherapy. Peter et al[25] published the results of Paclitaxel and Carboplatin chemotherapy plus radiation prior to surgery. It showed 50 months survival with trimodality therapy as compared to 24 months with surgery alone. The data suggest synergistic benefit utilizing neoadjuvant chemoradiotherapy in EC. The meta-analysis showed that preoperative chemoradiation significantly increased the rates of R_0 resection (89% vs 77%) and complete pathological response (22% vs 3.7%).

Chemotherapy for Metastatic Esophageal Cancer

Invariably many patients with EC have metastatic disease at onset. Many patients with localized disease also progress to develop distant metastasis. Treatment at this stage is designed to improve local and distant tumor control, quality of life and increase the chance of survival. The optimum treatment requires more than one therapeutic approach along with multimodality treatment. The number of treatment options are utilized alone or in combination to achieve relief from symptoms. Single agent chemotherapy like Cisplatin, 5FU, Methotrexate, Oxaliplatin can lead to clinical remission in approximately 20–40%; however, the benefit is short-lasting.

Recently, Paclitaxel or Docetaxel in combination with Cisplatin have shown complete remission in up to 15% of patients. The meta-analysis by Wagner et al[26] that chemotherapy does improve survival and quality of life as compared to symptom directed therapy. Usually, combination of platinum analogue (Cisplatin or Oxaliplatin) in combination with 5FU and Capecitabine are used. Addition of Docetaxel may further increase the efficacy. The knowledge about newer targeted therapies directed against growth factor receptors, pathways, tumor angiogenesis and tumor invasion and metastasis is showing new pathway to combine these agents with cytotoxic chemotherapy and radiation. Her-2 receptor overexpression is seen in 25% of the esophageal cancer and use of Trastuzumab has produced improved results.[27] Similarly, epidermal growth factor receptors (EGFR) expression is observed in 60–70% of squamous cell carcinomas and is associated with poor prognosis. EGFR manipulation can be approached extracellularly by (Cetuximab) monoclonal antibody or intracellularly by tyrosine kinase inhibitors (TKI).[28] Anti PD-1[29] check point immunotherapy is approved for patients with advanced GE junction cancer expressing PD-L1.[30] Similarly, RAINBOW study[31] demonstrated that antiangiogenic therapy with Ramucirumab in combination with Paclitaxel improved the survival by 2 months. Further input from molecular and biological data will help in future to achieve exciting results in EC.

REFERENCES

1. Stewart B, Wild CP. World Cancer Report 2014. IARC Non serial publication 2014;630.
2. Enzinger PC, Mayer RJ. Esophageal cancer. N Engl J Med 2003;349:2241–52.
3. Jemal A, Siegel R, Xu J, et al. Cancer Statistics, 2010.CA Cancer J Clin 2010;60:277–300.
4. Zhang HZ, Jin GF, Shen HB. Epidemiologic differences in esophageal cancer between Asian and Western populations. Chin J Cancer 2012.
5. Pennathur A, Gibson MK, LOBE BA, Luketich JD Oesophageal carcinoma Lancet 2013;381: 400–12.
6. Van Hagen P, Huslof M, Van Lanschot J, et al. Preoperative chemoradiotherapy for Esophageal or Junctional cancer. N Engl J Med 2012;366 2074–84.
7. David H Ilson. Esophageal cancer chemotherapy: Recent advances Gastrointestinal cancer Res 2008;2(2):85–92.
8. Muro K, Hamaguchi T, Ohtsu A, et al. A phase II study of single agent docetaxel in patients with metastatic esophageal cancer. Ann Oncol 2004; 15:955–9.

9. Kelsen DP, Magill GB, Cheng E, et al. Phase II trial of etoposide in adenocarcinoma of upper gastrointestinal tract cancer treat Rep 1983;67: 509–10.

10. Tepper J, Krasna MJ, Niedzwiecki D, Hollis D, Reed CE, Goldberg R, et al. Phase III trial of trimodality therapy with Cisplatin, Fluorouracil radiotherapy, and surgery compared with surgery alone for esophageal cancer: CALGB 9781. J Clin Oncol 2008;26:1086–92.

11. Roth DA, Maibach R, Falk S, et al. Docetaxel-Cisplatin-5FU (TCF) Versus Docetaxel- Cisplatin (TC) versus Epirubicin-Cisplatin-5FU (ECF) as systemic treatment for advanced gastric cancer. A randomized phase II trial of the Swiss group for clinical cancer Research (SAKK) Proc Am Soc clinic.oncol 2004;22:317.

12. Boonstra JJ, KoK TC, Wijnhoven BP, et al. Chemotherapy followed by surgery versus surgery alone in patients with resectable esoohageal squamous cell carcinima: long term results of a randomized control trial BMC Cancer 2011;11:181.

13. Allum WH, Stenning SP, Bancewicz J, Clark PI, Langley RE. Long-term results of a randomized trial of surgery with or without preoperative chemotherapy in esophageal cancer. J Clin Oncol 2009;27:5062–7.

14. Kelsen DP, Winter KA, Gunderson LL, et al. Radiation Therapy Oncology group; USA Intergroup. Long-terms results of RTOG trial 8911 (USA Intergroup 113): A random assignment trial comparison of chemotherapy followed by surgery compared with surgery alone for esophageal cancer. J Clin Oncol 2007;25:3719–25.

15. Medical Research council Oesophageal cancer working group. Surgical resection with or without preoperative chemotherapy in esophageal cancer: A randomize controlled trial. Lancet 2002;359(9319):1727–33.

16. Cunningham D, Allum WH, Stenning SP, et al. MAGIC Trial Participants. Perioperative chemotherapy versus surgery alone for resectable gastroesophageal cancer. N Engl J Med 2006; 355(1):11–20.

17. Ychou M, Boige V, Pignon JP, et al. Perioperative chemotherapy compared with surgery alone for resectable gastroesophageal adenocarcinoma: FNCLCC and FFCD multicenter phase III trial. J Clin Oncol 2011;29:1715–21.

18. Advani SH, Saikia TK, Swaroop S, Ramakrishnan G, Nair CN, Dinshaw KA, Sharma SS, Vyas JJ, Desai PB. Anterior chemo-

therapy in esophageal cancer. Cancer 1985;56(7): 1502–6 Europepmc.org.

19. Desai PB, Vyas JJ, Sharma S, Advani SH , Gopal R, Saikia TK, Dinshaw KA, Pinto JM, Swaroop VS. The impact of combined therapeutic modalities in head, neck and esophageal cancer. Semin Surg Oncol 1985;1(3):116–31.

20. Bosset JF, Gignoux M, Triboulet JP, Tiret E, Mantion G, Elias D, et al. Chemoradiotherapy followed by surgery compared with surgery alone in squamous-cell cancer of the esophagus. N Engl J Med 1997;337:161–67.

21. Burmeister BH, Smithers BM, Gebski V, Fitzgerald L, Simes RJ, Devitt P, Ackland S, Gotley DC, Joseph D, Millar J, et al. Surgery alone versus Chemoradiotherapy followed by surgery for resectable cancer of the oesophagus: a randomised controlled phase III trial. Lancet Oncol 2005;6:659–68.

22. Walsh TN, Noonan N, Hollywood D, et al. A comparison of multimodal therapy and surgery of esophageal adenocarcinoma. N Engl J Med 1996;335:462–7.

23. Shapiro J, van Lanschot JJB, Hulshof MC, et al. Neoadjuvant chemoradiotherapy plus surgery versus surgery alone for oesophageal or junctional cancer (CROSS): long-term results of a randomised controlled trial. Lancet Oncol 2015;16:1090-8.10.1016/S1470-2045(15) 00040-6.

24. Deng HY, Wang WP, Wang YC, et al. Neo-adjuvant chemoradiotherapy or chemotherapy? A Comprehensive systemic review and metanalysis of the options of Neoadjuvant therapy for treating esophageal cancer; Eur J Cardiothoracic surg 2016;10,1093.

25. Banciewicz P, Clark P, Smith R, Donnelly, Peter Fayers, Weeden S, Girling DJ, Hutchinson TA Harvey, Lyddiard J. Med Res Council Oesophageal Canc. Surgical resection with or without preoperative chemotherapy in oesophageal cancer: a randomised controlled trial. The Lancet Oncol 2002;359(9319):1727–33.

26. Wagner AD, Grothe W, Haerting J, Kleber G, Grothey A, Fleig WE. Chemotherapy in advanced gastric cancer: A systematic review and meta-analysis based on aggregate data. J Clin Oncol 2006;24(18):2903–9.

27. Ashwini Gowryshanker, et al. Her2 status in Barrett's esophagus and esophagus and esophageal cancer a meta analysis. J Gastrointest oncol 2014;5(1):25–35.

28. Lee MS, Mamon HJ, et al. Pre-operative Cetuximab, Irinotecan, Cisplatin and Radiation therapy for patients with locally advanced esophageal cancer. The Oncologist 2013;18:281–7.

29. Kudo T, Hamamoto Y, Kato K, Ura T, Kojima T, Tsushima T, Hironaka S, Hara H, Satoh T, Iwasa S, Muro K, Yasui H, Minashi K, Yamaguchi K, Ohtsu A, Doki Y, Kitagawa Y. Nivolumab treatment for oesophageal squamous-cell carcinoma: an open-label, multicentre, phase 2 trial: Lancet Oncol 2017;18(5):631–9.

30. Raufi AG, Klempner SJ. Immunotherapy for advanced gastric and esophageal cancer: preclinical rationale and ongoing clinical investigations: J Gastrointest Oncol 2015;6:561–9.

31. Wilke H, Muro K, Van Cutsem E, et al. Ramucirumab plus paclitaxel versus placebo plus paclitaxel in patients with previously treated advanced gastric or gastro-oesophageal junction adenocarcinoma (RAINBOW): A double-blind, randomised phase 3 trial. Lancet Oncol 2014;15:1224–35.

13

Radiation Therapy for Esophageal Cancer

Sarbani Ghosh Laskar, Jai Prakash Agarwal, Shyam Kishore Shrivastava

Esophageal cancer is divided into two distinct varieties. Squamous cell carcinoma involves cervical esophagus, upper, middle and lower thoracic esophagus. The adenocarcinoma involves the lower thoracic esophagus and gastroesophageal junction. The incidence of the latter has been persistently rising over the last decade.[1]

Treatment Recommendations

- Lesion within 5 cm of the cricopharynx, is generally treated with definitive chemoradiation as surgery entails resection of entire larynx, part of pharynx, the thyroid gland with proximal esophagus. Because of significant morbidity with surgery, it is preferable to treat with chemoradiation.[2] (Level 3, Grade B).
- Surgery is the treatment of choice for resectable esophageal cancer in the middle, lower third and at the esophagogastric junction[3] (Level 1b, Grade A).
- Early lesions can be treated with a single modality—Surgery $(T_1/T_2,N_0)$[4] (Level 3, Grade B).
- Locally advanced disease $(T_3/T_{4a}/Node$ positive) should receive multimodality treatment. Neoadjuvant chemotherapy/ chemoradiotherapy followed by surgery has superior outcomes than surgery alone. There is insufficient evidence to suggest any superiority of one neoadjuvant treatment over the other. (Level 1, Grade A).
- Patients having metastatic disease should receive treatment which best palliates their symptoms as palliative radiotherapy/esophageal stenting and palliative chemotherapy. (Level 2, Grade B).

The overall management of carcinoma esophagus will depend on the location, the stage of the disease and the overall condition based on pretherapy investigation of the patient.

The standard of care for radiotherapy technique in esophageal cancer was conventional 2-dimensional treatment planning till the 1990's.[5,6] From 1990's 3-dimensional conformal radiotherapy techniques gradually took over and is the standard of care at present along with Intensity Modulated Radiotherapy (IMRT) and Image Guided Radiotherapy Techniques (IGRT).[7,8]

Even with combined chemoradiotherapy relapses are local within the radiation field in majority of cases. Future efforts at reducing these local in-field relapses are needed in the form of dose escalation or selective tumor sensitization.[9] In the past three decades IMRT and IGRT techniques have been explored in various studies in an effort to improve target dosage as well as sparing of normal tissues. Inverse planning IMRT, Volumetric Modulated Arc Therapy (VMAT), IGRT including respiratory gated treatments, Proton Beam Therapy (PBT), etc. are the newer techniques. Dose escalation may be facilitated by the use of advanced radiotherapy techniques which better protect the normal tissues which are dose limiting constraints at present.

Radiotherapy Planning

Historically, two-dimensional based radiation planning has been carried out using anatomical landmarks such as bone and carina. Fluoroscopic barium swallow is also used to delineate the field borders. However, lately CT based planning is routinely used. The CT-based planning ensures improved visualization of target structure and organs at risk. Modern techniques such as three-dimensional reconstruction, beam's eye-view and Multi-Leaf Collimator (MLC) allows conformity of the target and spares the normal-tissue. The use of Dose-Volume Histogram (DVH) has been very useful in radiation planning. However, it is important to take into account the findings of endoscopic evaluation during planning, as superficial mucosal disease is often not discernable on routine radiological investigation.

Image Acquisition and Basics of Simulation

For planning radiation therapy for esophageal cancer, simulation is employed to ascertain the extent of the disease for radiation therapy by imaging (barium swallow, CT or PET simulation). CT simulation is appropriate for treatment planning. During simulation appropriate patient position is necessary (preferably supine) using immobilization devices (Vaclok vacuum cushion, body-fix, alpha cradle, etc.). Arms are generally kept over the head and knee support is used underneath the legs. Palpable neck nodes, if any, are demarcated with radiopaque wire. Oral contrast is used during simulation to delineate the esophagus. For upper esophagus a thermoplastic immobilization mask will help in daily reproducibility.

Patient is placed in the CT-simulator in the treatment position and a scan of the entire area with margins is taken at 3 to 5 mm slice thickness. Tomography (CT) scans has reduced the use of fluoroscopy in radiotherapy planning.[10] The planning CT should encompass the entire thoracic cavity and the abdomen to a level below the lower end of the kidneys. An arterial phase intravenous contrast is generally used to delineate mediastinal and abdominal vascular and nodal structures. Three fiducials are placed at the level of the nipple. Esophageal oral contrast may be used during simulation but is optional if a diagnostic CT scan with contrast was performed.[11]

Some investigators practice the delineation of the esophageal Gross Tumor Volume (GTV) on CT or routine MRI using Diffusion weighted MR images.[12] Cine-MRI has been used to quantify the movement of esophageal tumor and visualize tumor movement directly throughout multiple breathing cycles.[13] However, this is not routinely practiced in majority of institutions.

The 18-Fluoro Deoxy Glucose (18-FDG) PET-CT is used in esophageal cancer as a routine for initial staging for detection of distant metastases. Also, the use of PET-CT for tumour delineation results in increase accuracy of the target volume when compared to CT and EUS. There are contradictory findings regarding the use of 18-FDG PET-CT in decreasing intra- and interobserver variability. Therefore, standard implementation of PET-CT in tumour delineation process for radiation treatment planning remains a subject of debate and requires further clinical validation.[14]

As with other thoracic tumours, the esophagus also moves with respiration and cardiac motion.[15] This has been quantified using 4-D CT and attempts have been made to quantify the errors and generate appropriate Internal Target Volume (ITV) margins. Motion was greatest in the transverse (right-left) direction above the carina. However, there is no evidence available to demonstrate the clinical benefit of using 4-D CT in radiotherapy treatments. This may have a role in the planning of tumors, especially of the lower third esophagus and cardioesophageal junction.

Target volumes are contoured on the planning CT scan as per International Commission on Radiation Units and Measurements (ICRU). Reports 50 and 62 recommendations using endoscopic findings, endoscopic ultrasonography (EUS), and/or barium swallow findings in addition to the information from a diagnostic CT.[11] Initially, the margin of 5 cm above and below the GTV is recommended to cover the subclinical and nodal disease and 1.5 cm radial margin to be given depending on the individual case. An additional margin is to be given to set-up uncertainty and physiological internal organ motion to include in the planning target volume (PTV). However, the PTV is institution-specific but may incorporate physiological motion. For the lower third esophagus and gastroesophageal junction (GEJ) tumors the European consensus guidelines can be followed.[16] Several institutes have their own guidelines for delineation. During delivery of radiation therapy Image-Guidance Radiation Therapy (IGRT), including cone-beam CT may also be useful in localizing the tumor. The final boost volume encompasses a longitudinal margin of 3 cm to the gross disease, editing from bone and lung as appropriate. The circumferential margin usually remains the same.

There is controversy regarding the volume of lymph nodal irradiation elective versus involved. Only grossly involved nodes are included in the target volume. The CTV should include the celiac axis in tumours of the GEJ and lower esophagus. In patients treated with 3-Dimensional Conformal Radiation Therapy (3D-CRT) for esophageal squamous carcinomas, the omission of elective nodal irradiation was not associated with a significant amount of failure in lymph node regions not included in the planning target volume. Local failure and distant metastases remained the predominant problems.[17]

Field design: The radiation treatment for upper esophagus has been challenging because of changing contour from the neck to the thoracic inlet. The treatment of lesions of upper one-third esophagus treated from laryngopharynx to the carina depends on the extent of the disease. Supraclavicular and superior mediastinal nodes are irradiated electively.

The radiation field for adenocarcinoma of the esophagus is similar to that of lower thoracic squamous cell carcinoma. However, for these periesophageal lymph nodes are generally included in all patients. Generally, GE junction carcinomas are more advanced and to include celiac group of lymph nodes may be worthwhile.

Dose Prescription

When feasible, external Radiotherapy can be combined with Intraluminal Radiotherapy (ILRT) as a boost (especially when the treatment is radiotherapy alone). ILRT is usually avoided with concurrent chemotherapy. For definitive radiotherapy alone, higher doses of external Radiotherapy (RT), 60–64 Gy in 30–32 fractions with reducing fields or combination of external RT and intraluminal brachytherapy (external RT–50.4 Gy in 28 fractions with reducing fields and Intraluminal brachytherapy (high dose rate) 6 Gy per fraction X 2 fractions, once weekly, or low dose rate-20 Gy single fraction) may be considered.

For definitive concurrent chemoradiation, 50 Gy has been described. There was no evidence for dose escalation as evidenced in the INT 0123 trial.[3] Therefore 50Gy in 25 fractions over 5 weeks, plus cisplatin 75–100 mg/m^2

intravenously on the first day of weeks 1, 5, 8, and 11, and fluorouracil, 750–1000 mg/m^2 per day by continuous infusion on the first 4 days of weeks 1, 5, 8, and 11—RTOG regimen[5] is used. Other concurrent chemoradiation regimen includes Paclitaxel 50 mg/m^2 and carboplatin at AUC 2 weekly for 5 to 6 weeks-CROSS regimen.[18]

a. Dose Escalation: The predominant pattern of failure in esophageal cancer treated with definitive chemoradiation continues to be local in-field recurrence. This led to efforts to escalate dose to the gross tumour. The INT0123 trial[6] was one such initial effort, which has set the standard of care at 50.4 Gy/28 fractions. However, INT0123 utilised conventional planning techniques which are much inferior to conformal techniques in sparing of Organs At Risks (OARs). The use of advanced radiotherapy techniques like IMRT, VMAT, PET-CT based radiotherapy and adaptive radiation therapy may help in dose escalation by providing more conformal dose distributions to the target and better sparing of organs at risk. Although there are several dosimetric studies demonstrating this, robust clinical data is still being generated.[19–21] A single phase I study from China reports successful dose escalation to 70 Gy using PET-based delineation and Simultaneous Integrated Boost (SIB) with no dose limiting acute toxicity. However, late toxicity outcomes are still awaited.[22]

b. Altered Fractionation: Accelerated hyperfractionation has been tried in esophageal cancer without benefit in control rates and higher normal tissue toxicity.[23]

Treatment Delivery Techniques

a. 3D-CRT is the present standard of care in treatment of esophageal cancer as per all recent Radiation Therapy Oncology Group (RTOG) studies. Conformal radiotherapy techniques offer the potential for a 5–10 Gy escalation in dose delivered to the esophagus, without increasing the mean lung dose. This is expected to increase local tumor control by 15–25% using Tumour Control Probability-Normal Tissue Complication Probability (TCP-NTCP) calculations.[24] Conformal radiotherapy reduces cardiac doses especially for lower third and cardioesophageal junction tumors.[25] (Fig. 13.1)

b. IMRT: Five field IMRT plans are better than 3D-CRT plans in terms of the dose conformity and homogeneity in targets and the dose to OARs. The dose distributions changed little when the beam number increased from five to seven and nine.[26] IMRT provides superior target volume coverage and conformality, with decreased dose to normal structures such as spinal cord, brainstem and parotid glands.[27] However the low dose spill in the adjacent lungs need to be monitored carefully.

Several retrospective series reporting institutional experience and outcomes with IMRT have been reported, including the MD Anderson and Memorial Sloan Kettering Cancer Centres.[28,29] These show comparable outcomes in terms of local control and survival[26,30] as 3D-CRT with reduced toxicity. The MD Anderson Cancer Centre however reported a decreased risk of dying in patients treated with IMRT as compared with 3D-CRT.[31] However there is no randomized clinical data to show superiority of IMRT over 3D-CRT in terms of clinical outcome. Another option may be hybrid radiotherapy technique, in a phased manner, incorporating both 3D-CRT and IMRT to exploit the beneficial parameters of the technique.

c. VMAT: Compared with conformal-IMRT, VMAT, especially using 2 arcs slightly improves the OAR dose sparing, such as lungs and heart, and reduces NTCP and monitor units with a better PTV coverage.[32] A greater proportion of the body received low doses (V_5 was 18% greater) with VMAT compared to IMRT.[33] VMAT combined with Active Breath Control (ABC) to achieve moderate Deep Inspiratory Breath

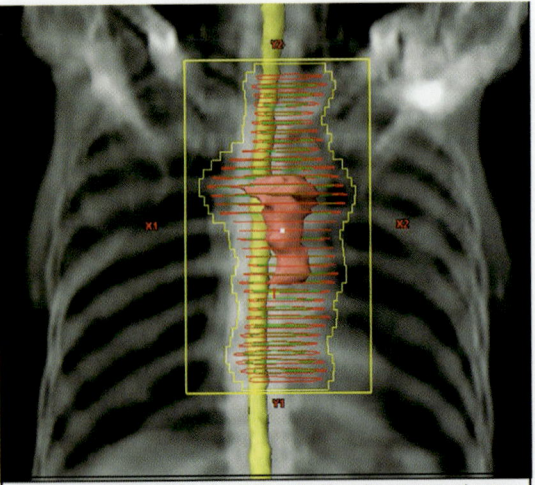

Beam's Eye View (BEV) of an AP portal with various target volumes
Solid red: GTV
Green line: CTV
Red line: PTV

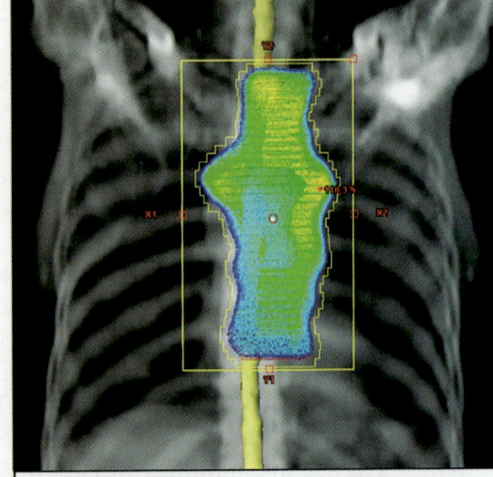

Frontal projection: 3DCRT plan showing 95% isodose coverage of the PTV

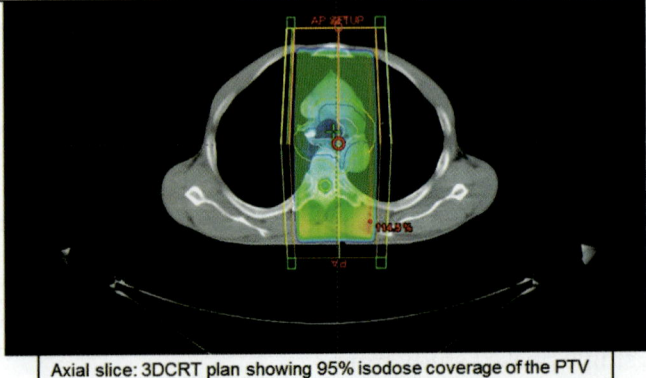

Axial slice: 3DCRT plan showing 95% isodose coverage of the PTV

Fig. 13.1: Treatment plan for 3D-conformal radiation therapy

Hold (mDIBH-representing 80% of peak DIBH value) is a feasible approach for radiotherapy of thoracic esophagus and has the potential to effectively reduce lung dose in a shorter treatment time and with better targeting accuracy. VMAT combined with DIBH reduced mean lung doses as well as V_{20}, V_{30}, V_{40} significantly and also had shorter treatment times.[34]

d. Respiratory Motion Management: Conformal radiotherapy with respiratory gating for esophageal cancer decreases the radiation doses to OARs such as heart, ipsilateral lung and spinal cord.[35] (Fig. 13.2).

Planning

1. Prescription: in 3D-CRT, target doses are prescribed to the isocentre of PTV as per ICRU 50 and 62.
2. Critical structures are delineated as per RTOG atlas—both lungs, heart, spinal cord, liver, brachial plexus (for upper esophageal tumors) and kidneys (especially in lower esophageal tumors).[36]

Plan Evaluation and Dose Constraints

⇒ Target Coverage: >95% of the PTV should receive 100% of the dose, with maximum dose ≤110% of the prescribed dose.[11]

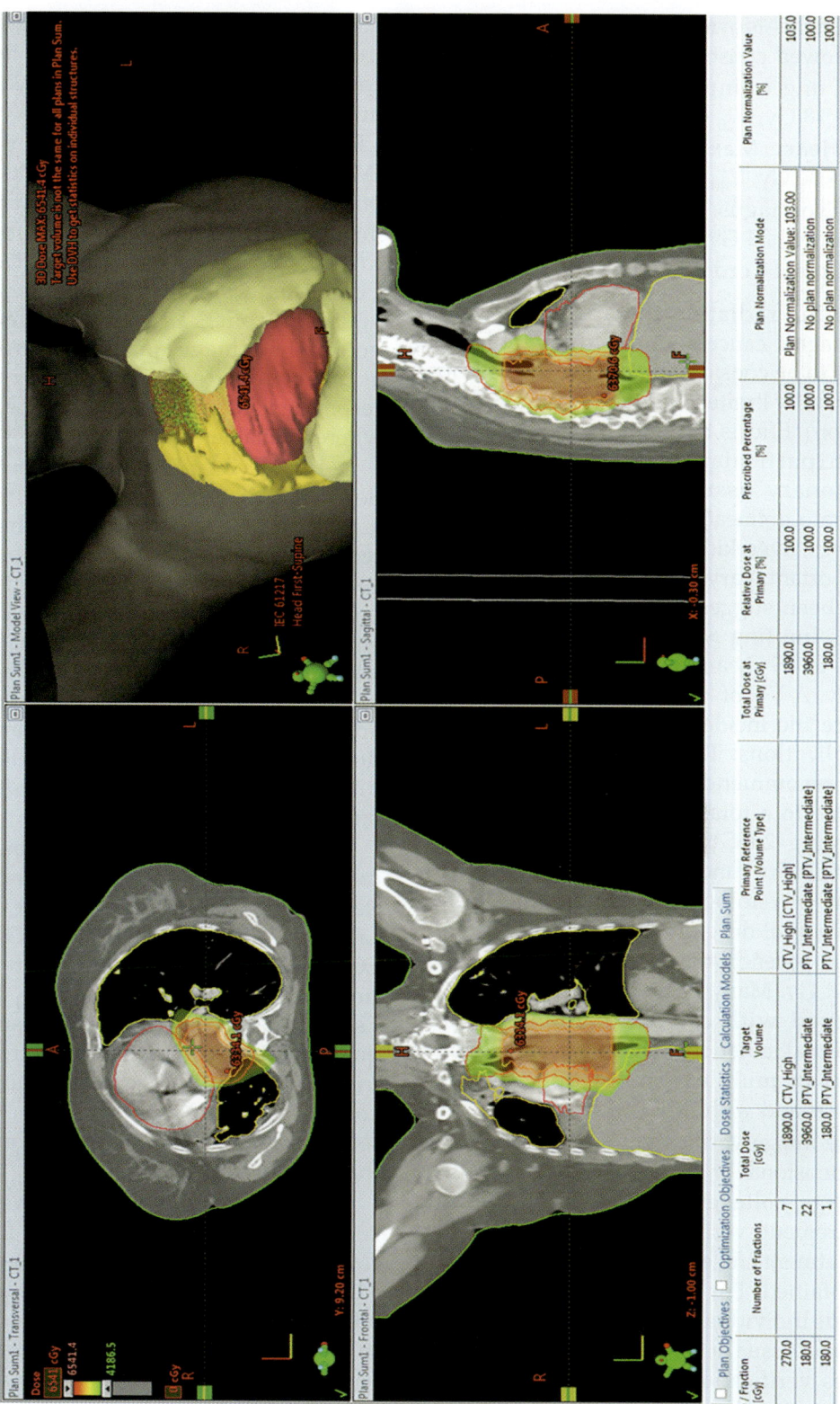

Fig. 13.2: Treatment plan with IMRT showing less dose to normal structures comparing 3D-CRT

⇒ Critical Normal Tissues: Commonly followed constraints include:

- Lung (minus PTV): Mean lung dose $\leq$18 Gy, $V_{20} \leq$25%, $V_5 \leq$50%
- Heart: Max dose $\leq$52Gy, mean dose $\leq$30 Gy, $V_{40} \leq$50%
- Esophagus: Max dose $\leq$74 Gy, mean dose $\leq$34 Gy
- Spinal Cord: Max dose $\leq$45 Gy

During radiation therapy planning for esophageal cancers, normal-tissue tolerance needs to be considered. The spinal cord dose is generally limited to 45 Gy (using 1.8 Gy per fraction). Efforts to minimize the dose to the heart (particularly left ventricle) and to pulmonary tissues should be exercised. Accurate delineation of normal organs such as lungs, liver, kidneys, heart and spinal cord is important. Varying dose volume constraints have been suggested such as a lung V_{20} of <20%, limiting >2,300 cm^3 of normal lung tissue to <5 Gy and using mean lung dose of <18Gy. A V_{10} of <60% has been proposed to reduce the incidence of postoperative lung complications. The heart constraints have been recommended to be <30% of cardiac volume to a total dose of 40 Gy and <50% receiving 25 Gy minimizing dose to left ventricle. For functioning kidney at least 70% of one physiologically functioning kidney receive total dose of <20 Gy. Generally, 70% of liver parenchyma should be kept to a dose of <30 Gy. Many of these constraints can be achieved with careful planning for 3D-conformal radiation (3D-CRT) using shielding blocks or multileaf collimation and DVH analysis and with IMRT in select cases.

The image verification may be done with 2-dimensional or 3-dimensional kilo voltage or mega voltage imaging. As a minimum requirement, verification images at the start of treatment and each week thereafter should be obtained. For 3D-CRT this imaging can include individual portal views; however, the poor soft tissue detail obtained in these images makes verification difficult. Consequently, bone anatomy is used as a surrogate to verify treatment position and tumour location is confirmed by extrapolation. Twice weekly imaging can consist of portal views for 3D-CRT and isocenter verification images. For IMRT orthogonal images verifying isocenter position are required. More frequent (daily) imaging is preferred, particularly for patients treated with motion management techniques. Cone Beam Computed Tomography (CBCT) verification offers an adequate 3-dimensional volumetric image quality to improve the accuracy of treatment delivery and is recommended to be used for image guidance where available.[37]

A larger volume of lung receives lower doses of radiation because of multiple beam arrangement and a smaller volume of lung receives higher doses because of better dose conformity in conformal plans. Acute pneumonitis correlates more with V_{30} values, whereas chronic pneumonitis was predominantly seen in patients with higher V_{20} values.[38] Patients with metastatic disease and adverse Dose-Volume Histogram (DVH) doses were more likely to develop severe pneumonitis independent of other risk factors.[39]

Quality of Life assessment may be routinely carried out using European Organisation for Research and Treatment of Cancer Quality of Life Questionnaire (EORTC QOLQ-C30), EORTC QLQ-OES18 questionnaire or Functional Assessment of Cancer Therapy-Esophageal Cancer (FACT-E) score. The quality-of-life score deteriorates from before treatment to end of treatment due to acute complications of chemo-radiotherapy, but recovers at 4 or 5 months and becomes better than before treatment.[40]

Protons and Heavy Particles: Welsh et al[41] compared dosimetric parameters for photon IMRT with Intensity-Modulated Proton Therapy (IMPT) for unresectable, locally advanced distal esophageal cancer. Relative to IMRT the IMPT plan with anteroposterior/left posterior oblique/right posterior oblique

(AP/LPO/RPO) beam arrangement led to considerable reductions in dose to the lung ($p \leq 0.005$), heart ($p \leq 0.003$), and liver ($p \leq 0.04$).

Follow up: Clinical evaluation, endoscopy, Contrast Enhanced Computed Tomography (CECT) and/or PET-CT. The intensity and frequency would be determined by intent of primary treatment and the scope for salvage therapy/effective palliation in the event of a recurrence.

Definitive Radiation and Chemoradiation Therapy

Concurrent chemoradiation is superior to radiation alone (Level 1A, Grade A). Two published (RTOG and ECOG) randomized trials have reported better overall survival with concomitant chemoradiation than radiation therapy alone.[5] However, increasing the dose of radiation therapy (50.4 versus 64.8) in concomitant chemoradiotherapy setting did not result in increased survival (Inter Group trial).[42]

Meta-analysis of 13 trials combining radiation with chemotherapy published in the Cochrane library has reported an absolute reduction in the mortality and local recurrence rate of 7% and 12% respectively in favour of combination therapy, at the cost of increased life-threatening toxicities (Level 1a, Grade A).[43] Two trials comparing surgery to radiation alone have reported better survival with surgery (Level 1b, Grade A).[44]

Based on the available evidence, if a patient is to be treated with definitive non-surgical treatment, it should be concomitant chemoradiotherapy, provided performance status is optimal. However, the issues of radiation volumes (margins to the gross tumor, elective nodal irradiation), total doses and optimal concurrent chemotherapy schedule still remain a matter of debate, with most practice being dictated by individual philosophy. If chemoradiation is used, 5FU with Cisplatin has the maximum evidence but due to logistic reasons, taxane with platinum is commonly used.[45,46] (Level 2b, Grade B).

Preoperative Radiotherapy

A meta-analysis as well as the five published randomized trials comparing preoperative radiation therapy to surgery alone has not shown benefit of preoperative radiation over surgery alone.[47] (Level 1a, Grade A).

Preoperative Concomitant Chemoradiation

There are three major trials and several smaller trials comparing preoperative concomitant chemoradiation to surgery alone. Of these, one trial has shown statistically improved survival with chemoradiation.[48]

• Meta-analysis of preoperative chemoradiation and surgery, to surgery alone (9 trials) has reported improved 3-year survival and reduced loco-regional recurrence.[49–52] (Level 1a, Grade A). However, combination treatment is associated with a trend towards increased treatment related morbidity and mortality.

• A recent randomized controlled trial (CROSS) comparing surgery alone to neo-adjuvant chemoradiotherapy followed by surgery showed improved R_0 resection, pathological response and significantly improved survival (49.4 versus 24 months) in the neo-adjuvant group, while the post-operative complications and mortality were similar in both groups.[53] (Level 1, Grade A).

Postoperative Radiotherapy

Three trials have compared surgery and postoperative radiation to surgery alone.

• The Chinese trial of 495 patients observed improved 5-year survival in patients with positive lymph nodes and stage III disease receiving postoperative radiation. However, the difference in the overall survival between the two groups was statistically not different.[54]

• The meta-analysis of all three trials also does not show benefit of postoperative radiotherapy.[55] Therefore, in the absence of Level 1 evidence postoperative radiotherapy is indicated only for patients with positive margin and residual disease.

- For lower third and GE junction adeno-carcinomas with multiple lymph nodes, positive margins, T_3 tumors; adjuvant CTRT may be considered with the increased incidence of treatment related toxicity.[56] (Level 1, Grade A).

Brachytherapy

Apart from the external beam therapy, Brachytherapy (intraluminal) can be used with curative or palliative intent. Brachy-therapy has an advantage of inverse-square law thereby quick dose fall off to reduce the dose to surrounding tissues. Majority of centres use High Dose Rate (HDR) techniques using ^{192}Ir source. The HDR source can deliver dose of 100–400 Gy per hour allowing treatment given in 5 to 10 minutes. (Fig. 13.3)

For intraluminal brachytherapy, an after-loading tube (catheter) is inserted through the nose into esophagus to the tumor site under fluoroscopic or endoscopic guidance. After localization films are taken and dosimetry is generated, the treatment can be delivered attaching the catheters to HDR machine. Dose of 5 to 12 Gy are usually prescribed at 1 cm from the center of catheter, when used as a boost during definitive treatment. Brachy-therapy boost is usually not preferred in combination with concurrent chemotherapy.

It has been observed that addition of intraluminal brachytherapy is found to be safe with low incidence of severe complications. The long-term relief from dysphagia has been good. Intraluminal brachytherapy is the best method of dose escalation in a subset of patients and has potential to improved outcome in esophageal cancers.[57–61]

Palliative Radiation

Palliative radiation is frequently used to control the symptoms due to primary disease or metastasis. Relief in symptoms especially pain and dysphagia can be achieved in large number of patients. The palliative treatment regimens vary from 20 Gy over one week or 30 Gy in two weeks. Intraluminal Radio-therapy (ILRT) can also serve as an effective modality for palliation in negotiable lesion. The usual schedule is 8 Gy in two fractions or 6 Gy in 3 fractions. In responders a combi-nation of external radiation therapy and ILRT may be employed. Self-expanding stents,[62] Laser ablation[63] and palliative chemotherapy can also be used. (Fig. 13.4)

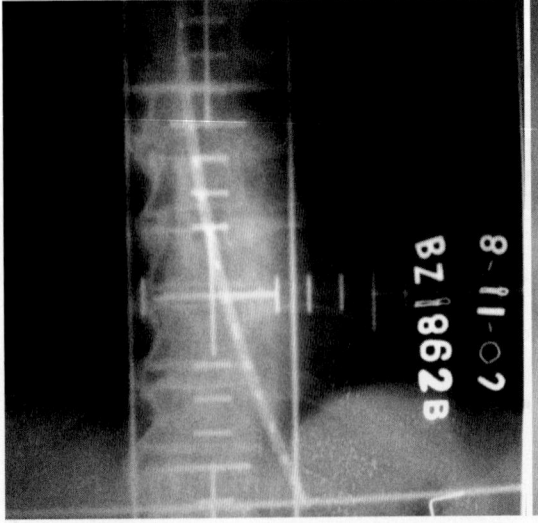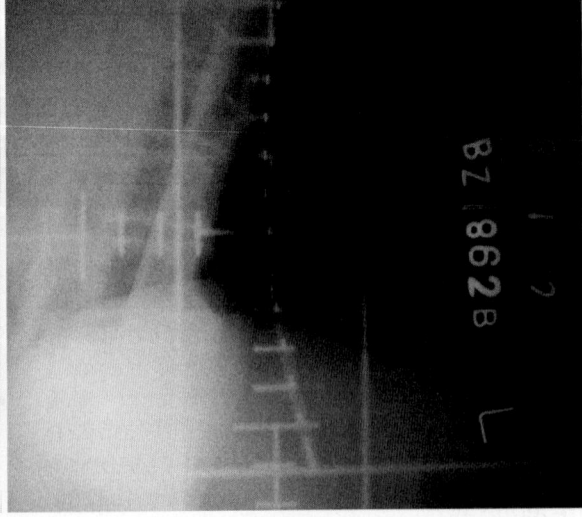

Fig. 13.3: Orthogonal X-rays with brachytherapy ILRT tube *in situ*

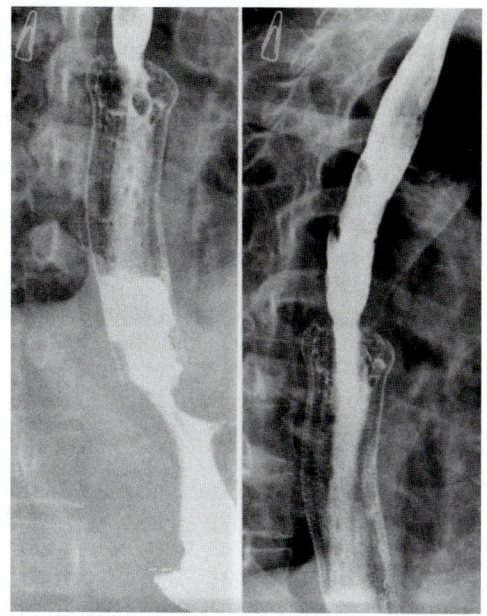

Fig. 13.4: Barium swallow X-ray with stent *in situ* as a palliative measure

For palliative radiotherapy the intent of treatment is to achieve quick and good palliation in the form of relief of dysphagia and pain.[64,65] The inclusion criteria are:

- Lesions in upper/mid/lower esophagus
- Lesion <10 cm long on barium swallow and esophagoscopy
- Histologically proven esophageal carcinoma
- Karnofsky performance status (KPS) of >50%.

Radiotherapy effectively relieves dysphagia in more than 90% patients. It improves the quality of life of these patients. However some of these patients will have persistent stricture, ulceration and residual disease.[66]

Treatment of Recurrent Disease

Salvage surgery for localized resectable failures is the treatment of choice. However, most of patients at recurrence may only be suitable for palliative treatment or supportive care alone as described before. Loco-regional chemoradiotherapy is given for localized failures, post-surgery. Following treatment may be offered for recurrent/metastatic disease.

- Dose (EBRT): 3000cGy/10 fractions/2 weeks portal: Esophageal lesion with 3 cm margin evaluation and response assessment is done after 2 weeks and further external radiotherapy or brachytherapy boost may be delivered.
- Reduced field/boost: 2000cGy/10 fractions/2 weeks, using oblique portals.
- Palliative radiation can also be delivered in the form of ILRT alone or in combination with EBRT. Suggested dose per fraction: 8 Gy, in 2 fractions, one week apart.
- There is no difference in local control or survival between high dose rate brachytherapy compared with external beam radiation.
- Various schedules of brachytherapy have been compared and two fractions of 8 Gy are found to be equivalent to three fractions of 6 Gy.[67] (Level 1, Grade A).
- Addition of EBRT to ILRT improves the dysphagia free survival.[68] (Level1, Grade A).

REFERENCES

1. Crew KD, Neugut AI. Epidemiology of upper gastrointestinal malignancies. Semin Oncol 2004; 31(4):450–64. [PMID:15297938]
2. Tong DK, Law S, Kwong DL, et al. Current management of cervical esophageal cancer. World J Surg 2011;35:600–7.
3. Wright CD. Esophageal cancer surgery in 2005. Minerva Chir 2005;60:431–44. Review.
4. Grotenhuis BA, van Heijl M, Zehetner J, et al. Surgical management of submucosal esophageal cancer: extended or regional lymphadenectomy? Ann Surg 2010;252(5):823–30.
5. Cooper JS, Guo MD, Herskovic A, Macdonald JS, Martenson JA Jr, Al-Sarraf M, Byhardt R, Russell AH, Beitler JJ, Spencer S, Asbell SO, Graham MV, Leichman LL. Chemoradiotherapy of locally advanced esophageal cancer: long-term follow-up of a prospective randomized trial (RTOG 85-01). Radiation Therapy Oncology Group. JAMA 1999;281(17):1623–7. [PMID: 10235156]

6. Minsky BD, Pajak TF, Ginsberg RJ, Pisansky TM, Martenson J, Komaki R, Okawara G, Rosenthal SA, Kelsen DP. INT0123 (Radiation Therapy Oncology Group 94-05) phase III trial of combined-modality therapy for esophageal cancer: high-dose versus standard-dose radiation therapy. J Clin Oncol 2002;20(5):1167–74. [PMID:11870157]

7. Rich T. Changing role of radiotherapy in the management of cancer of the esophagus. South Med J 1999;92(11):1054–63. [PMID:10586830]

8. Yang GY, McLosky A, Khushalani NI. Principles of Modern Radiation Techniques for Esophageal and Gastroesophageal Junction Cancers. Gastrointest Cancer Res 2009;3(Suppl 1):S6–10. [PMID:19461922]

9. Button MR, Morgan CA, Croydon ES, Roberts SA, Crosby TD. Study to determine adequate margins in radiotherapy planning for esophageal carcinoma by detailing patterns of recurrence after definitive chemo-radiotherapy. Int J Radiat Oncol Biol Phys 2009;73(3):818–23. [PMID:18718726]

10. Hishikawa Y, Taniguchi M, Kamikonya N, Tanaka S, Miura T. New technique of determining the irradiated field for esophageal cancer by using an endoscope and a simulator. Radiat Med 1988;6(1):46–7. [PMID:3413288]

11. Radiation Therapy Oncology Group. Protocol of RTOG 1010: A phase III trial evaluating the addition of Trastuzumab to tri-modality treatment of HER2- overexpressing esophageal adenocarcinoma. [Internet]. Available from http://www.rtog.org/ Clinical Trials/ Protocol Table.aspx accessed on 14 Nov 2014.

12. Hou DL, Shi GF, Gao XS, Asaumi J, Li XY, Liu H, Yao C, Chang JY. Improved longitudinal length accuracy of gross tumor volume delineation with diffusion weighted magnetic resonance imaging for esophageal squamous cell carcinoma. Radiat Oncol 2013;8:169. [PMID:23829638]

13. Lever FM, Lips IM, Crijns SP, Reerink O, van Lier AL, Moerland MA, van Vulpen M, Meijer GJ. Quantification of esophageal tumor motion on cine-magnetic resonance imaging. Int J Radiat Oncol Biol Phys 2014;88(2):419–24. [PMID:24321785]

14. van Rossum PS, van Lier AL, Lips IM, Meijer GJ, Reerink O, van Vulpen M, Lam MG, van Hillegersberg R, Ruurda JP. Imaging of oesophageal cancer with FDG-PET/CT and MRI. Clin Radiol 2015;70(1):81–95. [PMID:25172205]

15. Cohen RJ, Paskalev K, Litwin S, Price Jr. R, Feigenberg SJ, Konski A. Esophageal Motion During Radiotherapy: Quantification and Margin Implications. Dis Esophagus 2010;23(6):473–9. [PMID:20095993]

16. Matzinger O, Gerber E, Bernstein Z, Maingon P, Haustermans K, Bosset JF, Gulyban A, Poortmans P, Collette L, Kuten A. EORTC-ROG expert opinion: Radiotherapy volume and treatment guidelines for neoadjuvant radiation of adenocarcinomas of the gastroesophageal junction and the stomach. Radiother Oncol 2009; 92(2):164–75. [PMID: 19375186]

17. Zhao KL, Ma JB, Liu G, Wu KL, Shi XH, Jiang GL. Three-dimensional conformal radiation therapy for esophageal squamous cell carcinoma: is elective nodal irradiation necessary? Int J Radiat Oncol Biol Phys 2010;76(2):446–51. [PMID: 20004527]

18. van Hagen P, Hulshof MC, van Lanschot JJ, et al. CROSS Group. Preoperative chemo-radiotherapy for esophageal or junctional cancer. N Engl J Med 2012;31(366):2074–84.

19. Fakhrian K, Oechsner M, Kampfer S, Schuster T, Molls M, Geinitz H. Advanced techniques in neoadjuvant radiotherapy allow dose escalation without increased dose to the organs at risk: Planning study in esophageal carcinoma. Strahlenther Onkol. 2013 Apr;189(4):293–300. [PMID:23443611]

20. Welsh J, Palmer MB, Ajani JA, Liao Z, Swisher SG, Hofstetter WL, Allen PK, Settle SH, Gomez D, Likhacheva A, Cox JD, Komaki R. Esophageal cancer dose escalation using a simultaneous integrated boost technique. Int J Radiat Oncol Biol Phys 2012;82(1):468–74. [PMID:21123005]

21. Nkhali L, Thureau S, Edet-Sanson A, Doyeux K, Benyoucef A, Gardin I, Michel P, Vera P, Dubray B. FDG-PET/CT during concomitant chemo radiotherapy for esophageal cancer: Reducing target volumes to deliver higher radiotherapy doses. Acta Oncol 2015 Jun;54(6):909-15. doi: 10.3109/0284186X.2014.973062. Epub 2014 Nov 24. (PMID: 25417733).

22. Yu W, Cai XW, Liu Q, Zhu ZF, Feng W, Zhang Q, Zhang YJ,Yao ZF, Fu XL. Safety of dose escalation by simultaneous integrated boosting radiation dose within the primary tumor guided by 18FDG-PET/CT for esophageal cancer. Radiother Oncol. 2015 Jan 10. doi: 10.1016/j.radonc.2014.12.007. [Epub ahead of print]. [PMID:25586952]

23. Wang JH, Lu XJ, Zhou J, Wang F. A randomized controlled trial of conventional fraction and late course accelerated hyperfraction three-dimensional conformal radiotherapy for esophageal cancer. Cell Biochem Biophys 2012 Jan;62(1): 107–12. [PMID: 21858589]

24. Bedford JL, Viviers L, Guzel Z, Childs PJ, Webb S, Tait DM. A quantitative treatment planning study evaluating the potential of dose escalation in conformal radiotherapy of the oesophagus. Radiother Oncol 2000;57(2):183–93. [PMID: 11054522]

25. Mukherjee S, Aston D, Minett M, Brewster AE, Crosby TD. Clin Oncol (R CollRadiol). The significance of cardiac doses received during chemoradiation of oesophageal and gastro-oesophageal junctional cancers 2003;15(3):115–20. [PMID:12801047]

26. Fu WH, Wang LH, Zhou ZM, Dai JR, Hu YM, Zhao LJ. Comparison of conformal and intensity-modulated techniques for simultaneous integrated boost radiotherapy of upper esophageal carcinoma. World J Gastroenterol. 2004;10(8): 1098–102. [PMID:15069706]

27. Fenkell L, Kaminsky I, Breen S, Huang S, Van Prooijen M, Ringash J. Dosimetric comparison of IMRT vs. 3D conformal radiotherapy in the treatment of cancer of the cervical esophagus. Radiother Oncol 2008;89(3):287–91. [PMID: 18789828]

28. Roeder F, Nicolay NH, Nguyen T, Saleh-Ebrahimi L, Askoxylakis V, Bostel T, Zwicker F, Debus J, Timke C, Huber PE. Intensity modulated radiotherapy (IMRT) with concurrent chemotherapy as definitive treatment of locally advanced esophageal cancer. Radiation Oncology 2014;9:191. [PMID:25175056]

29. Li JC, Liu D, Chen MQ, Wang JZ, Chen JQ, Qian FY, Chen C, Zhang HP, Pan JJ. Different radiation treatment in esophageal carcinoma: a clinical comparative study. J BUON 2012;17(3): 512–6. [PMID:23033291]

30. Yu WW, Zhu ZF, Fu XL, Zhao KL, Mao JF, Wu KL, Yang HJ, Fan M, Zhao S, Welsh J. Simultaneous integrated boost intensity-modulated radiotherapy in esophageal carcinoma: Early results of a phase II study. Strahlenther Onkol 2014;190 (11):979–86. [PMID: 24609941]

31. Lin SH, Wang L, Myles B, Thall PF, Hofstetter WL, Swisher SG, Ajani JA, Cox JD, Komaki R, Liao Z. Propensity score-based comparison of long-term outcomes with 3-dimensional conformal radiotherapy vs intensity-modulated radiotherapy for esophageal cancer. Int J Radiat Oncol Biol Phys 2012;84(5):1078–85. [PMID: 22867894]

32. Yin L, Wu H, Gong J, Geng JH, Jiang F, Shi AH, Yu R, Li YH, Han SK, Xu B, Zhu GY. Volumetric-modulated arc therapy vs c-IMRT in esophageal cancer: A treatment planning comparison. World J Gastroenterol 2012;18(37):5266–75. [PMID: 23066322]

33. Van Benthuysen L, Hales L, Podgorsak MB. Volumetric Modulated arc therapy vs. IMRT for the treatment of distal esophageal cancer. Med Dosim 2011;36(4):404–9. [PMID: 21377864]

34. Gong G, Wang R, Guo Y, Zhai D, Liu T, Lu J, Chen J, Liu C, Yin Y. Reduced lung dose during radiotherapy for thoracic esophageal carcinoma: VMAT combined with active breathing control for moderate DIBH. Radiat Oncol 2013;8:291. [PMID: 24359800]

35. Lorchel F, Dumas JL, Noël A, Wolf D, Bosset JF, Aletti P. Dosimetric consequences of breath-hold respiration in conformal radiotherapy of esophageal cancer. Phys Med 2006;22(4):119–26. [PMID:17643895]

36. Kong FM, Ritter T, Quint DJ, Senan S, Gaspar LE, Komaki RU, Hurkmans CW, Timmerman R, Bezjak A, Bradley JD, Movsas B, Marsh L, Okunieff P, Choy H, Curran WJ Jr. Consideration of dose limits for organs at risk of thoracic radiotherapy: atlas for lung, proximal bronchial tree, esophagus, spinal cord, ribs, and brachial plexus. Int J Radiat Oncol Biol Phys 2011;81(5): 1442–57. [PMID: 20934273]

37. Hawkins MA, Aitken A, Hansen VN, McNair HA, Tait DM. Set-up errors in radiotherapy for oesophageal cancers—is electronic portal imaging or cone-beam more accurate? Radiother Oncol 2011;98(2):249–54. [PMID:21144607]

38. Kumar G, Rawat S, Puri A, Sharma MK, Chadha P, Babu AG, Yadav G. Analysis of dose-volume parameters predicting radiation pneumonitis in patients with esophageal cancer treated with 3D-conformal radiation therapy or IMRT. Jpn J Radiol 2012;30(1):18–24. [PMID:22160648]

39. Nomura M, Kodaira T, Furutani K, Tachibana H, Tomita N, Goto Y. Predictive factors for radiation pneumonitis in oesophageal cancer patients treated with chemoradiotherapy without prophylactic nodal irradiation. Br J Radiol 2012;85(1014):813–8. [PMID:22253344]

40. Yamashita H, Omori M, Okuma K, Kobayashi R, Igaki H, Nakagawa K. Longitudinal assessments of quality of life and late toxicities before

and after definitive chemoradiation for esophageal cancer. Jpn J Clin Oncol 2014;44(1):78–84. [PMID: 24220801]

41. Welsh J, Gomez D, Palmer MB, Riley BA, Mayank kumar AV, Komaki R, Dong L, Zhu XR, Likhacheva A, Liao Z, Hofstetter WL, Ajani JA, Cox JD. Intensity-modulated proton therapy further reduces normal tissue exposure during definitive therapy for locally advanced distal esophageal tumors: A dosimetric study. Int J Radiat Oncol Biol Phys 2011;81(5):1336–42. [PMID: 21470796]

42. Bruce D Minsky, Thomas F Pajak, Robert J Ginsberg, et al. INT 0123 (Radiation Therapy Oncology Group 94-05) Phase III Trial of Combined-Modality Therapy for Esophageal Cancer: High-Dose Versus Standard-Dose Radiation Therapy: Journal of Clinical Oncology 2002;20:1167–74.

43. Rebecca Wong, Richard Malthaner. Combined chemotherapy and radiotherapy (without surgery) compared with radiotherapy alone in localized carcinoma of the esophagus (Cochrane Review). The Cochrane Library, Issue 4, 2003.

44. Badwe RA, Sharma V, Bhansali MS, et al. The quality of swallowing for patients with operable esophageal carcinoma: A randomized trial comparing surgery with radiotherapy. Cancer. 1999;15;85:763.

45. Hainsworth JD, Meluch AA, Greco FA. Paclitaxel, carboplatin, and long-term continuous 5-fluorouracil infusion in the treatment of upper aerodigestive malignancies: preliminary results of phase II trial. Semin Oncol 1997;24:S19–42.

46. Kim DW, Blanke CD, Wu H, et al. Phase II study of preoperative paclitaxel/cisplatin with radiotherapy in locally advanced esophageal cancer. Int J Radiat Oncol Biol Phys 2007;1(67): 397–404.

47. Arnott SJ, Duncan W, Gignoux M, et al. Preoperative radiotherapy in esophageal carcinoma: A meta-analysis using individual patient data (Oesophageal Cancer Collaborative Group). Int J Radiat Oncol Biol Phys 1998;1;41: 579–83.

48. Walsh TN, Noonan N, Hollywood D, et al. A comparison of multimodal therapy and surgery for esophageal adenocarcinoma. N Engl J Med 1996;335:462–7.

49. Urschel JD, Vasan H. Am. A meta-analysis of randomized controlled trials that compared neoadjuvant chemoradiation and surgery to surgery alone for resectable esophageal cancer. J Surg 2003;185:538–4.

50. Fiorica F, Di Bona D, Schepis F, et al. Preoperative chemoradiotherapy for oesophageal cancer: a systematic review and meta-analysis. Gut 2004;53:925–30.

51. Sarah E Greer, Philip P Goodney, John E Sutton, et al. Neoadjuvant chemoradiotherapy for esophageal carcinoma: A meta-analysis. Surgery 2005;137:172–7.

52. Gebski Val, Burmeister Bryan, Smithers B Mark, Foo K, Zalcberg J, Simes J. Australasian Gastro-Intestinal Trials Group. Survival benefits from neoadjuvant chemoradiotherapy or chemotherapy in oesophageal carcinoma: a meta-analysis. Lancet Oncol. 2007 Mar;8(3):226–34. doi:10.1016/S1470-2045(07)70039-6(PMID: 17329193)

53. van Hagen P, Hulshof MC, van Lanschot JJ, et al. CROSS Group. Preoperative chemo-radiotherapy for esophageal or junctional cancer. N Engl J Med 2012;31(366):2074–84.

54. Xiao ZF, Yang ZY, Liang J, et al. Value of radiotherapy after radical surgery for esophageal carcinoma: a report of 495 patients. Ann Thorac Surg 2003;75:331–6.

55. Malthaner RA, Wong RK, Rumble RB, et al. Neoadjuvant or adjuvant therapy for resectable esophageal cancer: A systematic review and meta-analysis. BMC Med 2004;2:35.

56. Macdonald JS, Smalley SR, Benedetti J, et al. Chemoradiotherapy after surgery compared with surgery alone for adenocarcinoma of the stomach or gastroesophageal junction. N Engl J Med 2001;345:725–30.

57. Sharan K, Fernandes DJ, Prakash Saxena PU, Banerjee S, Sathian B. Treatment outcomes after intraluminal brachytherapy following definitive chemoradiotherapy in patients with esophageal cancer. J Cancer Res Ther 2014;10(2):337–41. doi: 10.4103/0973-1482.136623. PMID: 25022388

58. Sharma V, Mahantshetty U, Dinshaw KA, Deshpande R, Sharma S. Palliation of advanced/recurrent esophageal carcinoma with high-dose-rate brachytherapy. Int J Radiat Oncol Biol Phys. 2002;52(2):310–5. Review. PMID:11872275.

59. Vivekanandam S, Reddy KS, Velavan K, Balasundaram V, Ranga Rao S, Subba Rao KS, Nachiappan M. External beam radiotherapy and intraluminal brachytherapy in advanced in operable esophageal cancer: JIPMER experience. Am J Clin Oncol 2001;24(2):128–30. PMID: 11319284.

60. Sharma V, Agarwal J, Dinshaw K, Nehru RM, Mohandas M, Deshpande R, Rayabhattnavar S. Late esophageal toxicity using a combination of external beam radiation, intraluminal brachytherapy and 5-fluorouracil infusion in carcinoma of the esophagus. Dis Esophagus 2000;13(3): 219–25. PMID: 11206636.

61. Dinshaw KA, Sharma V, Pendse AM, Telang CS, Vege SS, Malliat MK, Deshpande R, Desai PB. The role of intraluminal radiotherapy and concurrent 5-fluorouracil infusion in the management of carcinoma esophagus: a pilot study. J Surg Oncol 1991;47(3):155–60. PMID:2072698.

62. Won JH, Lee JD, Wang HJ, Kim GE, Kim BW, Yim H, Han SK, Park CH, Joh CW, Kim KH, Park KB, Shin KM. Self-expandable covered metallic esophageal stent impregnated with beta-emitting radionuclide: an experimental study in canine esophagus. Int J Radiat Oncol Biol Phys 2002;53(4):1005–13. PMID:12095570

63. Wayman J, Irving M, Russell N, Nicoll J, Raimes SA. Intraluminal radiotherapy and Nd:YAG laser photoablation for primary malignant melanoma of the esophagus. Gastrointest Endosc 2004;59(7):927–9. No abstract available. PMID:15173820

64. Sur RK, Didcott CC, Levin CV, Kulhavy M, Donde B, Schafer M, Gavenescu J. Palliation of carcinoma of the oesophagus with brachytherapy and the Didcott dilator. Ann R Coll Surg Engl 1996;78(2):124–8. PMID: 8678445

65. Brewster AE, Davidson SE, Makin WP, Stout R, Burt PA. Intraluminal brachytherapy using the high dose rate microselectron in the palliation of carcinoma of the oesophagus. Clin Oncol (R Coll Radiol) 1995;7(2):102–5. PMID:7542470

66. Prasad NR, Karthigeyan M, Vikram K, Parthasarathy R, Reddy KS. Palliative radiotherapy in esophageal cancer. Indian J Surg 2015;77(1):34–8. doi: 10.1007/s12262-013-0817-4. Epub 2013 Jan 26. PMID:25829709

67. Sur RK, Levin CV, Donde B, et al. Prospective randomized trial of HDR brachytherapy as a sole modality in palliation of advanced esophageal carcinoma—an International Atomic Energy Agency study. Int J Radiat Oncol Biol Phys 2002;1;53:127–33.

68. Eduardo Rosenblatt, Glenn Jones, Ranjan K Sur, et al. Adding external beam to intraluminal brachytherapy improves palliation in obstructive squamous cell oesophageal cancer: A prospective multi-centre randomized trial of the International Atomic Energy Agency. Radiotherapy and Oncology 2010:97;488–94.

14

Immunotherapy–Channeling A Novel Approach to Treat Esophageal Carcinoma

Purvish Parikh, RK Deshpande, Aagre Suhas Vilasrao

Introduction

Patients with advanced esophageal cancer have poor prognosis. This has not changed significantly despite new developments in chemotherapy; driver mutation based targeted therapy and combination therapies. Hence the emergence of immunotherapy is like a ray of hope that is steadily increasing in radiance and relevance. In fact, it has also found place in the new molecular classification of gastric cancers, with Esophageal Squamous Cell Carcinomas (ESCC) being divided into three subtypes based on primary pathway affected by mutations.[1]

Group 1 involves NRF2 pathway, Group 3 is associated with phosphoinositide 3-kinase (PI3K) pathway. The middle group (ESCC2), on the other hand, is a basket of mutations affecting NOTCH1, PTEN, PIK3R1, KDM6A, KDM2D, ZNF750, and/or CDK6. Unfortunately, their prognostic implications have not translated into predictive value.[2] Hence there is special interest in the evaluation of MSI, PD-L1 and even PD1 parameters.

Selecting Esophageal Cancer Patients for Immunotherapy

There is a lot of controversy regarding the best way of selecting cancer patients for immunotherapy.[3,4] Till such time as we develop more robust data and novel biomarkers, we have to rely on Tumor Mutation Burden (TMB) and PD-L1 expression. Detection of PD-L1 in esophageal tumors shows great heterogeneity. It fluctuates with stage of the disease (*de novo* vs recurrent), prior treatment (if any; line(s) and combination of chemotherapy drugs), methods of PD-L1 testing (PCR vs IHC) and even the antibody/kit used. On top of this is the confusion regarding what cut-off to use for defining a patient as PD-L1 positive. It is 1%, 49% or 99%. And like other molecular mutations, there are ethnic variations too.

The expression of PD-L1 in esophageal cancer is different from that seen in other solid malignancies. In esophageal cancer the PD-L1 staining is less in the malignant cells as opposed to that in the infiltrating myeloid cells at the invasive margin of the tumor. One study amongst 378 advanced ESCC patients documented the PD-L1 expressed as seen in 29.9% (113/378) tumor cells as compared to 40.2% (152/378) tumor-infiltrating cells. This expression also correlated with age, level of differentiation, TNM stage and presences/absence of metachronous hematogenous metastasis. They also concluded that those with high PD-L1 expression in tumor cells had poor prognosis (P = 0.009).[5]

The exception is when the patient tumor is also EBV positive, in which case it is the tumor cells that express high PD-L1. Such patients seem to respond better and have relatively good prognosis. High levels of PD-L1 expression go hand in hand with High Microsatellite Instability (MSI-H). This is logical since the later leads to higher neoantigen expression which would facilitate interaction with T lymphocytes.[6] There are interesting observations regarding value of PD-L1 when patients are receiving conventional therapy. For patients treated with RT, its expression seems to increase with the total dose of radiation given.[7] Additionally, PD-L1 expression seems to correlate with the response to neoadjuvant chemoradiotherapy and may be used to select patients who could potentially be spared from surgery after neoadjuvant chemoradiotherapy.[8]

Common conventional chemotherapy drugs effective in esophageal cancer include platinum compounds (cisplatin, carboplatin, oxaliplatin), anthracyclines (doxorubicin, epirubicin), taxanes (paclitaxel, docetaxel) and antimetabolites (5-fluorouracil, capecitabine). Platinum compounds and anthracyclines seem to reduce PD-L1 expression whereas taxanes and antimetabolites increase its level.[9,10] Does this mean that patient selection for immunotherapy will be based on what chemotherapy drug(s) have been used previously? Hopefully we will get the answer in the future. These potentially immunogenic tumors represent about one-third of all cases.

The role of MSI phenotype was investigated in a phase I clinical trial where 15 tumor types were treated by pembrolizumab with promising results. The FDA has approved pembrolizumab based on this clinical trial for gastric cancer tumors with MSI-H phenotype. Researchers have also studied the other biomarkers. For instance, studies have shown that NY-ESO-1, LAGE-1, MAGE-A, and TTK can be overexpressed leading to induction of specific CTL cells and potential to enhance tumor cell kill.[11] Also unknown is the value

of studying the level of PD-L2 expression– which is high in about half (51.7%) of the patients with esophageal adenocarcinomas.

PD-L1 Inhibitors in Management of Esophageal Cancers[4,12–14]

Nivolumab

ATTRACTION-2 was a double-blind, multicentric, randomized phase III study in patients with unresectable gastric or Gastroesophageal Junction (GEJ) cancer who had failed at least two prior lines of chemotherapy. It demonstrated the role of nivolumab in heavily pretreated cases, as the Overall Survival (OS) improved with an immunotherapy agent inhibiting PD-L1. The 12-month OS was 26.6% in the study are as compared to 10.9% in the control arm. The Overall Response Rate (ORR) was 11.2% with nivolumab versus 0% with placebo. This benefit was significant in patients with PD-L1 positive and well as PD-L1 negative tumors. Based on this trial, nivolumab has gained approval in Japan.

ATTRACTION-3 (ONO-4538-24/CA209-473) study's have been recently disclosed. Here also nivolumab demonstrated a significantly better OS as compared to chemotherapy in previously treated unresectable advanced or recurrent esophageal cancer. Thus, nivolumab is the first checkpoint inhibitor to have documented a statistically significant improvement in OS, and that too in PD-L1-unselected cases.[15,16] CheckMate-032 compared single agent nivolumab versus its combination with ipilimumab. The study population was 160 cases who had progressed on standard chemotherapy. A total of 154/160 (96%) were evaluable. The ORR was 14% (nivolumab alone) versus 26% for N1 plus I3 arm. Among the PD-L1+ tumors (greater than 1% positive cells) the response rate with nivolumab was 27% (4/15) versus 44% (4/9) with N1/I3. There is also data for advanced squamous cell carcinoma of esophagus. A total of 65 cases were included in nivolumab ONO-4538-12 study. Of these, 17.2% achieved an objective response with a median OS of 12.1 months. CheckMate-577 study is evaluating the role of nivolumab in the adjuvant setting amongst resected stage II/III esophageal cancer (adenocarcinoma and squamous cell carcinomas). Involving 760 patients, this will be the largest adjuvant study of a checkpoint inhibitor in esophageal cancers.

Pembrolizumab

KEYNOTE-012, a multicenter, nonrandomized, open-label, phase Ib study used single-agent pembrolizumab in patients with PD-L1+ recurrent or metastatic gastric/GEJ adenocarcinoma. Amongst the 36/39 evaluable patients, ORR was 22% (8/36). It was tolerated well with 13% of patients experiencing grade 3–4 toxicity.

KEYNOTE-028 study used pembrolizumab in PD-L1+ advanced solid tumors including esophageal cancers. In 23 enrolled cases, the ORR was 30% and 12 months PFS was 21.7%. Interestingly this study included as many as 74% patients with squamous histology.[17]

KEYNOTE-059 is a first-line study where pembrolizumab is combined with chemotherapy and also includes maintenance therapy. OF the 259 patients enrolled, 55% (143/259) had tumors expressing PD-L1 (IHC 22C3 pharmDx Kit companion diagnostics). Here positivity was as per the combined positive score (CPS) ≥ 1 (staining in tumor cells, lymphocytes and macrophages) divided by total number of tumor cells evaluated and then multiplied by 100. For the positive patients, the ORR was 13.3% and interestingly 1.4% actually achieved complete response. Based on its first cohort, pembrolizumab received FDA approval in previously treated PD-L1 positive cases as identified by its companion diagnostic kit.

However, optimism was cooled by the results of the Keynote-061 trial randomizing patients between pembrolizumab and an active comparator paclitaxel which did not show any significant benefit. This is especially important since paclitaxel is no longer standard of care in the second line setting-comparison should have been with combination of paclitaxel and ramucirumab.

KEYNOTE-062 is an ongoing phase III trial evaluating pembrolizumab alone versus its combination with chemotherapy (cisplatin plus 5-FU).

KEYNOTE-180 is a phase 2, open-label, single-arm study that has enrolled 121 patients up to March 21, 2017. Eligibility was presences of advanced, metastatic esophageal cancer that had progressed after 2 or more lines of chemotherapy. Of these, 58 (47.9%) had tumors positive for PD-L1, (score of 10 or higher–a new cut-off) assessed by immunohistochemistry. Objective response rate was 13.8% (8/58) among the PD-L1-positive patients. 5 patients (4.1%) discontinued treatment because of adverse events.[18,19]

Other studies are evaluating pembrolizumab with radiation therapy. One is for *de novo* metastatic patients along with brachytherapy whereas another one is along with palliative teleradiation therapy. In summary, pembrolizumab is active in esophageal cancer patients whose tumors overexpress PD-L1. Response rates are higher in adenocarcinoma (40.0%) as compared to squamous cell carcinoma (29.4%). About half will show some amount of tumor reduction with manageable side effects.

Avelumab

JAVELIN studies are evaluating the role of another immunotherapy agent, Avelumab in several settings–including recurrent, locally advanced, or metastatic cases. This includes as maintenance phase following chemotherapy or in the second line or later stages.

Durvalumab

NCT02639065 study is evaluating durvalumab in 26 patients with persistent residual esophageal cancer after definitive therapy is completed. Durvalumab is also being studied in second and third line metastatic cases, both singly or in combination with the Anti CTLA4 agent tremelimumab. To complete the list of PD-L1 inhibitors, small phase I/II studies are also testing the value of nivolumab, pembro-lizumab, and durvalumab in the neoadjuvant setting (singly or in combination with neoadjuvant CT/CRT).

Other Immunotherapy Strategies

A complex vaccine (IMF-001; CHP-NY-ESO-1) having recombinant NY-ESO-1 protein plus cholesteryl hydrophobized pullulan (CHP) is being evaluated among patients with ESCC. Its use seems to be safe and does induce immunogenicity.[20]

A telomerase-specific oncolytic virus (OBP-301) is being tested by direct intratumoral administration followed by radiation therapy in elderly patients. Preliminary results indicate response in 3/6 (50%) with two achieving CR.[21] Endoscopic oncolytic virus injection in combination with locoregional radiotherapy was feasible and well-tolerated in patients with ESCC.

Adverse Effects

The field of immuno-oncology is currently brimming with hundreds of new drugs in discovery or development phase. In fact, the Nobel prize in medicine was given to two stalwarts in this field only last year (2018). Hence the field is rapidly evolving and so also are we discovering unexpected side effects. Besides the usual side effects of asthenia, fever, nausea, itching, rash, loss of appetite, pains/aches, constipation/diarrhea and infusion reactions, we have to be cautious of more ominous warning signs.

Respiratory symptoms like cough, short-ness of breath and hemoptysis are to be reported by patients promptly for necessary intervention. Lower respiratory tract infections, interstitial lung disease and resurgence of tuberculosis could occur and may rapidly progress with serious consequences. Endo-crine disorders and autoimmune effects in other parts of the body are also to be watched out for (especially liver, skin, mucosa, kidneys).[22]

Recently a severe case of esophageal stenosis was reported in a patient receiving nivolumab. Fortunately, it was reversed by the use of tocilizumab (An anti IL6 receptor MoAb).[23]

Such immune related adverse effects may require interruption of the PD-L1 blocker (temporarily or permanently) and may even need the use of high doses of corticosteroids.

CONCLUSIONS

Currently available data clearly indicates that immunotherapy has a vital emerging role in the management of esophageal cancers. Single-agent checkpoint inhibitors when used in the metastatic setting are expected to give an ORR of about 25% for those 40% who have PD-L1+ expression. In unselected patients this ORR can be expected to be 15%. Obviously, better biomarkers to enrich eligible patients will be required. In the meantime, higher the PD-L1 expression, better is the likely response rate. This is also true when using PD-1/CTLA-4 inhibitors. Response to combination immuno-oncology drugs is an avenue that needs to be explored systematically. For instance, nivolumab/ipilimumab combination has been shown to ORR of 21% even among heavily treated cases.

The answer lies in the various ongoing trials studying immune checkpoint inhibitors (anti-PD1, anti-PD-L1, Anti CTLA4 antibodies) in esophageal cancer-not only in advanced/metastatic disease setting, but also in adjuvant, neoadjuvant, or perioperative settings. ATTRACTION-3 data achieved a significant milestone wherein, for the first time, checkpoint inhibitor has shown clear overall survival benefit in heavily pretreated patients with esophageal cancer without any biomarker selection. However, a word of caution is necessary, as we understand the adverse consequences of playing with the immune system. Imbalance can lead to new and potentially life-threatening adverse effects. This is particularly important for developing countries where the incidence of latent or active tuberculosis may be high.

REFERENCES

1. Cancer Genome Atlas Research Network. Integrated genomic characterization of oesophageal carcinoma. Nature 2017;541:169–75.

2. Javadinia SA, Shahidsales S, Fanipakdel A, Mostafapour A, Joudi-Mashhad M, Ferns GA, Avan A: The Esophageal Cancer and the PI3K/AKT/mTOR signaling regulatory microRNAs; a novel marker for prognosis, and a possible target for immunotherapy. Curr Pharm Des 2019 Jan 10. doi: 10.2174138161282566190110143258. [Epub ahead of print]

3. Kosovec JE, Zaidi AH, Pounardjian TS, Jobe BA: The Potential Clinical Utility of Circulating Tumor DNA in Esophageal Adenocarcinoma: From Early Detection to Therapy. Front Oncol. 2018;8:610.

4. Kelly RJ. Immunotherapy for Esophageal and Gastric Cancer. Am Soc Clin Oncol Educ Book. 2017;37:292–300. doi:10.14694/EDBK_175231. (https://meetinglibrary.asco.org/record/138299/edbook#fulltext)

5. Rong L, Liu Y, Hui Z, Zhao Z, Zhang Y, Wang B, Yuan Y, Li W, Guo L, Ying J, Song Y, Wang L, Zhou Z, Xue L, Lu N. PD-L1 expression and its clinicopathological correlation in advanced esophageal squamous cell carcinoma in a Chinese population. Diagn Pathol 2019;14(1):6.

6. Kim JH, Park HE, Cho NY, Lee HS, Kang GH. Characterisation of PD-L1-positive subsets of microsatellite-unstable colorectal cancers. Br J Cancer 2016;115:490–6.

7. Minsky BD, Pajak TF, Ginsberg RJ, Pisansky TM, Martenson J, Komaki R, Okawara G, Rosenthal SA, Kelsen DP. INT 0123 (Radiation Therapy Oncology Group 94-05) phase III trial of combined-modality therapy for esophageal cancer: High-dose versus standard-dose radiation therapy. J Clin Oncol 2002;20:1167–74.

8. Tang Y, Li G, Wu S, Tang L, Zhang N, Liu J, Zhang S, Yao L. Programmed death ligand 1 expression in esophageal cancer following definitive chemoradiotherapy: Prognostic significance and association with inflammatory biomarkers. Oncol Lett 2018;15:4988–96.

9. Yang JH, Kim H, Roh SY, Lee MA, Park JM, Lee HH, Park CH, Lee HH, Jung ES, Lee SH, et al. Discordancy and changes in the pattern of programmed death ligand 1 expression before and after platinum-based chemotherapy in metastatic gastric cancer. Gastric Cancer 2018:1–8. doi: 10.1007/s10120-018-0842-x. [PubMed] [CrossRef]

10. Min Z, Yibo F, Xiaofang C, Kezuo H, Xiujuan Q. 5-Fluorouracil induced up-regulation of exosomal PD-L1 causing immunosuppression in gastric cancer patients. Ann. Oncol. 2018;29 doi: 10.1093/annonc/mdy268.043. [CrossRef]

11. Zhang Y, Zhang Y, Zhang L: Expression of cancer-testis antigens in esophageal cancer and their progress in immunotherapy. J Cancer Res Clin Oncol. 2019 Jan 17. doi:10.1007/s00432-019-02840-3. [Epub ahead of print]

12. Tanaka T, Nakamura J, Noshiro H. Promising immunotherapies for esophageal cancer. Expert Opin Biol Ther 2017;17(6):723–33.

13. Kojima T, Doi T. Immunotherapy for Esophageal Squamous Cell Carcinoma. Curr Oncol Rep 2017;19:33.

14. Vrána D, Matzenauer M, Neoral Č, Aujeský R, Vrba R, Melichar B, Rušarová N, Bartoušková M, Jankowski J. From Tumor Immunology to Immunotherapy in Gastric and Esophageal Cancer. Int J Mol Sci. 2018;20(1):pii: E13. doi: 10.3390/ijms20010013.

15. Opdivo® (Nivolumab) Demonstrates a Significant Extension in Overall Survival Versus Chemotherapy in Patients with Unresectable Advanced or Recurrent Esophageal Cancer in Phase III Clinical Study. ONO Pharmaceutical Co., LTD. Published January 10, 2019. https://bit.ly/2D2P3bX?rel=0". Accessed February 7, 2019.

16. https://www.epgonline.org/uk/news/opdivo-success-in-phase-iii-attraction-3-study-to-treat-oesophageal-cancer--bms---ono.html

17. Doi T, Sarina Anne Piha-Paul, Shadia Ibrahim Jalal, Hieu Mai-Dang, Sammy Yuan, et al. Pembrolizumab (MK-3475) for patients (pts) with advanced esophageal carcinoma: Preliminary results from KEYNOTE-028. J Clin Oncol, 2015;33(Suppl; abstr 4010).

18. Shah MA, Kojima T, Hochhauser D, Enzinger P, Raimbourg J, Hollebecque A, Lordick F, Kim SB, Tajika M, Kim HT, Lockhart AC, Arkenau HT, El-Hajbi F, Gupta M, Pfeiffer P, Liu Q, Lunceford

J, Kang SP, Bhagia P, Kato K. Efficacy and Safety of Pembrolizumab for Heavily Pretreated Patients With Advanced, Metastatic Adenocarcinoma or Squamous Cell Carcinoma of the Esophagus: The Phase 2 KEYNOTE-180 Study. JAMA Oncol. 2018 Dec 20. doi: 10.1001/ jamaoncol.2018.5441. [Epub ahead of print]

19. Parikh PM, Sahoo TP, Singh R, Bahl A, Talwar V, et al. Practical consensus recommendations— current role of iRECIST in the management of cancer patients receiving immunotherapy. Intl J Mol Immuno Oncol 2019;4:21–23.

20. Kageyama S, et al. Dose-dependent effects of NY-ESO-1 protein vaccine complexed with cholesteryl pullulan (CHP-NY-ESO-1) on immune responses and survival benefits of esophageal cancer patients. J Transl Med 2013; 11:246.

21. Tanabe S, Shunsuke Kagawa HT, Kazuhiro Noma, KiyotoTakehara, Takeshi Koujima, et al. Phase I/II trial of endoscopic intratumoral administrationof OBP-301, a novel telomerase-specific oncolytic virus, with radiation in elderly esophageal cancer patients. Cancer Res, 2015; 75(15 Suppl): Abstract nr CT123.

22. Parikh PM, Jhaveri K, Bahl A, Talwar V, Gandhi P, Singh R, et al. Special considerations for consent in immune-oncology: Medic LAWgic recommendations. Intl J Mol Immuno Oncol 2019;4:6–8.

23. Horisberger A, La Rosa S, Zurcher JP, Zimmermann S, Spertini F, et al. A severe case of refractory esophageal stenosis induced by nivolumab and responding to tocilizumab therapy. J Immunother Cancer 2018;6(1):156. doi: 10.1186/s40425-018-0481-0.

15

Therapeutic Endoscopy in Esophageal Cancer
(Prevention, Treatment and Palliation)

Samir Parikh, Anuj Parikh

Therapeutic endoscopy is of vital importance in the management of esophageal cancer. Premalignant lesions like Barrett's esophagus (BE) with dysplasia can be eradicated with a high success rate. The ability of endoscopic ultrasound to identify the depth of early esophageal cancer allows endoscopic resection of mucosal tumors. Surgical palliation for locally advanced incurable tumors is largely replaced by endoscopic local therapy to effectively reduce morbidity and improve the quality of life. The ability of an endoscopist to treat a few complications of surgery and radiotherapy makes him a useful team member in the overall care of esophageal cancer patients.

The role of therapeutic endoscopy includes:

1. Palliation of advanced inoperable cancer
2. Treatment of mucosal cancer
3. Treatment of premalignant lesions
4. Treatment of complications following surgery and chemoradiotherapy

Endoscopic Palliation of Esophageal Cancer

Most esophageal cancer patients present at a late stage of the disease when surgical cure is hardly possible (Fig. 15.1). Compared to surgical palliation, endoscopic palliation is simple, quick and is associated with lower morbidity and mortality. Even in the presence of marked weight loss, poor nutrition, history of aspiration and tracheoesophageal fistula, endoscopic palliation can be offered with relative ease in a cost-effective manner. Endoscopic palliation aims to improve oral intake and relieve pain. Various methods of palliating dysphagia includes esophageal dilation, laser therapy, absolute alcohol injection, intraluminal injection of cisplatin/epinephrine gel, photodynamic therapy (PDT), argon plasma coagulation, cryospray ablation, placement of stents and brachytherapy. Selection of palliative therapy is often determined by patient and tumor characteristics, clinicians preference, goals of therapy

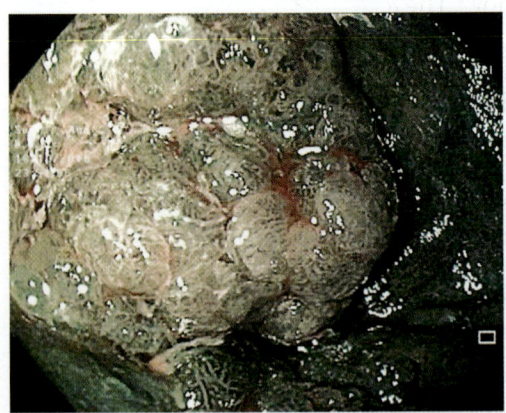

Fig. 15.1: Advanced inoperable esophageal cancer in the lower third occupying almost the entire lumen, narrow band imaging (NBI)

and cost-effectiveness.[1,2] Currently majority of centers prefer to place self-expandable metal stents to relieve dysphagia.[1-3]

Esophageal Dilation

Gradual dilation of the esophageal lumen over a guide wire, using Controlled Radial Expansion (CRE) balloons or bougies can relieve dysphagia for a short period. An effective luminal diameter of >13 mm can be achieved by dilating the lumen to 15–17 mm.[4] Dilatation may be required once in 15 days and carries a small risk of perforation.[5]

Laser Therapy

Neodymium: Yttrium-Aluminum-Garnet (Nd:YAG) laser fulgurates voluminous tumors to restore luminal patency. Therapy is performed every 48 hours over a week and effects last for a few months.[6] Relief of dysphagia for a few months is possible in majority.[6] Technically it is difficult to use laser for tortuous strictures, at the esophagogastric junction and near the cricopharynx. Need for repeated sessions, prolonged hospital stay, risk of perforation and high cost are disadvantages of the therapy.

Absolute Alcohol Injection

Tumor injection with absolute alcohol produces chemical ablation of voluminous tumor.[7] The technique is not standardized nor validated. Its popularity in developing countries is due to low cost, easy availability and small learning curve. However, it can produce mediastinitis, chest pain, tracheo-esophageal fistula and perforation. Relief in dysphagia is for a few weeks and alcohol injections often need to be repeated.[8]

Intraluminal Injection of Cisplatin/ Epinephrine Gel

After some success with local brachytherapy two studies have attempted injection of chemotherapy containing gel to relieve dysphagia with variable success.[9,10] However, this newer therapy needs to be evaluated in a prospective method and standardized.

Photodynamic Therapy (PDT)

The technique includes use of photosensitizing agent (Porfimer) intravenously with endoscopic laser to ablate malignant tumor. On laser application porfimer produces singlet oxygen which damages microvasculature of the tumor producing its necrosis.[11] It is most useful for treating tumor recurrences, residual tumor, in and overgrowth of tumor post stents and tumors close to cricopharynx and cardia.[12-14] Photosensitization of skin limits outdoor activities for 4–6 weeks.

Argon Plasma Coagulation

Argon plasma coagulation (APC) uses monopolar, noncontact, high frequency electrocautery that uses argon gas to cause coagulation and tumor necrosis. It has an overall success in relieving dysphagia in >90% with minor risk of bleeding.[15] Using APC with brachytherapy or PDT provides longer relief of dysphagia.[16] It is a simple, cost-effective therapy with no special space requirement and is available in most endoscopy units.

Cryospray Ablation

Cryospray ablation (CSA) uses supercoiling non-contact method to induce tumor necrosis. Relief of dysphagia occurred in about 60% patients where other methods had failed.[17] Post CSA therapy strictures occurred in about 10% patients.[18]

Endoscopic Stenting

Placement of self-expandable stents has replaced most other forms of palliating dysphagia.[19] They are most often used for thoracic and lower esophageal cancers, patients with tracheoesophageal fistula, post-neoadjuvant chemoradiotherapy strictures and recurrence of tumor at the local site (Fig. 15.2). Smaller diameter stents can be placed in cervical tumors 2 cm away from crico-

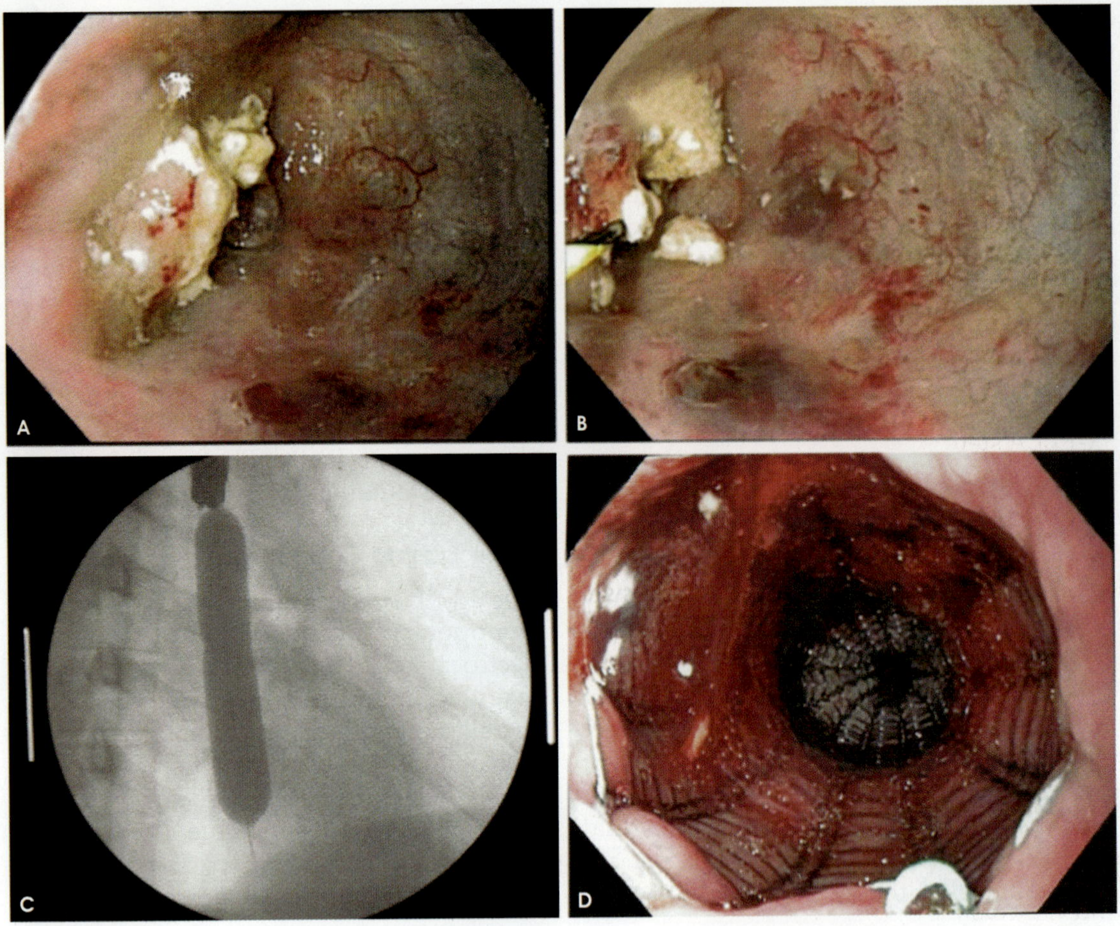

Fig. 15.2: (A) Recurrence of malignant stricture post therapy. (B) Guide-wire placed across the stricture. (C) CRE balloon dilation. (D) Partially covered 10 cm long wall stent placed

pharynx.[20,21] Stents are less effective when extraluminal nodal mass produces dysphagia.[22]

Types of Stents: Three types of expandable stents are available, viz. metal, plastic and biodegradable (Fig. 15.3).

Self-Expandable Metallic (SEM) Stents: They are composed of nitinol an alloy of nickel and titanium. SEM stents are available in various sizes, shapes and lengths. The three varieties include uncovered, partially covered and fully covered. Fully covered stents are used to treat tracheoesophageal fistula and resistant post-radiation strictures. They can be removed, resist tumor ingrowth but are more expensive and have a higher rate of migration.[23] Partially

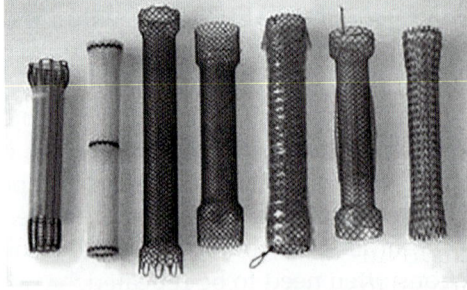

Fig. 15.3: Types of self-expandable stents

covered stents get embedded in the tissue and resist migration but are subject to tumor ingrowth resulting in recurrence of dysphagia in few months (4–6). Stents with larger proximal flare prevent migration. Antireflux stents are used when tumor is across the cardia and Niti-S stents are placed through the scope with a larger working channel.

Self-Expandable Plastic Stents: The polyflex stent is made of polyester and is fully covered with silicone. Though self-expandable plastic stents relieve dysphagia in cancer esophagus.[24] Its higher cost, complications and rate of migration limits its routine use.[25] They are occasionally used for short duration to improve nutrition prior to surgery or neoadjuvant therapy.[26]

Self-Expandable Biodegradable Stents: The SX-ELLA stent is made from a woven surgical suture material polydioxanone. It is an uncovered stent which degrades in three months. It is used to relieve dysphagia during neoadjuvant therapy but only outside USA.[27]

Method of Placement: Malignant stricture is first dilated to 8–10 mm, length of stricture is assessed, stent of appropriate length (stricture length + 4 cm) is selected, external markers are placed and stent is placed under fluoroscopy-control. For cervical esophageal, cancer a distal release stent and for cardia lesions a proximal release stent is preferred. Once stent is deployed assembly is withdrawn slowly and contrast check is performed. We start liquid diet within 2–4 hours and patient is advised to have small frequent meals and avoid fibrous foods. The average patency rates are 94%, 78% and 67% at 30, 90 and 180 days respectively.[28] SEM stents are safer, more effective, have lesser incidence of recurrent dysphagia and procedure related mortality compared to rigid plastic stents.[29] SEM stents produced quicker relief of dysphagia compared to laser or brachytherapy. Double layered Niti-S stent have lower failure rate compared to covered Niti-S stent as they have better radial expansion strength.[30,31] Stent placement along with neoadjuvant chemotherapy aims to relieve dysphagia quickly and improve nutrition. However, it is associated with higher migration rates, poor oncologic outcomes and even higher toxicities.[32,33] Recurrence of tumor postesophagectomy or

development of fistula can be effectively treated by placing SEM stents.[34] SEM stents related adverse events may occur during procedure, immediate postprocedure and delayed postprocedure in a few with overall mortality <2%.[35–37] Intraprocedural complications include perforation, aspiration and malpositioning. Immediate postprocedure complications include bleeding, chest pain, incomplete expansion and tracheal compression. Delayed postprocedural complications include tracheoesophageal fistula formation, gastroesophageal reflux, dysphagia recurrence due to tumor ingrowth or overgrowth.[36,38] High-risk patients for SEM stent placement include advanced tumor stage,[39] tumor invading aorta,[39] prior chemotherapy[40–42] and post placement chemotherapy.[36] Tumor ingrowth or overgrowth is best treated by placement of a second stent.[43] The efficacy of anti-reflux stent in preventing reflux when placed for cardia lesion extending into the stomach is only marginal.[29] Most SEM stents are MRI compatible.[36] In very advanced cancers with severe malnutrition or recurrence after esophagectomy a nasojejunal tube can be placed to improve nutrition (Fig. 15.4).

Brachytherapy

Brachytherapy technique includes placing a radioactive iridium in the esophageal lumen to provide higher doses of radiation to the tumor. It provides long-term relief in dysphagia with lower side-effects. This form of therapy is yet to become popular and need validation.

Endoscopic Treatment of Superficial Esophageal Cancer

Endoscopic resection (ER) is an esophagus sparing approach for M_1, M_2, M_3 intramucosal tumors without lymphovascular invasion (Fig. 15.5). ER may be preferred over esophagectomy in high-risk elderly patients with multiple co-morbidities. When preformed in high-risk patients with M_3 stage and

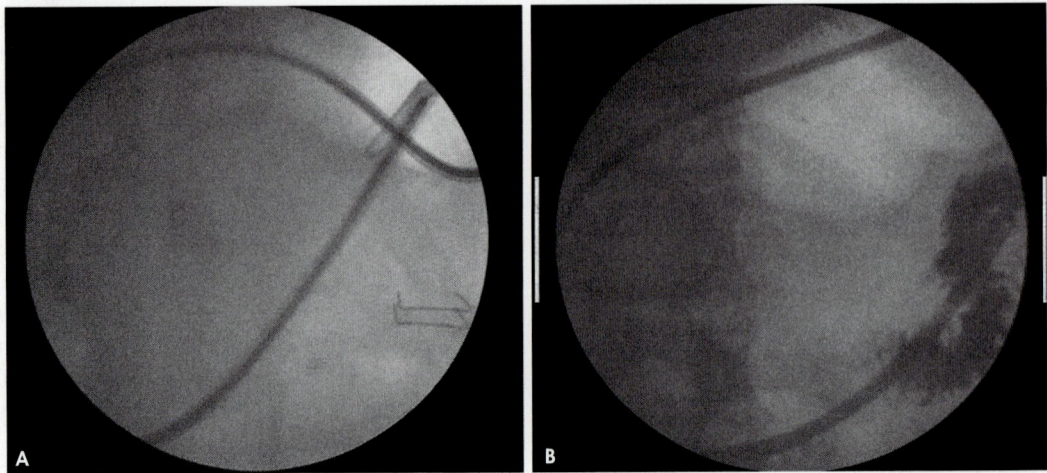

Fig. 15.4: (A) 14 Fr nasojejunal tube placed across the duodenojejunal flexure for postoperative recurrence to maintain nutrition. (B) Check enterogram showing contrast opacification of the jejunum

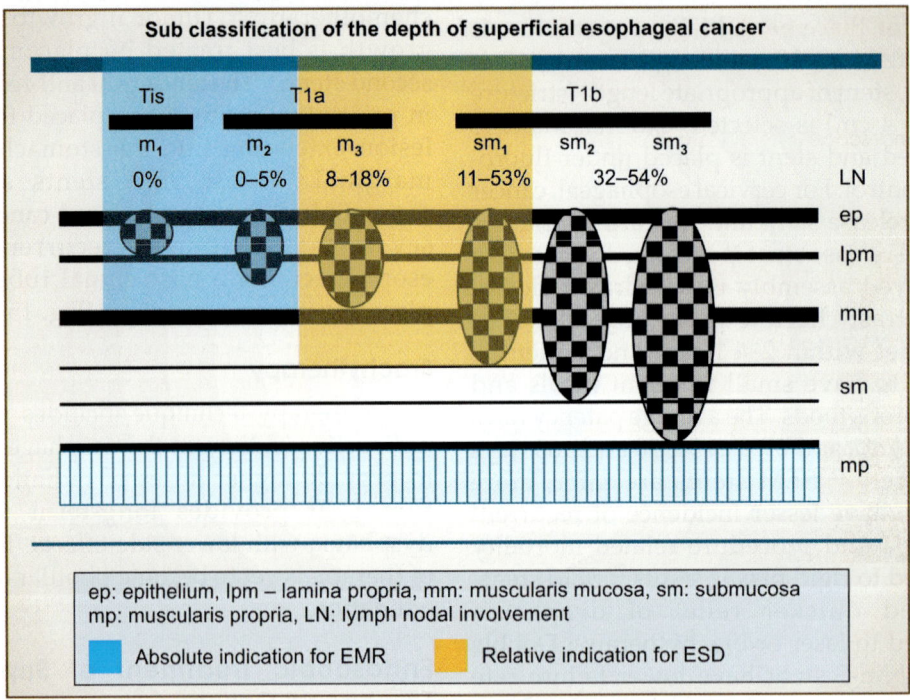

Fig. 15.5: Superficial esophageal cancer

lymphovascular invasion endoscopic resection is combined with photodynamic or radiofrequency ablation. Though ER is commonly performed, it is not universally accepted and have only a few long-term data and fewer randomized trials.[44,45] An ideal lesion for ER is a small (<2 cm diameter), single, flat mucosal tumor within short segments of Barrett's esophagus, with a negative no lift sign and lesion that can be easily sucked into the endoscopic cap (both later suggestive of no submucosal involvement). ER involves excision of neoplastic mucosa allowing a complete histological evaluation akin to surgical specimen. ER includes Endoscopic Mucosal Resection (EMR) wherein post-lift, tissue is excised with a snare (Fig. 15.6). In Endoscopic Submucosal Dissection (ESD) post-lift, neoplastic tissue of size >2 cm is excised using special endoscopic equipment and electrocautery (Fig. 15.7). EMR had a success rate of >95%. When used to treat High Grade Dysplasia (HGD) of BE, recurrence rates were 20% at 5 years, 4% required surgery and no deaths were reported due to esophageal cancer.[46] When larger lesions were treated with ESD R_0 resection was reported in about

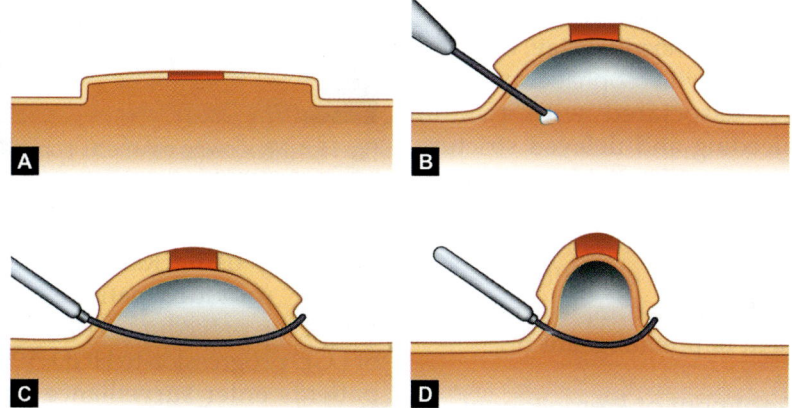

Fig. 15.6: Endoscopic mucosal resection. (A) Intramucosal tumor. (B) Tumor lifted up. (C) Snare applied. (D) Snare resection done

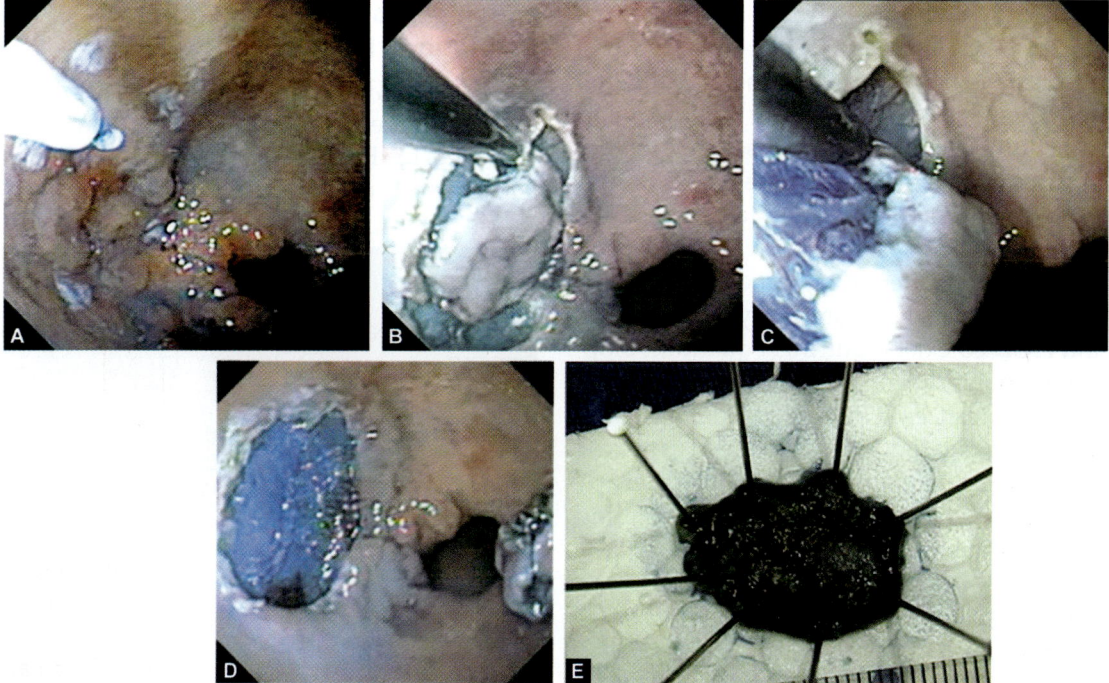

Fig. 15.7: Endoscopic submucosal dissection. (A) Intramucosal tumor markings done 2–3 mms away. (B) Tumor lifted up. (C) Submucosal dissection. (D) Post dissection ulcer. (E) Tumor removed and sent for histology

90% with 2–5% incidence of stricture.[47] The resected lesions should have approximately a 2 mm clear margin and no lymphovascular invasion to achieve ideal long-term results. Recurrence rates with Squamous Cell Carcinoma (SCC) were higher than with Esophageal Adenocarcinoma (EAC).[48] Patients with ER need to have closer follow-up compared to those with esophagectomy as the recurrence rates with ER are higher.[49,50] However, the complication rate, hospital stay, cost and morbidity are higher with esophagectomy.[49,50] ER therapy is associated with risk of perforation, bleeding and delayed stricture formation in about 15%.[51] Most of these complications and even recurrences can be treated endoscopically.[50] Post ER addition of photodynamic therapy or balloon radiofrequency ablation allows complete treatment of larger segment of premalignant BE.[52,53]

Endoscopic Treatment of Premalignant Lesion

Barrett's esophagus (BE) is a premalignant metaplastic change which increases the risk of EAC. Unlike the past, occurrence of dysplasia is now treated endoscopically and not by surgery. Endoscopic ablation and resection are increasingly used to prevent progression of dysplastic tissue to malignancy. Presence of dysplasia needs to be confirmed by a second experienced pathologist.[54] Often in a segment of BE areas of no dysplasia, Low Grade Dysplasia (LGD) and HGD co-exist requiring 4 quadrant biopsies at an interval of 1–2 cm (Flowchart 15.1). The risk of cancer in BE is reduced if the entire BE is eradicated not just the dysplastic mucosa. Endoscopic eradication therapy often includes combination of ablation and resection therapies.

Barrett's Esophagus with Low Grade Dysplasia

LGD in BE (Fig. 15.8) once confirmed by another pathologist is eradicated endo-

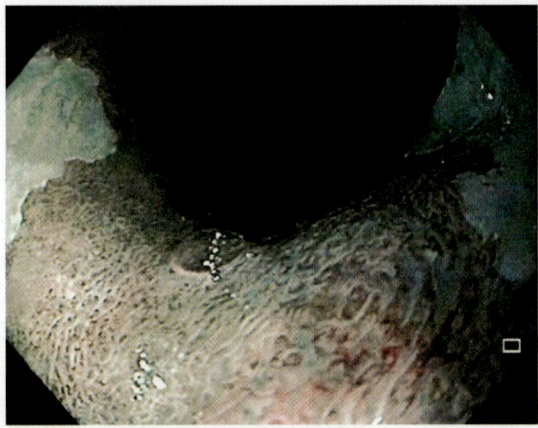

Fig. 15.8: NBI showing disturbed intrapapillary capillary loop with mild irregularity suggesting dysplasia on underlying Barrett's esophagus

scopically using Radiofrequency Ablation (RFA)[55] provided patients understand the risk of the procedure.[56] RFA reduces the risk of LGD progression to HGD.[56,57] Once ablated patients enter surveillance protocol as the duration of ablative benefits are not known.[58,59]

Barrett's Esophagus with High Grade Dysplasia or Intramucosal Cancer

Areas of HGD or intramucosal cancer and mucosal irregularity (Fig. 15.9) must be removed by ER. Entire metaplastic tissue is subsequently ablated by RFA. Though follow-

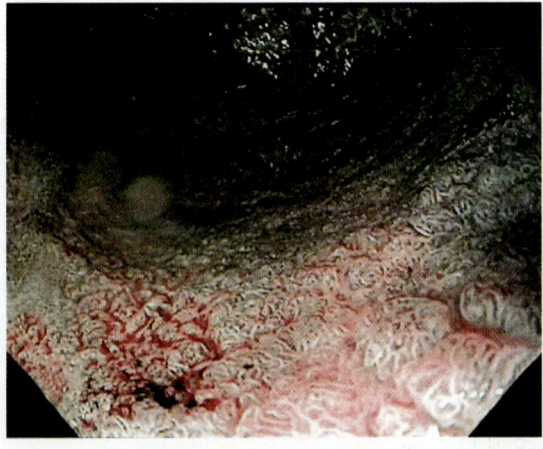

Fig. 15.9: NBI showing disturbed intra papillary capillary loop (IPCL) with mucosal irregularity suggesting HGD

Flowchart 15.1: Surveillance of Barrett's esophagus

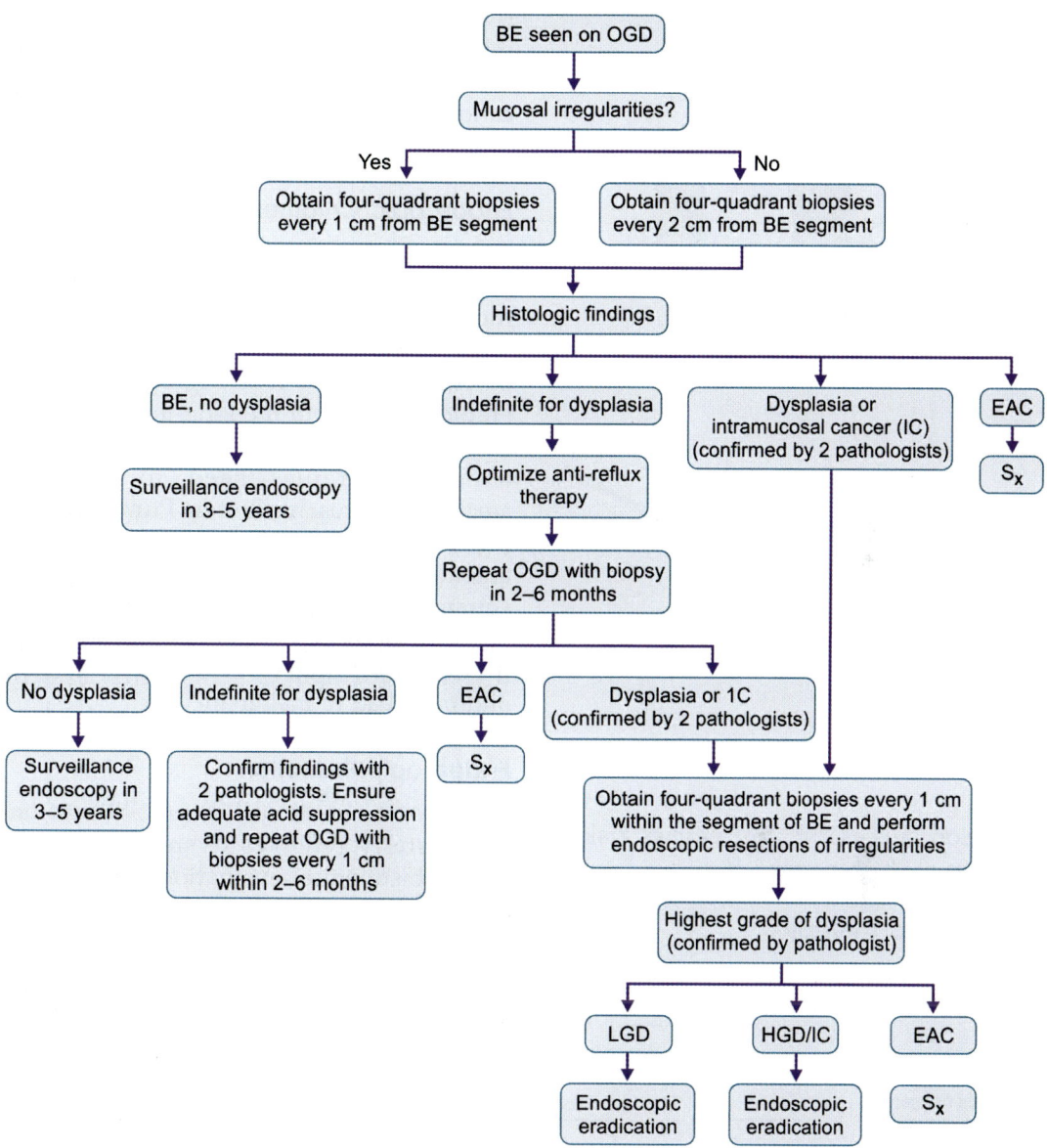

up of successfully treated patients are not available beyond 5 years they enjoy the longest quality adjusted life expectancy.[60, 61]

Endoscopic Ablation

Ablative treatments use thermal to photochemical or radiofrequency energy to ablate BE.[62–65] Contact RFA is most preferred but PDT and cryoablation are often used in tortuous and stricturous esophagus.

Radiofrequency Ablation

In this technique radiofrequency energy is applied using a balloon or paddle to ablate BE (Fig. 15.10).[64] RFA ablates BE, prevents progression to malignancy with >90%

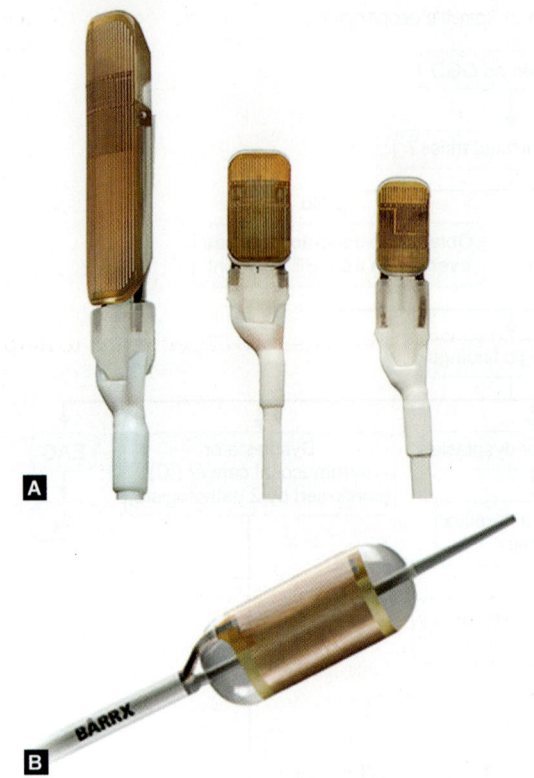

Fig. 15.10: Radiofrequency ablators: (A) Barrx focal ablation catheters. (B) Halo 360 ablation catheter

eradication success[65,66] but carries risk of recurrence at 9% per year.[67,68]

Photodynamic Therapy

Photodynamic therapy (PDT) involves use of photosensitizers that induce cytotoxicity when exposed to light of certain wavelength (Fig. 15.11). PDT is better than proton pump inhibitor (PPI) therapy but serious side-effects like stricture formation, development of cancer in treated patients and skin sensitivity limits its use.

Endoscopic Cryotherapy

It uses application of cryogen like nitrous oxide endoscopically for patients with BE. It induces freezing and thawing for patients with BE inducing apoptosis and thrombosis of blood vessels. It is highly effective to eradicate HGD but the long-term results are not known.[69–71] All patients who undergo ablative therapies need to be under surveillance yearly. Proton Pump Inhibitor (PPI) therapy is started within 24 hours of ablation and continued for life. Newly formed squamous epithelium on PPI therapy may have metaplastic remnant mucosa under it (buried BE). Buried BE is difficult to diagnose and may lead to malignancy.[72]

Endoscopic Resection

Endoscopic resection (ER) post-lift not only successfully removes dysplastic tissue it allows histological evaluation. Patients with submucosal invasion or lymphovascular involvement can be subjected to esophagectomy. At the time no more than 75% of circumferential BE is removed to avoid

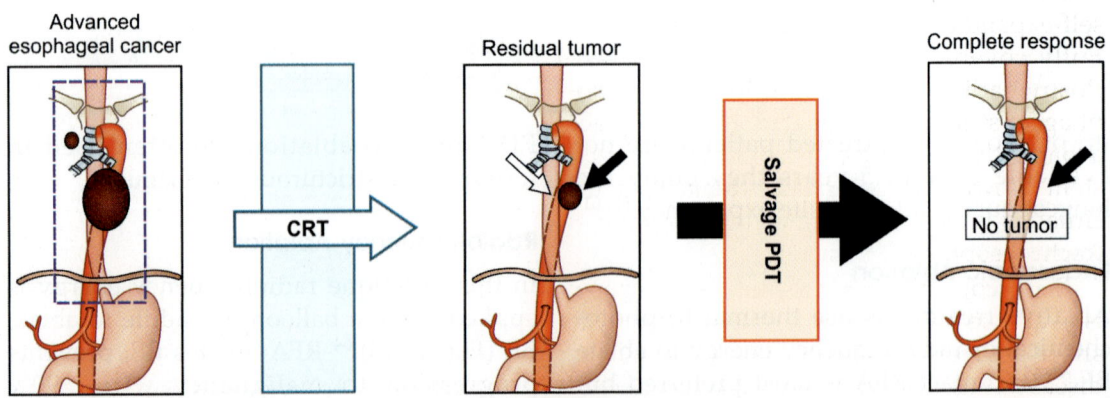

Fig. 15.11: Photodynamic therapy

stricture formation. In BE >5 cm length, ER is often performed at weekly interval in a piecemeal fashion. It is highly effective[66] and often combined currently with RFA.[73] Unlike RFA, ER requires very high skill and is operator dependent.

Endoscopic Treatment of Complications of Surgery and Neoadjuvant Therapy

Postoperative leak is a troublesome complication of esophagectomy for esophageal cancer. It occurs in about 4–20% with an associated mortality up to 80%. Endoscopic insertion of vicryl mesh with fibrin glue avoids repeat surgery in such patients.[74] Placement of fully covered self-expandable metal stents allow complete healing of leaks in about two-thirds with considerable reduction in mortality.[75] Application of Over The Scope Clip (OTSC) allows complete closure of leaks provided the esophageal mucosa with the opening can be sucked into the cap attached to the tip of the scope.[76] Endoscopic treatment of postoperative leaks is evolving. Most often patients' characteristics, size of leak, associated comorbidities and availability of endoscopic skill determine the type and the time of therapy offered.

Postoperative anastomotic strictures occur in less than 5% of patients. Balloon dilation with CRE balloon to about 12 mm is sufficient for most. Postdilation the stricture is evaluated for histological diagnosis. Recurrent/resistant strictures are treated with covered self-expandable stents for about 2–3 months. Fully covered stent can then be removed. Postneoadjuvant chemoradiotherapy esophageal strictures are dilated gently to place a partially covered self-expandable metal stent. However, placing SEM stents in such a situation is often complicated by formation of tracheoesophageal fistula.

Endoscopic treatment of esophageal cancer is available for all stages of the disease. One should carefully assess the stage of the disease, consider locally available technology and expertise in an attempt to offer cure or

reduce the morbidity associated with esophageal cancer. In India SCC still dominates all types of esophageal cancer where guidelines for surveillance of high-risk cases are not available. High index of suspicion, low threshold for biopsy and careful evaluation of esophageal mucosa may increase the detection of early esophageal cancers. Endoscopic ablation and resection therapy are now widely accepted and are promising. The cost of SEM stents need to be regulated to help the poorest of the poor in palliation of esophageal cancer. Therapeutic endoscopists are now important members of the team for evaluating and treating esophageal cancer. Thus, therapeutic endoscopy helps in preventing esophageal cancer (ablation/resection of BE), treatment of intramucosal esophageal cancer (endoscopic resection) and palliation of advanced cancer (self-expandable metal stents) to improve the quality of life. We believe therapeutic endoscopy is at the end of the beginning in the treatment of esophageal cancer.

REFERENCES

1. Shenfine J, McNamee P, Steen N, et al. A randomized controlled clinical trial of palliative therapies for patients with inoperable esophageal cancer. Am J Gastroenterol 2009;104: 1674.
2. Evans JA, Early DS, et al. ASGE standards of practice committee. The role of endoscopy in the assessment and treatment of esophageal cancer. Gastrointest Endosc 2013;77:328.
3. Jacobson BC, Hirota W, Baron TH, et al. The role of endoscopy in the assessment and treatment of esophageal cancer. Gastrointest Endosc 2003;57:817.
4. Boyce HW Jr. Palliation of dysphagia of esophageal cancer by endoscopic lumen restoration techniques. Cancer control 1999;6:73.
5. Hernandez LV, Jacobson JW, Harris MS. Comparison among the perforation rates of Maloney, balloon and savary dilation of esophageal strictures. Gastrointest Endosc 2000;51:460.
6. Mellow MH, Pinkas H. Endoscopic laser therapy for malignancies affecting the esophagus and

gastro-esophageal junction. Analysis of technical and functional efficacy. Arch Intern Med 1985;145:1443.

7. Chung SC, Leong HT, Choi CY, et al. Palliation of malignant esophageal obstruction by endoscopic alcohol injection. Endoscopy 1994; 26:275.

8. Ramakrishnaiah VP, Ramkumar J, Pai D. Intraluminal injection of absolute alcohol in carcinoma of gastroesophageal junction for palliation of dysphagia. Ecancermedical science 2014;8:395.

9. Monga SP, Wadleigh R, Sharma A, et al. Intratumoral therapy of cisplatin/epinephrine injectable gel for palliation in patients with obstructive esophageal cancer. Am J Clin Oncol 2000;23:386.

10. Harbord M, Dawes RF, Barr H, et al. Palliation of patients with dysphagia due to advanced esophageal cancer by endoscopic injection of cisplatin/epinephrine injectable gel. Gastrointest Endosc 2002;56:644.

11. Marcon NE. Photodynamic therapy and cancer of the esophagus. Semin Oncol 1994;21:20.

12. McCaughan JS Jr, Ellison EC, Guy JT, et al. Photodynamic therapy for esophageal malignancy: A prospective twelve year study. Ann Thorac Surg 1996;62:1005.

13. Muto M, Yano T, Katada C, et al. Salvage photodynamic therapy for loco-regional failure after definitive chemo radiotherapy for esophageal cancer (abstract). Proc Am Soc Clin Oncol 2004;23:355.

14. Lightdale CJ, Heier SK, Marcon NE, et al. Photodynamic therapy with porfimer sodium versus thermal ablation therapy with Nd:YAG laser for palliation of esophageal cancer: a multicenter randomized trial: Gastrointest Endosc 1995;42:507.

15. Eickhoff A, Jakobs R, Schilling D, et al. Prospective non randomized comparison of two modes of argon beamer (APC) tumor desobstruction: effectiveness of the new pulsed APC versus forced APC. Endoscopy 2007:30;637.

16. Rupinski M, Zagorowicz E, Regula J, et al. Randomized comparison of three palliative regimens including brachytherapy, photodynamic therapy and APC in patients with malignant dysphagia (consort 1a) (revised II) Am J Gastroenterol 2011;106:1612.

17. Cash BD, Johnston LR, Johnston MH. Cyrospray ablation (CSA) in the palliative treatment of squamous cell carcinoma of the esophagus. World J Surg Oncol 2007;5:34.

18. Greenwald BD, Dumot JA, Abrams JA, et al. Endoscopic spray cryotherapy for esophageal cancer: safety and efficacy. Gastrointest Endosc 2010;71:686.

19. Kochar R, Shah N. Enteral stents from esophagus to colon. Gastrointest Endosc 2013;78:913.

20. Battaglia G, Antonello A, Realdon S, et al. Feasibility, efficacy and safety of stent insertion as a palliative treatment for malignant strictures of the esophagus and the hypopharynx. Surg Endosc 2016;30:159.

21. Speer E, Dunst CM, Shada A, et al. Covered stents in cervical anastomosis following esophagectomy. Surg Endosc 2016;30:3297.

22. Bethge N, Sommer A, Vakil N. Palliation of malignant esophageal obstruction due to intrinsic and extrinsic lesions with expandable metal stents. Am J Gastroenterol 1998;93:1829.

23. Sharma P, Kozarek R. Practice parameters and committee of American College of Gastroenterology. Role of esophageal stents in benign and malignant diseases. Am J Gastroenterol 2010;105:258.

24. Conio M, Repici A, Battaglia, et al. A randomized prospective comparison of self-expandable plastic stents and partially covered self-expandable metal stents in the palliation of malignant esophageal dysphagia. Am J Gastroenterol 2007;102:2667.

25. Verschuur EM, Repici A, Kuipers EJ, et al. New design esophageal stents for the palliation of dysphagia from esophageal or gastric cardia cancers: a randomized trial. Am J Gastroenterol 2008;103:304.

26. Brown RE, Abbas AE, Ellis S, et al. A prospective phase II evaluation of esophageal stenting for neo-adjuvant therapy for esophageal cancer: optimal performance and surgical safety. J Am Coll Surg 2011;212:582.

27. Tokar JL, Banerjee S, et al. ASGE Technology Committee. Drug eluting/biodegradable stents. Gastrointest Endosc 2011;74:954.

28. Im JP, Kang JM, Kim SG, et al. Clinical outcomes and patency of self-expanding metal stents in patients with malignant upper gastrointestinal obstruction. Dig Dis Sci 2008;53:938.

29. Dai Y, Li C, Xie Y, et al. Interventions for dysphagia in esophageal cancer. Cochrane database Sys Rev 2014;CD005048.

30. Battersby NJ, Bonney GK, Suber D, et al. Outcomes following esophageal stent insertion for palliation of malignant stricture. A large single center series. J Surg Oncol 2012;105:60.

31. Kim ES, Jeon SW, Park SY, et al. Comparison of double-layered and covered Niti-S stents for palliation of malignant dysphagia. J Gastroenterol Hepatol 2009;24:114.

32. Siddiqui AA, Sarkar A, Beltz S, et al. Placement of fully covered self-expandable metal stents in patients with locally advanced esophageal cancer before neoadjuvant therapy. Gastrointest Endosc 2012;76:44.

33. Francis SR, Orton A, Thorpe C, et al. Toxicity and outcomes in patients with and without esophageal stents in locally advanced esophageal cancer. Int J Radiat Oncol Biol Phys 2017;99:884.

34. Van Heel NC, Haringsma J, Spaander MC, et al. Esophageal stents for the palliation of malignant dysphagia and fistula recurrence after esophagectomy. Gastrointest Endosc 2010;72:249.

35. Medeiros VS, Martins BC, Lenz L, et al. Adverse events of self-expandable metallic stents in patients with long term survival from advanced malignant disease. Gastrointest Endosc 2017;86:299.

36. Baron TH. Expandable metal stent for the treatment of cancerous obstruction of the gastrointestinal tract. N Eng J Med 2001;344:1681.

37. Baron TH. Minimizing endoscopic complications endoluminal stents. Gastrointest Endosc Clin N Am 2007;17:83.

38. Burstow M, Kelly T, Panchani S, et al. Outcome of palliative esophageal stenting for malignant dysphagia: A retrospective analysis. Dis Esophagus 2009;22:519.

39. Sumiyoshi T, Gotoda T, Muro K, et al. Morbidity and mortality after self-expandable metallic stent placement in patients with progressive or recurrent esophageal cancer after chemoradiotherapy. Gastrointest Endosc 2003;57:882.

40. Fuccio L, Scagliarini M, Frazzoni L, et al. Development of a prediction model of adverse events after stent placement for esophageal cancer. Gastrointest Endosc 2016;83:746.

41. Park JY, Shin JH, Song HY, et al. Airway complications after covered stent placement for malignant esophageal stricture: special reference to radiation therapy. AJR Am J Roentgenol 2012;198:453.

42. Bick BL, Song LM, Buttar NS, et al. Stent associated esophago respiratory fistulas: incidence and risk factors. Gastrointest Endosc 2013;77:181.

43. Lagattolla NR, Row PH, Anderson H, et al. Restenting malignant esophageal stricture. Br J Surg 1998;85:261.

44. Bergman JJ. Endoscopic resection for treatment of mucosal Barrett's cancer: Time to swing the pendulum. Gastrointest Endosc 2007;65:11.

45. DeMeester SR. EMR for intramucosal adenocarcinoma of the esophagus: Does one size fit all? Gastrointest Endosc 2007;65:14.

46. Pech O, Behrens A, May A, et al. Long term results and risk factors analysis therapy in 349 patients with high grade intraepithelial neoplasia and mucosal adenocarcinoma in Barrett's esophagus. Gut 2008;57:1200.

47. Sun F, Yuan P, Chen T, et al. Efficacy and complication of endoscopic submucosal dissection for superficial esophageal carcinoma: a systemic review and meta-analysis. J Cardiothoracic Surg 2014;9:78.

48. Nakagawa K, Koike T, Lijima K, et al. Comparison of the long term outcomes of endoscopic resection for superficial squamous cell carcinoma and adenocarcinoma of the esophagus in Japan. Am J Gastroenterol 2014; 109:348.

49. Pech O, Bollschweiler E, Manner H, et al. Comparison between endoscopic and surgical resection of mucosal esophageal adenocarcinoma in Barrett's esophagus at two-high volume centers. Ann Surg 2011;254:67.

50. Prasad GA, Wu TT, Wigle DA, et al. Endoscopic and surgical treatment of mucosal (T_{1a}) esophageal adenocarcinoma in Barrett's esophagus. Gastroenterology 2009;137:815.

51. Peters FP, Kara MA, Rosmolen WD, et al. Stepwise radical endoscopic resection is effective for complete removal of Barrett's esophagus with early neoplasia: a prospective study. Am J Gastroenterol 2006;101:1449.

52. Sharma VK, Wang KK, Overholt BF, et al. Balloon based, circumferential, endoscopic radiofrequency ablation of Barrett's esophagus: 1 year follow up of 100 patients. Gastrointest Endosc 2007;65:185.

53. Bergman JJ. Radiofrequency energy ablation of Barrett's esophagus: The best is yet to come. Gastrointest Endosc 2007;65:200.

54. Shaheen NJ, Falk GW, Iyer PG, et al. ACG clinical guideline: Diagnosis and management of Barrett's esophagus. Am J Gastroenterol 2016; 111:30.

55. Wani S, Rubenstein JH, Vieth M, et al. Diagnosis and management of low grade dysplasia in Barrett's esophagus: Expert review from the clinical practice updates committee of the American Gastroenterology 2016;151:822.

56. Phoa KN, Van Vilsteren FG, Weusten BL, et al. Radiofrequency ablation vs endoscopic surveil-

lance for patients with Barrett's esophagus and low grade dysplasia: a randomized clinical trial. JAMA 2014:311:1209.

57. Pandey G, Mulla M, Lewis WG, et al. Systemic review and meta-analysis of the effectiveness of radio-frequency ablation in low-grade dysplastic Barrett's esophagus. Endoscopy 2018;50:953.

58. Gupta N, Waxman I, Sharma P. A critical look at endoscopic eradication therapy for Barrett's esophagus: are we putting the cart before the horse? Gastrointest 2011;73:659.

59. Spechler SJ. Barrett's esophagus without dysplasia: wait or ablate? Dig Dis Sci 2011;56: 1926.

60. Shaheen NJ, Inadomi JM, Overholt BF, et al. What is the best management strategy for high grade dysplasia in Barrett's esophagus? A cost effective analysis. Gut 2004;53:1736.

61. Vij R, Triadafilopoulos G, Owens DK, et al. Cost-effectiveness of photodynamic therapy for high grade dysplasia in Barrett's esophagus. Gastrointest Endosc 2004;60:739.

62. Van den Boogert J, Van Hiellegersberg R, Siersema PD, et al. Endoscopic ablation therapy for Barrett's esophagus with high grade dysplasia: A review. Am J Gastroenterol 1999;94: 1153.

63. Sampliner RE. Endoscopic ablative therapy for Barrett's esophagus: current status. Gastrointest Endosc 2004;59:66.

64. Bright T, Watson DI, Tam W, et al. Randomized trial of argon plasma coagulation versus endoscopic surveillance for Barrett's esophagus after anti-reflux surgery: Late results. Ann Surg 2007; 246:1016.

65. Oman ES, Li N, Shaheen NJ, et al. Efficacy and durability of radiofrequency ablation for Barrett's esophagus: systemic review and meta-analysis. Clin Gastroenterol Hepatol 2013;11:1245.

66. Chadwick G, Groene O, Markar SR, et al. Systemic review comparing radio-frequency ablation and complete endoscopic resection in treating dysplastic Barrett's esophagus: a critical assessment of histologic outcomes and adverse events. Gastrointest Endosc 2014;79:718.

67. Small AJ, Sutherland SE, Hightower JS, et al. Comparative risk of recurrence of dysplasia and carcinoma after endoluminal eradication therapy of high grade dysplasia versus intra-mucosal carcinoma in Barrett's esophagus. Gastrointest Endosc 2015;81:1158.

68. Guthikonda A, Cotton CC, Madanick RD, et al. Clinical outcomes following recurrence of intestinal metaplasia after successful treatment of Barrett's esophagus with Radiofrequency ablation. Am J Gastroenterol 2017;112:87.

69. Shaheen NJ, Greenwald BD, Peery AF, et al. Safety and efficacy of endoscopic spray cryotherapy for Barrett's esophagus with high grade dysplasia. Gastrointest Endosc 2010; 71:680.

70. Gosain S, Mercer K, Twaddell WS, et al. Liquid nitrogen spray cryotherapy in Barrett's esophagus with high grade dysplasia: long term results. Gastrointest Endosc 2013;78:260.

71. Canto MI, Shin EJ, Khashab MA, et al. Safety and efficacy of carbon dioxide cryotherapy for treatment of neoplastic Barrett's esophagus. Endoscopy 2015;47:582.

72. Van Laethem JL, Peny MO, Salmon I, et al. Intramucosal adenocarcinoma arising under squamous re-epithelialization of Barrett's esophagus. Gut 2000;46:574.

73. Van Vilsteven FG, Pouw RE, Seewald S, et al. Step-wise radical endoscopic resection versus radiofrequency ablation for Barrett's esophagus with high grade dysplasia or early cancer: A multicenter randomized trial. Gut 2011;60:765.

74. Truong S, Bohm G, Klinge U, et al. Results after endoscopic treatment of post-operative gastrointestinal fistulas and leaks using combined vicryl plug and fibrin glue. Surgical Endoscopy 2004;18(7):1105–8.

75. Jean-Michel Gonzalez, C Servajean, B Aider, et al. Efficacy of the endoscopic management of post-operative fistulas of leakages after esophageal surgery for cancer: a retrospective series. Surgical Endoscopy 2016;30(11),4895–4903.

76. Rudolf Mennigen, Mario Colombo-Benkmann, Norbert S, et al. Endoscopic closure of post-operative gastrointestinal leakages and fistulas with the over-the-scope clip (OTSC). J of Gastrointest Surg 2013;17(6):1058–65.

16

Survival Rates

Praful Desai

Survival rates of patients with esophageal cancer, the world over, are poor and ranges from 5 to 90% depending on the stage of the disease. In patients undergoing resection, the 5 year survival rate ranges from 5 to 30%.[1-3] Stratification according to T and N stage will prove that survival rates increase significantly with earlier stage of the disease (Table 16.1). The Japanese group, identifying very early cancers in a field survey[4] has been able to record 90% five years survival after endoscopic mucosectomy.

The positive impact of three field radical lymphadenectomy on survival rates has not been universal. Apart from the heterogenecity of esophageal cancers, the results of surgery are not uniform across the globe as the surgical procedures are often performed by surgeons of varying expertise and experience, irrespective of T and N staging of a given tumor. There is however a consensus that very early or advanced lesions, are unlikely to benefit from such extensive procedures. Patients with $T_{1-2}N_1$ group up to 5–6 nodes will benefit with a proper nodal dissection and a likely increase in survival rates with decreased morbidity when surgery is performed by experienced surgeons. It is important however, to accept and realize that overall survivals from esophageal cancer are poor mainly due to late presentation and the complexity of the surgical procedure. In our personal series, 70% five year survivals are identified for $T_1N_0M_0$ lesions mainly due to early diagnosis.

REFERENCES

1. Fok M, Law S, et al. A comparison of trans-hiatal and trans-thoracic resections for esophageal cancer. Endoscopy 1993;56:838–46.
2. Goldminc M, Haddevor G, et al. Esophagectomy by a trans-hiatal approach or thoracotomy—a prospective randomized trial. Br J Surg 1993;80: 368–70.
3. Vigneswaran NT, Trartek VF, et al. Trans-hiatal esophagectomy for cancers of the esophagus. Ann Thorac Surg 1993;56:838–46.
4. Endo M. Endoscopic resection as local treatment of mucosal cancer of the esophagus. Endoscopy 1993;25:672.

Table 16.1	Five year survival rates in cancer of the esophagus (Desai et al Personal series. All resections as per stage)	
Pathological stage	No. resected N = 1072	5 year survival
$T_1 N_0 M_0$	13	70%
$T_2 N_0 M_0$	65	33.3%
$T_3 N_0 M_0$	287	22.4%
$T_2 N_1 M_0$	41	12.9%
$T_3 N_1 M_0$	666	3.2%

Epilogue

Praful Desai

In the entire field of oncology cancer of the esophagus is one of the more difficult cancers to manage and treat. In its therapeutic complexity, it rates along with cancers of the brain, the liver and probably also with that of the lung. The diagnosis is comparatively easy and straightforward with simple investigations like imaging, endoscopic assessment and a tissue biopsy of the lesion. Further investigations like imaging of the chest, abdomen and in the current era of PET-CT scan a near complete assessment of the extent of the disease is usually possible and mandatory. These pre-therapy evaluations and assessment constitute the cornerstone of planning an appropriate therapeutic approach. Though the etiological factors are well- defined; (Tobacco, Barrett's, GERD, etc.) prevention of this fatal disease is not easy.

Esophageal cancer is the 8th most common cancer with 4,81,000 new cases reported worldwide in 2008 and 6th most common cause of death from cancer with 4,06,000 deaths. This includes both adenocarcinoma and squamous cell carcinoma types. More than 80% of deaths occur in developing countries. Markedly higher incidences are reported from China, Japan, India, Iceland and UK. In India, there are estimated 29,000 new esophageal cancer cases and 26,000 deaths as per GLOBOCAN estimates. Esophageal cancer is the commonest malignancy in Kashmir, Karnataka, Kerala and Assam.

The incidence of esophageal cancer increases with age; patients with gastroesophageal reflux disease (GERD) of long duration are at a higher risk, as is Barrett's esophagus. Over a period of 1–12 years this can progress to epithelial metaplasia, dysplasia and subsequently carcinoma. Though screening for early diagnosis is not a practical proposition, selective screening approach in countries with high incidence is worthwhile. Population with the habit of chewing tobacco and alcohol addiction are at a major risk.

Apart from avoidance of tobacco and alcohol in any form, diets with high fruits and vegetables are known to reduce the risks. Overweight and obese population who are prone to esophageal reflux has a higher chance of developing adenocarcinoma of the esophagus. In a disease like esophageal cancer, where patients present late, it is technically difficult to treat them surgically with a high rate of mortality; it would be better to emphasize the importance of prevention by avoiding excess of tobacco and alcohol intake.

The overall prognosis and long-term results of esophageal cancer are admittedly poor since most patients present late for evaluation and treatment; most often with significant dysphagia and weight loss. Surgery, up until about 15 years ago, was the only curative approach with poor results (less than 5 to 8% survivors for 5 years); however, with the advent of chemo-radiotherapy the overall survival has improved. Besides the resection of the esophagus, lymphadenectomy which may be a two or three field should be performed by experienced surgeons. Adequate lymphadenectomy should be able to remove at least 12 to 15 lymph nodes. This requires a surgeon with adequate experience in this difficult procedure. Training for 5 years or more with an experienced esophageal surgeon is mandatory before embarking on esophageal surgery. The morbidity and mortality in inexperienced hands is significant; initially the procedure should be performed by young hands, only in the presence of a senior experienced esophageal surgeon to avoid major complications.

Index